Obesity

Guest Editors

DEREK LEROITH, MD, PhD
EDDY KARNIELI, MD

MEDICAL CLINICS
OF NORTH AMERICA

www.medical.theclinics.com

September 2011 • Volume 95 • Number 5

SAUNDERS an imprint of ELSEVIER, Inc.

W.B. SAUNDERS COMPANY
A Division of Elsevier Inc.

1600 John F. Kennedy Boulevard ● Suite 1800 ● Philadelphia, Pennsylvania 19103-2899

http://www.theclinics.com

MEDICAL CLINICS OF NORTH AMERICA Volume 95, Number 5
September 2011 ISSN 0025-7125, ISBN-13: 978-1-4557-2369-0

Editor: Rachel Glover

Medical Clinics of North America (ISSN 0025-7125) is published bimonthly by Elsevier Inc., 360 Park Avenue South, New York, NY 10010-1710. Months of issue are January, March, May, July, September, and November. Periodicals postage paid at New York, NY, and additional mailing offices. Subscription prices are USD 218 per year for US individuals, USD 404 per year for US institutions, USD 110 per year for US students, USD 277 per year for Canadian individuals, USD 525 per year for Canadian institutions, USD 173 per year for Canadian students, USD 336 per year for international individuals, USD 525 per year for international institutions and USD 173 per year for international students. To receive student/resident rate, orders must be accompanied by name of affiliated institution, date of term, and the *signature* of program/residency coordinator on institution letterhead. Orders will be billed at individual rate until proof of status is received. Foreign air speed delivery is included in all *Clinics* subscription prices. All prices are subject to change without notice. **POSTMASTER:** Send address changes to *Medical Clinics of North America*, Elsevier Health Sciences Division, Subscription Customer Service, 3251 Riverport Lane, Maryland Heights, MO 63043. **Customer Service: Telephone: 1-800-654-2452** (U.S. and Canada); **1-314-447-8871** (outside U.S. and Canada). **Fax: 1-314-447-8029. E-mail: journalscustomerservice-usa@elsevier.com** (for print support); **journalsonlinesupport-usa@ elsevier.com** (for online support).

Reprints. For copies of 100 or more of articles in this publication, please contact the Commercial Reprints Department, Elsevier Inc., 360 Park Avenue South, New York, NY 10010-1710. Tel.: 212-633-3812; Fax: 212-462-1935; E-mail: reprints@elsevier.com.

Medical Clinics of North America is also published in Spanish by McGraw-Hill Interamericana Editores S. A., P.O. Box 5-237, 06500 Mexico, D.F., Mexico.

Medical Clinics of North America is covered in *MEDLINE/PubMed (Index Medicus), Current Contents, ASCA, Excerpta Medica, Science Citation Index,* and *ISI/BIOMED.*

Printed in the United States of America.

GOAL STATEMENT

The goal of *Medical Clinics of North America* is to keep practicing physicians up to date with current clinical practice by providing timely articles reviewing the state of the art in patient care.

ACCREDITATION

The *Medical Clinics of North America* is planned and implemented in accordance with the Essential Areas and Policies of the Accreditation Council for Continuing Medical Education (ACCME) through the joint sponsorship of the University of Virginia School of Medicine and Elsevier. The University of Virginia School of Medicine is accredited by the ACCME to provide continuing medical education for physicians.

The University of Virginia School of Medicine designates this enduring material activity for a maximum of 15 *AMA PRA Category 1 Credit*(s)™ for each issue, 90 credits per year. Physicians should only claim credit commensurate with the extent of their participation in the activity.

The American Medical Association has determined that physicians not licensed in the US who participate in this CME enduring material activity are eligible for a maximum of 15 *AMA PRA Category 1 Credit*(s)™ for each issue, 90 credits per year.

Credit can be earned by reading the text material, taking the CME examination online at http://www.theclinics.com/home/cme, and completing the evaluation. After taking the test, you will be required to review any and all incorrect answers. Following completion of the test and evaluation, your credit will be awarded and you may print your certificate.

FACULTY DISCLOSURE/CONFLICT OF INTEREST

The University of Virginia School of Medicine, as an ACCME accredited provider, endorses and strives to comply with the Accreditation Council for Continuing Medical Education (ACCME) Standards of Commercial Support, Commonwealth of Virginia statutes, University of Virginia policies and procedures, and associated federal and private regulations and guidelines on the need for disclosure and monitoring of proprietary and financial interests that may affect the scientific integrity and balance of content delivered in continuing medical education activities under our auspices.

The University of Virginia School of Medicine requires that all CME activities accredited through this institution be developed independently and be scientifically rigorous, balanced and objective in the presentation/discussion of its content, theories and practices.

All authors/editors participating in an accredited CME activity are expected to disclose to the readers relevant financial relationships with commercial entities occurring within the past 12 months (such as grants or research support, employee, consultant, stock holder, member of speakers bureau, etc.). The University of Virginia School of Medicine will employ appropriate mechanisms to resolve potential conflicts of interest to maintain the standards of fair and balanced education to the reader. Questions about specific strategies can be directed to the Office of Continuing Medical Education, University of Virginia School of Medicine, Charlottesville, Virginia.

The faculty and staff of the University of Virginia Office of Continuing Medical Education have no financial affiliations to disclose.

The authors/editors listed below have identified no professional or financial affiliations for themselves or their spouse/partner:

Elliot M. Berry, MD, FRCP; Gal Dubnov-Raz, MD, MSc; Remco Franssen, MD; Emily Jane Gallagher, MRCPI; Rachel Glover (Acquisitions Editor); Eddy Karnieli, MD (Guest Editor); John J.P. Kastelein, MD, PhD; Anna Krook, PhD; L. Romayne Kurukulasuriya, MD; Guido Lastra, MD; Camila Manrique, MD; Peter A. McCullough, MD, MPH; Wendy M. Miller, MD; Houshang Monajemi, MD; Donal J. O'Gorman, PhD; Eric D. Peterson, MD, MPH; Gerald M. Reaven, MD; Brian R. Smith, MD; James R. Sowers, MD; Sameer Stas, MD; Erik S.G. Stroes, MD, PhD; Andrew Wolf, MD (Test Author); and Kerstyn C. Zalesin, MD.

The authors/editors listed below identified the following professional or financial affiliations for themselves or their spouse/partner:

George A. Bray, MD is on the Advisory Committee/Board for Herbalife Nutrition Institute and Takeda Pharmaceuticals, and has a Travel Grant with Vivus Pharmaceuticals.

Barry A. Franklin, PhD is on the Advisory Board for Smart Balance, Inc.

Derek LeRoith, MD, PhD (Guest Editor) is a consultant for Sanofi, BMS/AZ, and Merck.

Emily M. Lindley, PhD is an industry funded research/investigator for Synthes, Inc.

Ninh T. Nguyen, MD is on the Speakers' Bureau for Covidien and Ethicon.

Phil Schauer, MD receives grant support from Ethicon Endosurgery, Stryker Endoscopy, Bard-Davol, Gore, Baxter, Covidien, and Allergan; is on the Scientific Adviosry Board for Ethicon Endosurgery, Stryker Endoscopy, Bard-Davol, Barosense, Surgiquest, and Cardinal/Snowden Pincer; is a consultant for Ethicon Endosurgery, Bard-Davol, and Gore; and is on the Board of Directors for Remedy MD and Surgical Excellence LLC.

Brent Van Dorsten, PhD is on the Speakers' Bureau for Medtronic Corporation, Pearson Assessments, Inc., and Quest Laboratories.

Disclosure of Discussion of Non-FDA Approved Uses for Pharmaceutical Products and/or Medical Devices

The University of Virginia School of Medicine, as an ACCME provider, requires that all faculty presenters identify and disclose any off-label uses for pharmaceutical and medical device products. The University of Virginia School of Medicine recommends that each physician fully review all the available data on new products or procedures prior to clinical use.

TO ENROLL

To enroll in the Medical Clinics of North America Continuing Medical Education program, call customer service at 1-800-654-2452 or visit us online at http://www.theclinics.com/home/cme. The CME program is available to subscribers for an additional fee of USD 228.

RELATED INTEREST

Psychiatric Clinics of North America, December 2011 (Volume 34, Issue 4)
Obesity and Associated Eating Disorders: A Guide for Mental Health Professionals
Thomas A. Wadden, PhD, G. Terence Wilson, PhD, Albert J. Stunkard, MD,
Robert I. Berkowitz, MD, *Guest Editors*

VISIT US ONLINE!
Access your subscription at:
www.theclinics.com

Contributors

GUEST EDITORS

DEREK LEROITH, MD, PhD
Chief, Division of Endocrinology, Diabetes, and Bone Diseases, Department of Medicine, Mount Sinai Medical Center, New York, New York

EDDY KARNIELI, MD
Director and Associate Professor, Institute of Endocrinology, Diabetes, and Metabolism, Rambam Medical Center; and R.B. Rappaport Faculty of Medicine, Technion–Israel Institute of Technology, Haifa, Israel

AUTHORS

ELLIOT M. BERRY, MD, FRCP
Department of Human Nutrition and Metabolism, The Braun School of Public Health and Community Medicine, Hadassah-Hebrew University Medical Center, Jerusalem, Israel

GEORGE A. BRAY, MD
Boyd Professor, Pennington Biomedical Research Center, Baton Rouge, Louisianna

GAL DUBNOV-RAZ, MD, MSc
Pediatric Obesity, Exercise and Sport Medicine, Department of Pediatrics, Mount Scopus, Hadassah-Hebrew University Medical Center, Jerusalem, Israel

BARRY A. FRANKLIN, PhD
Director, Cardiac Rehabilitation and Exercise Laboratories, William Beaumont Hospital, Royal Oak, Michigan

REMCO FRANSSEN, MD
Department of Vascular Medicine, Academic Medical Center, Amsterdam, The Netherlands

EMILY JANE GALLAGHER, MRCPI
Division of Endocrinology, Diabetes, and Bone Diseases, Department of Medicine, Mount Sinai Medical Center, New York, New York

EDDY KARNIELI, MD
Director and Associate Professor, Institute of Endocrinology, Diabetes, and Metabolism, Rambam Medical Center; and R.B. Rappaport Faculty of Medicine, Technion–Israel Institute of Technology, Haifa, Israel

JOHN J.P. KASTELEIN, MD, PhD
Department of Vascular Medicine, Academic Medical Center, Amsterdam, The Netherlands

ANNA KROOK, PhD
Associate Professor, Department of Physiology and Pharmacology, Karolinska Institutet, Stockholm, Sweden

L. ROMAYNE KURUKULASURIYA, MD
Assistant Professor of Clinical Medicine, Department of Internal Medicine; Cosmopolitan International Diabetes and Endocrinology Center, University of Missouri-Columbia School of Medicine, Columbia, Missouri

GUIDO LASTRA, MD
Resident Physician in Internal Medicine, Department of Internal Medicine; Cosmopolitan International Diabetes and Endocrinology Center, University of Missouri-Columbia School of Medicine, Columbia, Missouri

DEREK LEROITH, MD, PhD
Chief, Division of Endocrinology, Diabetes, and Bone Diseases, Department of Medicine, Mount Sinai Medical Center, New York, New York

EMILY M. LINDLEY, PhD
Research Instructor, Department of Orthopedics, University of Colorado Denver, Aurora, Colorado

CAMILA MANRIQUE, MD
Resident Physician, Department of Internal Medicine; Cosmopolitan International Diabetes and Endocrinology Center, University of Missouri-Columbia School of Medicine, Columbia, Missouri

PETER A. MCCULLOUGH, MD, MPH, FACC, FACP, FAHA, FCCP
Consultant Cardiologist, Chief Academic and Scientific Officer, St John Providence Health System, Providence Park Heart Institute, Novi, Michigan

WENDY M. MILLER, MD
Medical Director, Weight Control Center, Division of Nutrition and Preventative Medicine, William Beaumont Hospital, Royal Oak, Michigan

HOUSHANG MONAJEMI, MD
Department of Vascular Medicine, Academic Medical Center, Amsterdam, The Netherlands

NINH T. NGUYEN, MD, FACS
Associate Professor of Surgery and Chief, Division of Gastrointestinal Surgery, University of California, Irvine Medical Center, Orange, California

DONAL J. O'GORMAN, PhD
Lecturer, School of Health and Human Performance, Dublin City University, Dublin, Ireland

ERIC D. PETERSON, MD, MPH
Duke Clinical Research Institute, Duke University School of Medicine, Durham, North Carolina

GERALD M. REAVEN, MD
Professor of Medicine (Active Emeritus), Division of Cardiovascular Medicine, Stanford University School of Medicine, Stanford Medical Center, Stanford, California

PHIL SCHAUER, MD
Professor of Surgery and Director, Bariatric and Metabolic Institute, Cleveland Clinic, Cleveland, Ohio

BRIAN R. SMITH, MD
Assistant Clinical Professor of Surgery, University of California, Irvine Medical Center, Orange; Chief, Division of General Surgery, Veterans Affairs Healthcare System Long Beach, Long Beach, California

JAMES R. SOWERS, MD
Professor of Medicine, Pharmacology, and Physiology; Thomas W. and Joan F. Burns Chair in Diabetes and Director of the Missouri University Diabetes and Cardiovascular Center, Departments of Internal Medicine and Medical Pharmacology and Physiology, Thomas W. Burns Center of Diabetes and Cardiovascular Research; Harry S. Truman Veterans Affairs Medical Center, University of Missouri-Columbia School of Medicine, Columbia, Missouri

SAMEER STAS, MD
Assistant Professor of Clinical Medicine, Department of Internal Medicine; Cosmopolitan International Diabetes and Endocrinology Center, University of Missouri-Columbia School of Medicine, Columbia, Missouri

ERIK S.G. STROES, MD, PhD
Department of Vascular Medicine, Academic Medical Center, Amsterdam, The Netherlands

BRENT VAN DORSTEN, PhD
Associate Professor, Department of Physical Medicine and Rehabilitation, University of Colorado Denver, Aurora, Colorado

KERSTYN C. ZALESIN, MD
Division of Nutrition and Preventative Medicine, Department of Medicine, William Beaumont Hospital, Royal Oak, Michigan

Contents

In today's society with the escalating levels of obesity, diabetes, and cardiovascular disease, the metabolic syndrome is receiving considerable attention and is the subject of much controversy. Greater insight into the mechanism(s) behind the syndrome may improve our understanding of how to prevent and best manage this complex condition.

Insulin-mediated glucose disposal varies at least sixfold in apparently healthy individuals. The adverse effect of decreases in the level of physical fitness on insulin sensitivity is comparable to the untoward impact of excess adiposity, with each accounting for approximately 25% of the variability of insulin action. It is the loss of insulin sensitivity that explains why obese individuals are more likely to develop cardiovascular disease, but not all overweight/obese individuals are insulin resistant. At a clinical level, it is important to identify those overweight individuals who are also insulin resistant and to initiate the most intensive therapeutic effort in this subgroup. Finally, it appears that the adverse impact of overall obesity, as estimated by body mass index, is comparable to that of abdominal obesity, as quantified by waist circumference.

The alarming and still increasing prevalence of obesity and associated cardiovascular risk raises much concern. The increase in cardiovascular risk depends to a significant extent on the changes in lipid profiles as observed in obesity. These changes are decreased high-density lipoprotein cholesterol and increased triglyceride levels. Much effort has already been expended into the elucidation of the mechanisms behind these obesity-associated lipid changes. Insulin resistance certainly plays a central role and, in addition, both hormonal and neurologic pathways have recently been found to play an important role. This article focuses on the mechanisms involved in the development of the proatherogenic lipid changes associated with obesity.

Hypertension and obesity are major components of the cardiometabolic syndrome and are both on the rise worldwide, with enormous consequences to global health and the economy. The relationship between hypertension and obesity is multifaceted; the etiology is complex and it is not well elucidated. This article reviews the current knowledge on obesity-related hypertension. Further understanding of the underlying mechanisms of this epidemic will be important in devising future treatment avenues.

The epidemiology of cardiovacular disease risk factors is changing rapidly with the obesity pandemic. Obesity is independently associated with the risks for coronary heart disease, atrial fibrillation, and heart failure. Intra-abdominal obesity is also unique as a cardiovascular risk state in that it contributes to or directly causes most other modifiable risk factors, namely, hypertension, dysmetabolic syndrome, and type 2 diabetes mellitus. Obesity can also exacerbate cardiovascular disease through a variety of mechanisms including systemic inflammation, hypercoagulability, and activation of the sympathetic and reninangiotensin systems. Thus, weight reduction is a key strategy for simultaneous improvement in global cardiovascular risk, with anticipated improvements in survival and quality of life.

Dietary modulation is an essential part of weight loss and maintaining its reduction. Although simple in behavioral terms (eat less, exercise more), the tremendous difficulty of weight loss and maintenance has inspired many different diet regimens, in search of an easier, more efficient way to lose weight. Contemporary issues in this matter are the composition of diets (low fat versus low carbohydrate), the choice of carbohydrate (the glycemic index), and the role of calcium and dairy products. This article discusses the scientific evidence of the various dietary manipulations for weight loss and the challenges of maintaining a reduced obese state.

Lifestyle intervention programs encompassing exercise and healthy diets are an option for the treatment and management of obesity and type 2 diabetes and have long been known to exert beneficial effects on whole-body metabolism, in particular leading to enhanced insulin-sensitivity. Obesity is associated with increased risk of several illnesses and premature mortality. However, physical inactivity is itself associated with a number of similar risks, independent of body-mass index, and is an independent risk factor for more than 25 chronic diseases, including type 2 diabetes and cardiovascular disease. This article addresses the debate regarding the relative effects of physical exercise itself and the effect of exercise-induced weight loss.

Cognitive behavioral interventions have formed the cornerstone of obesity treatment for the past two decades. These techniques, often combined with diet and exercise strategies, have been shown to produce weight losses of sufficient magnitude so as to reduce health risks. Though success in producing short-term weight loss is improving, many factors, including a metabolic energy gap, continue to challenge long-term weight maintenance results. This article reviews the unique influence of cognitive, behavioral, and metabolic factors on weight loss and weight-loss maintenance, and how future treatment packages might be modified to improve long-term weight loss outcomes.

Only two drugs are currently approved for long-term use in the treatment of obesity, and four others for short-term use. Evaluating the risk-benefit profile is an essential first step. For individuals who have a low body mass index for whom the risk is small, the risk profile must make the drug acceptable for almost everyone. For higher-risk patients, such as those planning intestinal bypass or who have sleep apnea, a wider range of drugs may be considered. Obesity is a chronic disease that has many causes. Treatment is aimed at palliation—that is, producing and maintaining weight loss. Regardless of the primary site of action, the net effect must be a reduction in food intake or increase in energy expenditure.

As bariatric surgery for the treatment of morbid obesity enters its sixth decade, much has been and continues to be learned from the results of several key bariatric operations, particularly the Roux-en-Y gastric bypass. Because of the obesity epidemic and development of the laparoscopic approach, bariatric procedures have increased exponentially in the past decade and are now among the more commonly performed gastrointestinal operations. Emerging data support the role of bariatric surgery as an effective treatment for improvement or remission of type 2 diabetes, hypertension, dyslipidemia, and multiple other comorbid conditions that accompany obesity. The mechanisms involved in the remission of these conditions, however, remain poorly understood and constitute an exciting area of research. This article delineates the current types of bariatric surgery, their respective outcomes, and their impact on obesity-related medical comorbidities.

Preface

Obesity

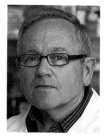 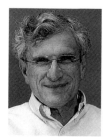

Derek LeRoith, MD, PhD   Eddy Karnieli, MD
Guest Editors

The articles that have been chosen for this issue represent clinical aspects of this very important disorder. Obesity, as everyone knows, has become an epidemic, not just in North America, but worldwide. The epidemic of obesity is also driving the marked increase in type 2 diabetes worldwide. While obesity is easily recognizable clinically and readily measurable in the United States, a feature that is not well recognized is the central adiposity that maybe the only or main feature in South East Asian communities, many of whom are highly represented in the United States. Thus, often, we as clinicians may not be screening for the obesity-related abnormalities that represent the metabolic syndrome, and therefore, preventative or therapeutic modalities are introduced very late in the disease process.

The first article describes the Metabolic Syndrome specifically. The Metabolic Syndrome includes obesity, hypertension, hyperlipidemia, and glucose intolerance, has insulin resistance as the underlying etiology, and is commonly seen in patients with type 2 diabetes. As described in this article by Gallagher, LeRoith, and Karnieli, it is extremely common in both developed countries as well as in third-world countries and is associated with visceral adiposity. While the exact definitions of the metabolic syndrome differ slightly between various organizational and governing bodies, its existence and its relationship to type 2 diabetes are unequivocal. The article also presents information on how insulin resistance is caused by obesity and how the insulin resistance causes the hypertension, hyperlipidemia, and glucose intolerance.

Gerald Reaven was one of the first investigators who described the Metabolic Syndrome (which he originally named "Syndrome X"); here he describes the relationship between obesity and cardiovascular disease. He initially presents the relationship between abdominal obesity and reduced insulin-mediated glucose uptake into muscle. This resultant insulin resistance and hyperinsulinemia lead to increased risk factors for cardiovascular disease. Today this cardio-metabolic syndrome is so common that major efforts are underway to attempt to reverse the abnormality, since heart attacks and strokes are the major causes of the high mortality rates in type 2 diabetic patients.

Med Clin N Am 95 (2011) xiii–xv
doi:10.1016/j.mcna.2011.06.011
0025-7125/11/$ – see front matter © 2011 Elsevier Inc. All rights reserved.

medical.theclinics.com

Obesity and dyslipidemia is another complication that is commonly appreciated in the medical community. The cardiovascular risk associated with obesity is mostly predicted by the dyslipidemia, characterized by increased triglyceride levels, decreased high-density lipoproteins levels, and a shift in low-density lipoproteins (LDL) to a more pro-atherogenic composition (small, dense LDL). These features are covered in the article by Franssen, Monajemi, Stroes, and Kastelein. They describe how the classic concept of insulin resistance, lipolysis, with excess free fatty acid (FFA) release leading to hypertriglyceridemia is still the central theme.

Obesity-related hypertension has many etiologies, as outlined by Kurukulasuriya, Stas, Lastra, Manrique, and Sowers. These include the well-known causes such as insulin resistance, activation of the renin-angiotensinogen-aldosterone system with renal sodium retention, and the sympathetic nervous system. More recent studies have demonstrated that adipocytokines, FFAs, and other molecules may cause endothelial dysfunction. More recently the effect of sleep deprivation on obesity and therefore on hypertension has been described. While the causes are being investigated, the need for intensive anti-hypertensive therapy is primarily to prevent the cardiovascular and renal complications that result.

The relationship between obesity and cardiovascular disease is further explored in the article by Zalesin, Franklin, Miller, Peterson, and McCullough. They address the increased risk factors and increased cardiac disease in obese individuals that cause heart attacks, atrial fibrillation, and heart failure. Importantly, they describe the epidemic of obesity and the increased rates of hypertension, hyperlipidemia, and glucose intolerance in the pediatric population and the eventual increase in cardiovascular disease that is bound to result at younger ages.

One of the most difficult topics in obesity is the issue of dietary management for both reducing weight and weight maintenance. Dubnov-Raz and Berry discuss this difficult topic by comparing the various well-studied diets involving low-calorie, low-fat, and many fad diets. While some diets such as Atkins, low calorie, Mediterranean, and low glycemic index diets have proven relatively effective, the most critical issue remains compliance, ie, the human element.

O'Gorman and Krook discuss the importance of exercise in the management of obesity and prevention of many of the complications associated with excess weight. There are apparently genetic determinants for the ability to respond to excess weight. There are a number of genetic and phenotypic effects of exercise, including changes in mitochondrial metabolism and switching of muscle fiber types. These and other changes are important for the improvements, not just in weight reduction, but also in reducing the negative effects on the cardiovascular system, associated with obesity.

As compliance of lifestyle modification is very important in managing obesity, Van Dorsten and Lindley pursue the issue of behavioral therapy in the lifestyle management of obesity, for both weight reduction and maintenance. Both the dietary and the exercise components of therapy require cognitive-behavioral elements to implement the lifestyle changes, thereby enhancing their effectiveness and avoiding relapses.

There is a large amount of interest in using medications to treat obesity. On the one hand, lifestyle intervention alone has been largely unsuccessful in reversing the obesity epidemic. On the other hand, bariatric surgery is reserved for morbid obesity and moderate obesity with comorbidities. As described in the article by Bray there are currently two drugs approved for treating obesity. Sibutramine is an appetite suppressant and orlistat interferes with fat digestion and absorption. Both are successful in helping produce weight reduction, but both have side effects. Cannabinoid receptor-1 antagonists such as rimonobant are being tested in clinical trials and may be useful in the future for moderate weight reduction, if the side-effect profile is limited.

Of note, the use of this drug was approved in many countries in the European Union, but subsequently removed due to excess side-effects.

Smith, Schauer, and Nguyen cover the very important topic of bariatric surgery. Over the past decade the techniques have evolved and the morbidity and mortality of the procedures have been reduced dramatically so that the value of this approach is now widely accepted for morbidly obese individuals (body mass index (BMI) >40) and obese individuals (BMI >35) with comorbid diseases such as diabetes. Interestingly, there is now interest in using these techniques for treating patients with uncontrolled type 2 diabetes as the primary disorder with mild obesity (BMI 28-35). While the first indication remains obesity, the more recent studies suggest that new indications such as diabetes may become realistic in the future once more studies have been presented.

These articles bring to the practicing physician knowledge about the basic pathophysiology and the clinical aspects of obesity, and we hope that the information is informative and practical.

Derek LeRoith, MD, PhD
Division of Endocrinology, Diabetes, and Bone Diseases
Department of Medicine
Mount Sinai Medical Center
One Gustave L. Levy Place, Box 1055
New York, NY 10029-6574, USA

Eddy Karnieli, MD
Institute of Endocrinology, Diabetes, and Metabolism
Rambam Medical Center
R.B. Rapaport Faculty of Medicine-Technion
12 Halia Street
Haifa 31096, Israel

E-mail addresses:
derek.leroith@mssm.edu (D. LeRoith)
eddy@tx.technion.ac.il (E. Karnieli)

The Metabolic Syndrome—from Insulin Resistance to Obesity and Diabetes

Emily Jane Gallagher, MRCPI[a], Derek LeRoith, MD, PhD[a],
Eddy Karnieli, MD[b],*

KEYWORDS

- Metabolic syndrome • Insulin resistance • Prediabetes
- Cardiometabolic risk factors • Obesity

The growing prevalence of obesity worldwide is increasing concern surrounding the rising rates of diabetes, coronary, and cerebrovascular disease with the consequent health and financial implications for the population.[1] The metabolic syndrome comprises an assembly of risk factors for developing diabetes and cardiovascular disease. Opinion varies with regard to the etiology of the metabolic syndrome and whether it should be defined as a syndrome of insulin resistance, the metabolic consequences of obesity, or risk factors for cardiovascular disease.[2] Some consider it not a to be a syndrome, but rather a collection of statistical correlations.[3] This article will try to unveil some of the molecular and physiologic mechanisms underlying the entities of insulin resistance and the metabolic syndrome. It will focus on their clinical relevance for the care of overweight and/or obese patients with or without diabetes as defined by the American Diabetes Association (ADA) criteria.[4]

HISTORIC OVERVIEW

The metabolic syndrome has undergone a host of incarnations in the medical literature since the clustering of metabolic risk factors for coronary artery disease, diabetes, and hypertension was described as "Syndrome X" by Reaven in 1988.[5] The initial factors described by Reaven included impaired glucose tolerance (IGT), hyperinsulinemia, elevated triglycerides (TG), and reduced high-density lipoprotein cholesterol (HDLc).

A version of this article appeared in the 37:3 issue of the *Endocrinology and Metabolism Clinics of North America*.

[a] Division of Endocrinology, Diabetes, and Bone Diseases, Department of Medicine, Mount Sinai Medical Center, One Gustave L. Levy Place, Box 1055, New York, NY 10029-6574, USA

[b] Institute of Endocrinology, Diabetes, and Metabolism, Rambam Medical Center and R.B. Rapaport Faculty of Medicine–Technion, 12 Halia Street, Haifa 31096, Israel

* Corresponding author.

E-mail address: eddy@tx.technion.ac.il

Subsequently, hyperuricemia and raised plasminogen activator inhibitor 1 (PAI-1) were suggested as components of the same syndrome.[5,6] Obesity was not included in Reaven's definition of Syndrome X, as he suggested that insulin resistance, rather than obesity, was the unifying feature. The core components of what we now call the metabolic syndrome: obesity, insulin resistance, dyslipidemia, and hypertension have remained since the World Health Organization (WHO) produced its definition in 1998. WHO published criteria to define the metabolic syndrome in an attempt to harmonize reporting of prevalence through epidemiologic studies. The criteria included a measure of insulin resistance, by a hyperinsulinemic euglycemic clamp, impaired fasting glucose (IFG), impaired glucose tolerance (IGT) or diabetes, obesity (BMI >30 kg/m^2), hypertension ($\geq$140/90 mm Hg), and microalbuminuria.[7] Critics of the WHO definition highlighted the impracticality of performing hyperinsulinemic clamp studies in epidemiologic research. They also pointed out that rather than measuring the waist-to-hip ratio, waist circumference measurement was more convenient and had a comparable correlation to obesity. In addition, some believed that microalbuminuria should not be included at all given the insufficient evidence of a close correlation with insulin resistance.[3] These opinions lead to the second definition in 1999, from the European Group for the Study of Insulin Resistance (EGIR). They renamed the syndrome, "insulin resistance syndrome" and excluded subjects with diabetes because of excessive complexities in measuring insulin resistance in these individuals. Insulin resistance remained an essential component, defined as a fasting insulin level above the 75th percentile for the population. Two of these other elements (criteria associated with increased risk of coronary artery disease from the Second Joint Task Force of European and other Societies on Coronary Prevention) were also required: obesity defined as waist circumference 94 cm (37 inches) or more for men and 80 cm (32 inches) or more for women, hypertension remained defined as 140/90 mm Hg or higher, and dyslipidemia with TG 180 mg/dL (2.0 mmol/L) or more, and/or HDLc less than 39 mg/dL (1.01 mmol/L).[3] In 2001, The National Cholesterol Education Program (NCEP) Adult Treatment Panel III (ATP III) changed the focus to cardiovascular risk factors and away from relying on measures of insulin resistance and possible etiologies; therefore, the title "The Metabolic Syndrome" was reassigned. The criteria were any three of the following: obesity (waist circumference $\geq$102 cm [40 inches] in males and $\geq$88 cm [35 inches] in females, based on the 1998 National Institutes of Health [NIH] obesity clinical guidelines), hypertension ($\geq$130/85 mm Hg based on Joint National Committee guidelines), fasting glucose more than 110 mg/dL (6.1 mmol/L, including diabetes), TG 150 mg/dL (1.69 mmol/L) or more, and HDLc less than 40 mg/dL (1.03 mmol/L) in men or less than 50 mg/dL (1.3 mmol/L) in women.[8] Waist circumference was not a required element as the NCEP/ATP III wished to include certain individuals and ethnic groups that have metabolic and blood pressure abnormalities associated with elevated cardiovascular risk, but do not meet the criteria for abdominal obesity. Subsequently, in 2003, the American Association of Clinical Endocrinologists (AACE) modified the ATP III criteria and renamed the disorder "Insulin Resistance Syndrome." The AACE did not set out stringent criteria to define the syndrome, but described it as a group of abnormalities associated with insulin resistance, including glucose intolerance (but not diabetes), abnormalities in uric acid metabolism, dyslipidemia (consistent with NCEP/ATP III criteria), hemodynamic changes, prothrombotic factors, markers of inflammation, endothelial dysfunction and elevated blood pressure (as NCEP/ATP III). This consensus also endeavored to identify individuals at increased risk of developing the insulin resistance syndrome in the future: BMI greater than 25 kg/m^2 (or waist circumference >40 inches in men and 35 inches in women), known cardiovascular disease, hypertension, polycystic ovarian syndrome (PCOS), nonalcoholic fatty liver disease (NAFLD), or acanthosis nigricans; family history of type 2 diabetes (T2DM), hypertension, or cardiovascular disease; history of gestational diabetes or glucose intolerance; non-Caucasian ethnicity; sedentary lifestyle; and age older than 40 years.[9] In parallel, the International Diabetes Federation (IDF) aimed to create a straightforward, clinically useful definition, to provide worldwide conformity for epidemiologic studies and identify those at greatest risk of developing diabetes and cardiovascular disease. To this end, the IDF proposed a new consensus definition of the metabolic syndrome in 2005. Obesity (BMI >30 kg/m^2 or if $\leq$30 kg/m^2 by ethnic-specific waist circumference measurements) was a prerequisite factor, as they felt it was a central etiologic component of the syndrome. Two of four other factors were also required: TG 150 mg/dL or higher, HDLc less than 40 mg/dL in men or less than 50 mg/dL in women, systolic blood pressure 130 mm Hg or higher or diastolic blood pressure 85 mm Hg or higher, fasting glucose more than 100 mg/dL (5.6 mmol/L, 2003 ADA definition of IFG[10]) including diabetes, and those with a previous diagnosis of or treatment for any of these conditions.[11]

DEFINITIONS

In this *Clinics of North America* series, we follow the 2005 American Heart Association (AHA)/National Heart, Lung and Blood Institute (NHLBI) criteria as shown in **Table 1**. The revised definition is based on the ATP III criteria, requires three of the five factors listed in **Table 1**[12] and primarily aims to diagnose those patients at increased risk of type 2 diabetes and cardiovascular disease. When using these criteria, the reader should take into account the updated differences relating to waist circumference measures by ethnic origin (as suggested by the IDF) as well as the revised criterion for impaired fasting glucose indicating those individuals at greater risk of developing the metabolic syndrome.[9,10,12]

Table 1
Criteria for diagnosis of the metabolic syndrome (American Heart Association/National Heart, Lung and Blood Institute) 2005

Any Three of the Following Criteria	Parameter
Elevated waist circumference	$\geq$102 cm ($\geq$40 inches) in men $\geq$88 cm ($\geq$35 inches) in women
Elevated triglycerides	$\geq$150 mg/dL (1.7 mmol/L)
Reduced HDLc	<40 mg/dL (1.03 mmol/L) in men <50 mg/dL (1.3 mmol/L) in women
Elevated blood pressure	$\geq$130 mm Hg systolic blood pressure OR $\geq$85 mm Hg diastolic blood pressure
Elevated fasting glucose	$\geq$100 mg/dL ($\geq$5.6 mmol/L)

International Diabetes Foundation ethnic-specific values for waist circumference:
Europoids: male $\geq$94 cm, female $\geq$80 cm; South Asians: male $\geq$90 cm, female $\geq$80 cm; Japanese: male $\geq$90 cm, female $\geq$80 cm. Ethnic south and central Americans use South Asian criteria until more specific criteria are available; sub-Saharan Africans, eastern Mediterranean, and Middle Eastern (Arab) populations use Europoid data at present.

Data from Grundy S, Cleeman J, Daniels S, et al. Diagnosis and management of the metabolic syndrome: an American Heart Association/National Heart, Lung, and Blood Institute scientific statement. Circulation 2005;112(17):2735–52.

Comparing the AHA/NHLBI to the IDF definition of the metabolic syndrome, blood pressure, lipid, and glucose ranges are the same; however, in contrast to the IDF, the AHA/NHLBI have not made obesity essential to the diagnosis but draw attention to the increased risk of insulin resistance and the metabolic syndrome in certain ethnic groups (ie, populations from South Asia, China, Japan, and other Asian countries) with only moderate increases in waist circumference. The IDF waist circumference cut-off values that define obesity for Europoids are 8 cm less for both males and females than those measurements in the AHA/NHLBI criteria, which were based on the National Health and Nutrition Examination Survey (NHANES).[11,12] The waist circumference cut-off measurements in the AHA/NHLBI definition approximate a BMI of 29.8 kg/m^2 in males and 24.9 kg/m^2 in females.[12,13]

It is likely that the definitions of the metabolic syndrome will continue to develop. Which definition is most useful will depend on its ability to predict cardiovascular outcomes in prospective studies.

PREVALENCE

Reported rates of prevalence vary widely with the criteria used, age of the population, gender, ethnic group, prevalence of obesity in the background population, and environment. Based on the NHANES 1999–2002, it is estimated that 34.6% of the US population meet the ATP III criteria for the metabolic syndrome. There is minimal gender difference: 34.4% of males and 34.5% of females. An increased prevalence has been shown with advancing age.[14–16]

Worldwide, prevalence rates of the metabolic syndrome were found to be similar irrespective of which set of criteria was applied, however different individuals were identified using different criteria.[17] The ATP III and IDF criteria similarly classified 92.9% of individuals in the NHANES. The IDF (with the lower waist circumference cut-off points) increased the overall age-adjusted prevalence estimate to 39.1% (40.7% in males and 37.1% in females).[18] However, concordance rates vary widely between studies. Both the Dallas Heart Study and the NHANES demonstrated the lowest concordance rate among Hispanic males. The PROCAM study from Germany, along with other European population studies, revealed low concordance rates.[19] Other European population studies have shown large differences in estimated prevalence.[20,21] In a northern Mexican population study the IDF criteria classified 94.4% of females as having obesity by waist circumference measurements (≥80 cm), which may suggest the waist circumference cut-off levels are inappropriately low for this population.[22] Of particular interest, the IDF criteria underestimate the metabolic syndrome prevalence in Asian populations, for example in Korea and China, as many individuals in these regions have metabolic risk factors without significant obesity.[23,24]

The NHANES study showed that with both the ATP III and IDF criteria, in males, the highest prevalence of the metabolic syndrome is in whites at 35% (IDF 42.6%). The lowest was in African American males, 21.6% (IDF 24.2%) despite the higher overall prevalence of hypertension and diabetes in this group. Mexican American women had the highest overall prevalence 37.8% (IDF 39.2%). White and African American women had similar prevalence, 33.7% and 33.8% respectively (36.9% and 35.8% by IDF).[18] The NHANES group had insufficient numbers of other ethnic groups to calculate their prevalence rates. Apart from the Mexican American population, other studies have shown that American Indians, Hawaiian, Filipino, and Polynesian populations have a higher incidence than those of European descent.[15,25–28]

Rural populations tend to have lower prevalence rates than urban populations, which have been demonstrated in multiple ethnic groups and studies of migrations to western society.[22,29] Western diet appears to bring with it increased risk of the metabolic syndrome particularly in Chinese, Indian, and Middle Eastern populations.[30–32] Arab populations living in the United States have been shown to have higher prevalence than those living in the Middle East.[22,29–33]

Low cardiorespiratory fitness in some studies correlates significantly with incidence of the metabolic syndrome in both men and women. In a Swedish study of healthy volunteers over age 60, metabolic syndrome prevalence was 24% and 19% in men and women, respectively. The adjusted odds ratio for having the metabolic syndrome in the high leisure-time physical activity group was 0.33, that of the low physical activity group.[34] A study of volunteers in Dallas, TX, with an age range of 20–80 years yielded similar results, showing a hazard ratio of 0.47 in men and 0.37 in the physically active women.[35]

PROGNOSIS

Equal to, if not exceeding, the importance of clinically practical definitions of the metabolic syndrome is having criteria that are pertinent for predicting the development of type 2 diabetes and cardiovascular disease. In the United States in 2003, the prevalence of cardiovascular disease was 34.2% and was a contributing or underlying cause of death in 37.3% of cases, which equates to 1 in every 2.7 deaths or 2500 deaths each day and a cost of $403.1 billion.[36] Data from the NHANES II show that combined, pre-existing cardiovascular disease and diabetes carry the greatest hazard for mortality from coronary artery disease (hazard ratio [HR] 6.25) and cardiovascular disease (HR 5.26).[37] Diabetes alone carries a HR of 2.87 for coronary artery disease mortality and 2.42 for all cardiovascular disease mortality.[37] Independent of the traditional Framingham risk factors (age, smoking, total cholesterol, HDLc levels, and systolic blood pressure), some researchers have found that the metabolic syndrome is associated with an increased probability of cardiovascular disease and conveys a higher risk than the Framingham risk score of developing type 2 diabetes.[38–45] However, the Framingham investigators report little or no increase in the predictive power for coronary heart disease by adding abdominal obesity, triglycerides, or fasting glucose to their 10-year risk algorithm (**Fig. 1**).[46,47] Debate surrounds which definition is the best predictor of diabetes, cardiovascular disease, and mortality.[24,48,49]

Three recent meta-analyses of prospective studies investigating the metabolic syndrome as a significant risk for cardiovascular disease and mortality show increased relative risk of both events.[50–52] One study demonstrated a relative risk of diabetes of 2.99[50] and all three analyses revealed more moderate increases in risk for cardiovascular events ranging from 1.53 to 2.7. All-cause mortality risk was estimated to be between 1.37 and 1.60 for those with the metabolic syndrome, depending on the criteria employed.[50,51] This greater probability of cardiovascular events and mortality has been shown to exist with the metabolic syndrome both in the presence and absence of diabetes; however, as in the NHANES II, the presence of diabetes, along with the metabolic syndrome, significantly increases this risk (HR 1.56 without diabetes, 1.82 with diabetes).[37,39,53] The increased risk of cardiovascular disease with the metabolic syndrome does not appear to be explained entirely by insulin resistance. In studies that calculate insulin resistance by the homeostasis model assessment of insulin resistance (HOMA-IR), the predictive power of the metabolic syndrome for diabetes and cardiovascular disease development has been demonstrated to be independent of the HOMA-IR.[39–41] There is also conflict regarding whether the metabolic syndrome as a whole confers a greater risk of cardiovascular disease and diabetes than its individual components.[49,53–55] In the Atherosclerosis

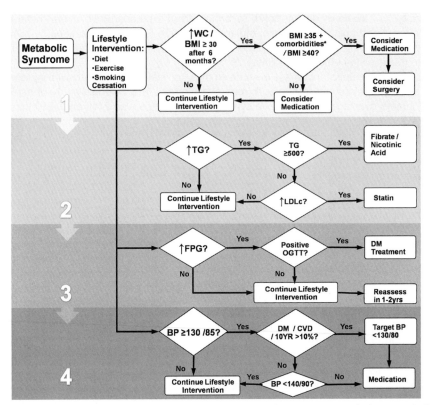

Fig. 1. Four-step algorithm for management of modifiable aspects of the metabolic syndrome. ↑WC, Waist Circumference >102 cm (men), >88 cm women; BMI, Body Mass Index in kg/m²; ↑TG, Elevated triglycerides; ↑LDLc, Elevated low-density lipoprotein cholesterol (see text); ↑FPG, Elevated fasting plasma glucose (>100 mg/dL); Positive OGTT, Oral glucose tolerance test (75 g) with 2-hour glucose of ≥200 mg/dL; DM, diabetes mellitus; BP, blood pressure: CVD, cardiovascular disease; 10YR, 10-year risk of CAD calculated by Framingham risk score. *Age >45 years (male), >55 years (female), cigarette smoking, dyslipidemia, hypertension, IFG, IGT, type 2 diabetes, family history of premature CVD in first-degree relative (male <55 years, female <65 years). (*Data from* Grundy SM, Brewer HB Jr, Cleeman JI, et al. Definition of metabolic syndrome: Report of the National Heart, Lung, and Blood Institute/American Heart Association Conference on scientific issues related to definition. Circulation 2004;109(3):433–8.)

Risk in Communities (ARIC) study, hypertension and low HDLc were found to be the strongest predictors of coronary heart disease; the metabolic syndrome as a whole was not found to have a greater prediction power than these individual elements.[53]

PATHOGENESIS

Whether the metabolic syndrome is an assortment of unrelated risk factors or allied traits attributable to a common mechanism is a matter of ongoing debate.[56,57] Although risk factors for the metabolic syndrome have been identified, the etiology remains incompletely understood.[9,12] As initially proposed by Reaven, it appears that insulin resistance is likely to be a significant link between the components of the metabolic syndrome.[5,58] Indeed, as mentioned previously, the metabolic syndrome is also known as the insulin resistance syndrome.[3,9] Many lifestyle, molecular, and genetic contributors[59] leading to the metabolic syndrome have been described; these include obesity and disorders of adipose tissue; physical inactivity; diet; insulin receptor and signaling anomalies[60,61]; inflammatory cascades; mitochondrial dysfunction[62]; molecules of immunologic, hepatic, or vascular origin (including adiponectin, leptin, PAI-1, resistin, angiotensinogen); endocannabinoid receptors; nuclear receptors; hormones; and polygenic variability in individuals and ethnic groups. Here, we will summarize how some of these factors contribute to the abnormalities within the metabolic syndrome.

In response to glucose stimulation, pancreatic β cells release insulin, leading to suppression of hepatic gluconeogenesis and increased glucose uptake and metabolism by the muscle and adipose tissue. Glucose transport into cells is mediated by glucose transporters (GLUT). One of the most important glucose transporters, GLUT4, is regulated by insulin. In response to insulin, GLUT4 is mobilized from intracellular storage vesicles and fuses to the cellular membrane to internalize glucose (see review[63]). This is the major rate-controlling step in insulin mediated glucose uptake and muscle glycogen synthesis.[60,64,65] GLUT4 cellular concentration in adipocytes is decreased with advancing age, obesity, and type 2 diabetes.[60] In skeletal muscle of obese and diabetic humans, GLUT4 is not decreased, but rather dysfunctional.[66] Exercise and adiponectin appear to increase the expression of GLUT4, coincident with insulin sensitivity. With insulin resistance, there is an initial loss of the immediate postprandial (first phase) response to insulin, leading to postprandial hyperglycemia. Subsequently, there is an exaggerated second-phase insulin response, which over time causes chronic hyperinsulinemia.[59] The resulting chronic hyperinsulinemia leads to resistance to the action of insulin (as further detailed).[1,67,68]

At a cellular level, insulin binds to the insulin receptor (IR) activating the tyrosine kinase pathway. This pathway stimulates the phosphorylation of receptor substrates and adaptor proteins, including insulin receptor substrates 1 and 2 (IRS1, IRS2), Gab1, Shc, and APS on selected tyrosine residues and these form docking sites for further downstream effectors.[69,70] There are then two major pathways in insulin-mediated activities: one is initiated by phosphatidylinositol 3-kinase (PI3K) and is the major channel of the metabolic effects of insulin; second is that downstream of mitogen-activated protein (MAP) kinase signaling, mostly involved in growth and mitogenesis.[69] Within the PI3K pathway, tyrosine-phosphorylated IRSs recruit and interact with the regulatory p85 subunit of PI3K, resulting in synthesis of phosphatidylinositol 3,4,5 phosphate (PIP3). Downstream kinases PDK (phosphoinositide dependent kinase) and Akt, bind to PIP3 and this results in their activation. Akt is known to mediate the effects of insulin on glucose transport and storage, protein synthesis, and prevention of lipid degradation. Some of these metabolic effects are mediated through Akt phosphorylation of FOXO (forkhead box class O) transcription factors.[61,71] FOXO1 plays a key role in hepatic gluconeogenesis. When phosphorylated it is sequestered in the cytoplasm and prevented from activating gluconeogenic genes.[72,73] It has also been shown in vitro to repress the transcription of peroxisome proliferator activated-receptor (PPAR)γ promoter genes.[73] PPARγ is one of a family of nuclear receptors, also including PPARα and PPARβ/d, which are key transcription factors involved in the regulation of glucose and lipid metabolism, along with insulin sensitivity. PPARγ is found in insulin-responsive tissues, whereas PPARα is expressed in hepatocytes, cardiac myocytes, and enterocytes, and PPARβ/d is ubiquitous. While PPARγ represses GLUT4 transcription,[71,74] its thiazoledinedione synthetic ligands enhance insulin sensitivity, probably by dismissal of co-repressor complexes, switching them with co-activator complexes[75,76] while concomitantly detaching PPARγ/RXR dimer from its DNA binding site on the GLUT4 gene promoter.[76] This, along with serine phosphorylation of IRS (and prevention of tyrosine phosphorylation) by hyperinsulinemia, cytokines (ie, tumor necrosis factor alpha [TNFα]), decreased PI3K activity and genetic defects (ie, Akt2) have been shown in vitro, in mouse models, and in humans to induce insulin resistance.[70,77] The result of deficits in the insulin-signaling pathway is increased nuclear activity of FOXO1 with greater expression of gluconeogenic genes, as well as induction of lipogenic transcription factor sterol regulatory element binding protein 1c (SREBPIc) and elevated expression of lipogenic genes and a rise in VLDL secretion.[60,78]

Obesity has an important role in insulin resistance.[2] Adipose tissue is not simply a storehouse for fat, but has been shown to be an endocrine organ producing many factors, including interleukin (IL)-6, TNFα, resistin, lipoprotein lipase, acylation stimulation protein, cholesteryl-ester protein, retinol binding protein-4 (RBP4), estrogens, leptin, angiotensinogen, adiponectin, insulin like growth factor-1 (IGF-1), and monobutyrin.[79] In this series of *Clinics of North America*, other articles will further discuss the adipose cell as an endocrine system as well as the mechanisms through which adipose tissue leads to insulin resistance.

Visceral adiposity is independently associated with insulin resistance; lower HDLc levels; higher apolipoprotein B, RBP4, and triglyceride levels; smaller LDLc particles; aortic stiffness; coronary calcification; and hypertension.[79–81] Obesity has been shown to contribute to the metabolic syndrome by increasing nonesterified fatty acids (NEFA) and production of inflammatory cytokines that result in insulin resistance, dyslipidemia, hypertension, and production of prothrombotic factors.

NEFA are fatty acids derived from lipolysis of adipose tissue triglycerides that are usually a source of energy in the fasting state. In obese subjects, NEFA levels are increased despite higher levels of insulin. In skeletal muscle, excess NEFA contribute to insulin resistance by increasing levels of diacylglycerol (DAG), which lead to serine phosphorylation of IRS, thereby inhibiting normal insulin signaling. In the liver, NEFA cause insulin resistance in a similar manner, leading to increased gluconeogenesis and accentuation of hyperglycemia by increasing hepatic glucose output resulting in nonalcoholic fatty liver disease (NAFLD). They also contribute to increased VLDL production and secretion by the liver, with increased triglycerides, apolipoprotein B (Apo-B), and small LDLc particles. In addition, NEFA lead to a decreased level of HDLc by increasing the hepatic exchange of VLDL for HDL along with increasing hepatic lipase, which degrades HDL. Other abnormalities associated with elevated levels of NEFA are endothelial dysfunction, beta cell apoptosis, and increased PAI-1.[2,60] In another article the role of fatty acids in obesity and insulin resistance will be further described.

Inflammatory cytokines such as TNFα and IL-1β are produced by macrophages in adipose tissue. They trigger proinflammatory cytokines c-jun N terminal kinase (JNK) and inhibitor of κB kinase β/nuclear factor κB (IKKβ/NF-κB) through classical receptor-mediated mechanisms. JNK leads to phosphorylation of c-jun compartment of activator protein complex 1 (APC1) transcription factor, which leads to serine phosphorylation of IRS, leading to impaired insulin signaling. JNK and IKKβ/NF-κB also, directly or indirectly, activate proinflammatory genes, leading to a self-perpetuating cycle of up-regulation of inflammatory cytokines and inadequate utilization of body energy. TNFα has also been shown to decrease endothelial nitric oxide synthase (eNOS), causing decreased expression of mitochondrial oxidative phosphorylation genes, leading to increased oxidative cellular stress, with the accumulation of reactive oxygen species (ROS), as well as increased endoplasmic reticulum stress and decreased half-life of nitric oxide (NO). Decreased expression of PPARγ co-activator 1α (PGC1α), an inducible co-regulator of nuclear receptors involved in the control of mitochondrial biogenesis and function, has also been found in subjects with insulin resistance and type 2 diabetes. These responses to cellular stress further increase IKKβ/NF-κB and thus the inflammatory process and well as PAI-1.[2,60,62,69] A perceived energy deficit may occur with obesity, because of decreased hepatic ATP, possibly because of impaired mitochondrial function, leading to central appetite stimulation. It is also associated with decreased exercise capacity and increased fatigability, possibly because of mitochondrial dysfunction.[82] The role of mitochondria in obesity and diabetes is also reviewed in this issue of the journal.

Retinol binding protein 4 (RBP4) is the transporter for vitamin A (retinol) in the blood. Serum levels and expression of RBP4 in adipose tissue were found to be increased in mice with adipose-specific knockout for GLUT4.[83] As mentioned above, decreased GLUT4 expression is a common feature of obesity, insulin resistance, and type 2 diabetes.[60] These mice develop impaired insulin action in the muscle, liver, and adipose tissue.[84] Injecting RBP4 into mice or transgenic overexpression of RBP4 leading to increased concentrations caused impaired insulin signaling and increased expression of the gluconeogenic enzyme phosphoenolpyruvate carboxylase in the liver.[83] Analogous to this, RPB4 knockout mice developed increased insulin sensitivity and glucose tolerance.[83] These findings led to interest in the possible causal role of RBP4 in insulin resistance. In humans, higher levels of RBP4 are found with obesity, type 2 diabetes, impaired glucose tolerance, and those with a strong family history of type 2 diabetes.[85] RBP4 is correlated with insulin resistance and has been shown in some studies to correlate more specifically with insulin resistance than leptin, adiponectin, IL-6, or C-reactive protein (CRP).[81,85] As RBP4 is the main transport protein for vitamin A, it has been postulated that the synthetic retinoid, fenretinide could lower RBP4 levels and improve insulin sensitivity, although this has yet to be determined.[85]

Hypertension is about 6 times more frequent in obese than in lean subjects. According to the NHANES III, hypertension is present in 15% of males and females with a BMI 25 kg/m² or less, and 42% of males and 38% of females with a BMI greater than 30 kg/m².[79,86] The mechanism behind hypertension is hypothesized to be a combination of the direct hemodynamic effects of obesity on cardiac output, which is increased, and normal or increased peripheral vascular resistance (PVR). The increased PVR is thought to be a result of sympathetic overactivity, volume expansion from the antinatiuretic effects of insulin, and increased angiotensinogen II and proinflammatory cytokine IL-6 with associated increased oxidative stress, leading to decreased NO and endothelial dysfunction.[79,80,87] PPARγ has been shown to be a major regulator of many of these components in adipocytes.[87] Weight loss improves hypertension in 50% of subjects.[79] Further consideration on the relationship between obesity and hypertension is also detailed in this issue.

Other factors involved in the metabolic abnormalities associated with obesity and cardiovascular risk include leptin, adiponectin, resistin, and adipocyte fatty acid binding protein (A-FABP). The absence of leptin leads to extreme obesity, as demonstrated in the ob/ob mice and humans with congenital leptin deficiency.[88,89] Most obese individuals will however have elevated leptin levels with resistance to its appetite-suppressing effects.[90] It is also linked to marked insulin resistance, but has mixed consequences on other cardiovascular abnormalities.[80] Leptin appears to work in adipocytes and augments the expression of PGC1α gene, which has been shown to increase mitochondrial biogenesis and potentially increased mitochondrial oxidation.[62] Adiponectin is an anti-inflammatory adipokine produced by adipocytes. Its expression is affected by insulin, glucocorticoids, β-adrenergic agonists, and TNFα. It is decreased in obesity and increased in lean persons. It appears to have a direct anti-atherogenic affect via its anti-inflammatory properties (reducing production of proinflammatory and increasing anti-inflammatory cytokines) or via its insulin sensitizing action. Adiponectin receptors 1 and 2 (Adipo R1 and adipo R2) are expressed in macrophages and modulated by PPAR ligands; adipo R2 is a more predominant receptor and is induced by PPAR α and PPARγ in primary and THP-1 macrophages. There is some evidence that adiponectin may in fact be a proinflammatory agent, but desensitizes macrophages to itself and other inflammatory stimuli; there is ongoing investigation into its mechanism of action.[91,92] Resistin, a hormone produced by adipocytes, appears to oppose the action of insulin; however, its functional significance in humans is not as yet known.[2] A-FABP is a cytosolic protein present in mature adipocytes, macrophages, and in the bloodstream. Elevated levels correspond with the features of the metabolic syndrome. Recently, subjects from the Nurses Health study and Health Professionals follow-up study[93] have been found to carry a functional genetic variant of A-FABP gene, resulting in decreased adipose tissue A-FABP expression, associated with reduced triglycerides and lower incidence of type 2 diabetes and coronary artery disease. Its proatherogenic activity is believed to be mediated by its direct affect in macrophages. A-FABP decreases PPARγ activity and cholesterol efflux in macrophages, thus leading to the formation of foam cells. A-FABP correlates with CRP levels. Its levels are inversely related to those of adiponectin.[94]

Recently, the cannabinoid system has received much interest because of its effects of cardiometabolic parameters and potential for pharmacologic manipulation. Two cannabinoid receptors (CB1 and CB2) have been identified to date. CB1 is found in the central nervous system (CNS), notably in the cerebral cortex, hypothalamus, reward circuits (nucleus accumbens and amygdala), and anterior pituitary.[95] It is also found in white adipose tissue, enteric nervous system, hepatocytes, and skeletal muscle myocytes.[96,97] The ligands for CB1 and CB2 are anandamide and 2-arachidonylglycerol (2-AG). The receptor is a G-protein coupled receptor, the activation of which leads to activation of inward-rectifying potassium (Kir) channels in the CNS and inhibition of voltage-gated calcium channels. The expression of CB1 and CB2 is down-regulated by glucocorticoids, leptin, and dopamine and up-regulated by glutamate.[96] Activation of CB1 receptors has been shown to have central effects on appetite stimulation as well as increasing hepatic lipogenesis (via increase in lipoprotein lipase and SREBP1c), increasing adipocyte tissue accumulation and decreasing muscle glucose uptake. Increased activation is also associated with decreased adiponectin levels. CB2 appears to be more prevalent in the immune system.[96,97] Antagonists of this endocannabinoid system have been shown to suppress appetite, induce weight loss, improve dyslipidemia, and improve glucose utilization.[98] At least one such drug (Rimonabant) has been approved for therapy in Europe.[95,96]

There appears to be a role of glucocorticoids, sex hormones, and growth hormone (GH) in the development of the metabolic syndrome. Adipocytes express the enzyme 11β-hydroxysteroid dehydrogenase (11β-HSD), which converts inactive cortisone to active cortisol, resulting in locally enhanced cellular glucocorticoid levels. The enzyme is particularly elevated in visceral adipose tissue from obese individuals.[99] Sex steroids have been implicated in the regulation of adiponectin expression/secretion. Testosterone has been shown to selectively inhibit high molecular weight adiponectin, believed to be associated with the higher risk of insulin resistance in men than women. Low adiponectin levels have been associated with development of the metabolic syndrome in postmenopausal women.[80] Growth hormone deficiency has also been related to an increased risk of metabolic syndrome.[100]

CLINICAL APPROACH TO A PATIENT WITH THE METABOLIC SYNDROME

Aggressive intervention to reduce the risk of cardiovascular disease and type 2 diabetes is recommended in individuals with the metabolic syndrome; therefore, long-term intervention and monitoring by their primary care physician is warranted. As an underlying mechanism has yet to be elucidated, treating the individual components is necessary at this time.

Identifying patients of having metabolic abnormalities and thus at high risk for CVD and diabetes is important. Overall, the metabolic syndrome is highest among Mexican American females[14]; however, it is worth noting that certain ethnic groups such as Southern Asian groups may have metabolic abnormalities without abdominal obesity.[29,30] It is recommended to monitor blood pressure, pulse rate, fasting glucose and insulin levels, lipid profile, and liver and kidney function tests together with body weight, height, and waist circumference. In certain individuals, a glucose tolerance test will be warranted as suggested by the ADA guidelines. Establishing a risk category for coronary artery disease can be done using an online risk calculator based on the Framingham heart study (http://hp2010.nhlbihin.net/atpiii/calculator.asp?usertype= prof).[101] As the Framingham heart study was based on a middle-aged white population, with a minority of individuals with diabetes, it should be used with a degree of caution in other ethnic groups, who may have a higher population prevalence of coronary disease and in those with diabetes.

The primary management is a healthy lifestyle. The Diabetes Prevention Program showed that lifestyle intervention reduced the incidence of metabolic syndrome by 41% compared with placebo.[102] Weight loss of the order of 7% to 10% body weight over 6 to 12 months is recommended.[103] This should be achieved through moderate calorie restriction (500–1000 kcal/day deficit), physical activity of ideally 30 to 60 minutes daily, supplemented by an increase in daily lifestyle activities. In the Diabetes Prevention Program and Finnish Diabetes Prevention Study, weight loss contributed to a 58% reduction in the development of diabetes.[104,105] Exercise is also associated with improvement in dyslipidemia independent of weight loss.[106] Exercise enhances the expression and translocation of GLUT4 and improves insulin sensitivity.[107,108] The composition of the diet should be altered to contain less than 200 mg/day of cholesterol, less than 7% saturated fat, with total fat of 25% to 35% of calories, low simple sugars, and increased intake of fruits, vegetables, and whole grains.[12] Smoking cessation should be implemented in all individuals with the metabolic syndrome. Low dose of aspirin is recommended in all cases of moderate to high risk of cardiovascular disease.[12]

For those in whom lifestyle change is not sufficient, pharmacotherapy is available for treatment of obesity, dyslipidemia, and hyperglycemia. Pharmacologic treatment for obesity includes sibutramine, a serotonin norepinephrine reuptake inhibitor; orlistat, which is an inhibitor of intestinal lipase; rimonabant, which is an endocannabinoid receptor-1 antagonist; and metformin, which reduces hepatic glucose production. Metformin was shown to induce weight loss and was associated with a 31% decreased incidence of diabetes when compared with placebo in the Diabetes Prevention Program.[104,109] It is worthy to note that some of the above-mentioned drugs have not yet been approved for the treatment of metabolic syndrome or prevention of diabetes. Individuals with morbid obesity (BMI >40 kg/m^2 or >35 kg/m^2 with major comorbidities) can be candidates for bariatric surgery or laparoscopic gastric banding.[110] The treatments of obesity are discussed in other chapters in this issue.

Drug therapy for dyslipidemia is very successful with the use of HMG Co-A reductase inhibitors (statins), niacin, fibrates, ezetimibe (with statins), and fish oils. LDLc lowering is the primary therapeutic target (<100 mg/dL [2.6 mmol/L] with a history of cardiovascular disease or diabetes and possibly <70 mg/dL [1.8 mmol/L] in the presence of both) with statins as the primary pharmaceutical treatment. The second target in lipid manipulation is to target the non-HDL cholesterol (30 mg/dL above the LDLc goal).[111] Presently, niacin is effective for HDLc raising as well as for lowering triglycerides and LDLc, however causes significant flushing. Fibrates act via the PPARα receptor and are more effective for lowering triglycerides but do not have the beneficial effects on HDLc or LDLc. The risk of myositis and rhabdomyolysis with statins is greater with gemfibrozil, which inhibits the glucouronidation of statins, therefore increasing the plasma levels of all except for fluvastatin.[112] Fenofibrate does not have this interaction and is preferred for combination therapy with statins. Omega-3 polyunsaturated fatty acids in fish oil lower triglycerides also by activating the PPARα receptor. Doses of 3000 mg of eicosapentaenoic acid (EPA) and docosahexaenoic acid (DHA) are required.

The 7th Joint National Committee guidelines require the blood pressure to be recorded as an average of two or more properly seated blood pressure measurements (with the patient on a chair with feet flat on the floor and the arm at the same level as the heart and a blood pressure cuff covering 80% of the upper arm) taken at two or more office visits. Treatment with lifestyle modification is first recommended, which if fails (blood pressure >140/90 or 130/80 in those with diabetes or chronic kidney disease) should be followed by addition of medication. First-line medication would be a thiazide diuretic in uncomplicated cases; angiotensin-converting enzyme (ACE) inhibitors or angiotensin receptor blockers (ARBs) in those with diabetes, congestive cardiac failure, or chronic kidney disease; and possibly beta blockers in those with angina.[113] Prevention of the development of diabetes in those with impaired fasting glucose has been studied in the Diabetes Prevention Program, Finnish Diabetes Prevention Study, and the DREAM trial.[104,105,114] The ADA currently recommends lifestyle modification rather than medication (metformin or thiazoledinediones) for the prevention of diabetes in view of the cost and potential side-effects, including possible cardiovascular risk associated with medication.[4,115] In those with diabetes, current guidelines include a target HbA1c of <7% aiming toward 6% (reference range 4%–6%), blood pressure goal of lower than 130/80 mm Hg, LDLc less than <100 mg/dL, triglycerides <150 mg/dL, and HDLc >40 mg/dL in men and >50 mg/dL in women.[4]

SUMMARY

In today's society with the escalating levels of obesity, diabetes, and cardiovascular disease, the metabolic syndrome is receiving considerable attention and is the subject of much controversy. Greater insight into the mechanism(s) behind the syndrome may improve our understanding of how to prevent and best manage this complex condition.

REFERENCES

1. Roth J, Qiang X, Marban SL, et al. The obesity pandemic: where have we been and where are we going? Obes Res 2004;12(Suppl 2):88S–101S.
2. Grundy SM. Obesity, metabolic syndrome, and cardiovascular disease. J Clin Endocrinol Metab 2004;89(6):2595–600.
3. Balkau B, Charles MA. Comment on the provisional report from the WHO consultation. European group for the study of insulin resistance (EGIR). Diabet Med 1999;16(5):442–3.

4. American Diabetes Association. Standards of medical care in diabetes–2008. Diabetes Care 2008;31(Suppl 1):S12–54.
5. Reaven GM. Banting lecture 1988. Role of insulin resistance in human disease. Diabetes 1988;37(12):1595–607.
6. Reaven GM. Role of insulin resistance in human disease (syndrome X): an expanded definition. Annu Rev Med 1993;44:121–31.
7. Alberti K, Zimmet P. Definition, diagnosis and classification of diabetes mellitus and its complications. Part 1: diagnosis and classification of diabetes mellitus. Provisional report of a WHO consultation. Diabet Med 1998;15:539–53.
8. Expert Panel on Detection, Evaluation, and Treatment of High Blood Cholesterol in Adults. Executive summary of the third report of the National Cholesterol Education Program (NCEP) expert panel on detection, evaluation, and treatment of high blood cholesterol in adults (Adult Treatment Panel III). J Am Med Assoc 2001;285(19):2486–97.
9. Einhorn D, Reaven GM, Cobin RH, et al. American college of endocrinology position statement on the insulin resistance syndrome. Endocr Pract 2003; 9(3):237–52.
10. Report of the expert committee on the diagnosis and classification of diabetes mellitus. Diabetes Care 2003;26(Suppl 1):S5–20.
11. Alberti KG, Zimmet P, Shaw J. The metabolic syndrome—a new worldwide definition. Lancet 2005;366(9491):1059–62.
12. Grundy S, Cleeman J, Daniels S, et al. Diagnosis and management of the metabolic syndrome: an American Heart Association/National Heart, Lung, and Blood Institute scientific statement. Circulation 2005;112(17):2735–52.
13. Ford ES. The metabolic syndrome and mortality from cardiovascular disease and all-causes: findings from the National Health and Nutrition Examination Survey II mortality study. Atherosclerosis 2004;173(2):307–12.
14. Ford ES, Giles WH, Dietz WH. Prevalence of the metabolic syndrome among US adults: findings from the third National Health and Nutrition Examination Survey. J Am Med Assoc 2002;287(3):356–9.
15. Maggi S, Noale M, Gallina P, et al. Metabolic syndrome, diabetes, and cardiovascular disease in an elderly Caucasian cohort: the Italian longitudinal study on aging. J Gerontol A Biol Sci Med Sci 2006;61(5):505–10.
16. Patel A, Huang KC, Janus ED, et al. Is a single definition of the metabolic syndrome appropriate? A comparative study of the USA and Asia. Atherosclerosis 2006;184(1):225–32.
17. Cameron AJ, Shaw JE, Zimmet PZ. The metabolic syndrome: prevalence in worldwide populations. Endocrinol Metab Clin North Am 2004;33(2):351–75, table of contents.
18. Ford ES. Prevalence of the metabolic syndrome defined by the International Diabetes Federation among adults in the US. Diabetes Care 2005;28(11):2745–9.
19. Assmann G, Guerra R, Fox G, et al. Harmonizing the definition of the metabolic syndrome: comparison of the criteria of the Adult Treatment Panel III and the International Diabetes Federation in United States American and European populations. Am J Cardiol 2007;99(4):541–8.
20. Adams RJ, Appleton S, Wilson DH, et al. Population comparison of two clinical approaches to the metabolic syndrome: implications of the new International Diabetes Federation consensus definition. Diabetes Care 2005;28(11):2777–9.
21. Athyros VG, Ganotakis ES, Elisaf M, et al. The prevalence of the metabolic syndrome using the national cholesterol educational program and International Diabetes Federation definitions. Curr Med Res Opin 2005;21(8):1157–9.

22. Lorenzo C, Serrano-Rios M, Martinez-Larrad MT, et al. Geographic variations of the International Diabetes Federation and the National Cholesterol Education Program-Adult Treatment Panel III definitions of the metabolic syndrome in non diabetic subjects. Diabetes Care 2006;29(3):685–91.

23. Yoon Y, Lee E, Park C, et al. The new definition of metabolic syndrome by the International Diabetes Federation is less likely to identify metabolically abnormal but non-obese individuals than the definition by the revised national cholesterol education program: the Korea NHANES study. Int J Obes (Lond) 2007;31(3):528–34.

24. Tong P, Kong A, So W, et al. The usefulness of the International Diabetes Federation and the National Cholesterol Education Program's Adult Treatment Panel III definitions of the metabolic syndrome in predicting coronary heart disease in subjects with type 2 diabetes. Diabetes Care 2007;30(5):1206–11.

25. Mancia G, Bombelli M, Corrao G, et al. Metabolic syndrome in the Pressioni Arteriose Monitorate e Loro Associazioni (PAMELA) study: daily life blood pressure, cardiac damage, and prognosis. Hypertension 2007;49(1):40–7.

26. Welty TK, Lee ET, Yeh J, et al. Cardiovascular disease risk factors among American Indians: the strong heart study. Am J Epidemiol 1995;142(3):269–87.

27. Araneta MRG, Wingard DL, Barrett-Connor E. Type 2 diabetes and metabolic syndrome in Filipina-American women: a high-risk nonobese population. Diabetes Care 2002;25(3):494–9.

28. Simmons D, Thompson CF. Prevalence of the metabolic syndrome among adult New Zealanders of Polynesian and European descent. Diabetes Care 2004; 27(12):3002–4.

29. Feng Y, Hong X, Li Z, et al. Prevalence of metabolic syndrome and its relation to body composition in a chinese rural population. Obesity 2006;14(11):2089–98.

30. Thomas GN, Ho SY, Janus ED, et al. The US National Cholesterol Education Programme Adult Treatment Panel III (NCEP ATP III) prevalence of the metabolic syndrome in a Chinese population. Diabetes Res Clin Pract 2005;67(3):251–7.

31. McKeigue PM, Ferrie JE, Pierpoint T, et al. Association of early-onset coronary heart disease in South Asian men with glucose intolerance and hyperinsulinemia. Circulation 1993;87(1):152–61.

32. Whincup PH, Gilg JA, Papacosta O, et al. Early evidence of ethnic differences in cardiovascular risk: cross sectional comparison of British South Asian and white children. BMJ 2002;324(7338):635–40.

33. Al-Lawati JA, Mohammed AJ, Al-Hinai HQ, et al. Prevalence of the metabolic syndrome among Omani adults. Diabetes Care 2003;26(6):1781–5.

34. Halldina M, Rosella M, de Fairea U, et al. The metabolic syndrome: prevalence and association to leisure-time and work-related physical activity in 60-year-old men and women. Nutr Metab Cardiovasc Dis 2007;17(5):349–57.

35. LaMonte MJ, Barlow CE, Jurca R, et al. Cardiorespiratory fitness is inversely associated with the incidence of metabolic syndrome: a prospective study of men and women. Circulation 2005;112(4):505–12.

36. Thom T, Haase N, Rosamond W, et al. Heart disease and stroke statistics—2006 update: a report from the American Heart Association Statistics Committee and Stroke Statistics Subcommittee. Circulation 2006;113(6):e85–151.

37. Malik S, Wong ND, Franklin SS, et al. Impact of the metabolic syndrome on mortality from coronary heart disease, cardiovascular disease, and all causes in United States adults. Circulation 2004;110(10):1245–50.

38. Girman CJ, Rhodes T, Mercuri M, et al. The metabolic syndrome and risk of major coronary events in the Scandinavian Simvastatin Survival Study (4S)

and the Air Force/Texas Coronary Atherosclerosis Prevention Study (AFCAPS/TexCAPS). Am J Cardiol 2004;93(2):136–41.

39. Saely CH, Aczel S, Marte T, et al. The metabolic syndrome, insulin resistance, and cardiovascular risk in diabetic and nondiabetic patients. J Clin Endocrinol Metab 2005;90(10):5698–703.

40. Rutter MK, Meigs JB, Sullivan LM, et al. Insulin resistance, the metabolic syndrome, and incident cardiovascular events in the Framingham offspring study. Diabetes 2005;54(11):3252–7.

41. Jeppesen J, Hansen TW, Rasmussen S, et al. Insulin resistance, the metabolic syndrome, and risk of incident cardiovascular disease: a population-based study. J Am Coll Cardiol 2007;49(21):2112–9.

42. Eberly LE, Prineas R, Cohen JD, et al. Metabolic syndrome: risk factor distribution and 18-year mortality in the multiple risk factor intervention trial. Diabetes Care 2006;29(1):123–30.

43. de Simone G, Devereux RB, Chinali M, et al. Prognostic impact of metabolic syndrome by different definitions in a population with high prevalence of obesity and diabetes: the strong heart study. Diabetes Care 2007;30(7):1851–6.

44. Anderson KM, Wilson PW, Odell PM, et al. An updated coronary risk profile. A statement for health professionals. Circulation 1991;83(1):356–62.

45. Wannamethee SG, Shaper AG, Lennon L, et al. Metabolic syndrome vs Framingham risk score for prediction of coronary heart disease, stroke, and type 2 diabetes mellitus. Arch Intern Med 2005;165(22):2644–50.

46. Grundy SM, Brewer HB Jr, Cleeman JI, et al. For the conference p: definition of metabolic syndrome: report of the National Heart, Lung, and Blood Institute/American Heart Association conference on scientific issues related to definition. Circulation 2004;109(3):433–8.

47. Wilson PW. Estimating cardiovascular disease risk and the metabolic syndrome: a Framingham view. Endocrinol Metab Clin North Am 2004;33(3):467–81, v.

48. Lorenzo C, Williams K, Hunt KJ, et al. The National Cholesterol Education Program-Adult Treatment Panel III, International Diabetes Federation, and World Health Organization definitions of the metabolic syndrome as predictors of incident cardiovascular disease and diabetes. Diabetes Care 2007;30(1): 8–13.

49. Wang JJ, Ruotsalainen S, Moilanen L, et al. The metabolic syndrome predicts cardiovascular mortality: a 13-year follow-up study in elderly non-diabetic Finns. Eur Heart J 2007;28(7):857–64.

50. Ford ES. Risks for all-cause mortality, cardiovascular disease, and diabetes associated with the metabolic syndrome: a summary of the evidence. Diabetes Care 2005;28(7):1769–78.

51. Gami AS, Witt BJ, Howard DE, et al. Metabolic syndrome and risk of incident cardiovascular events and death: a systematic review and meta-analysis of longitudinal studies. J Am Coll Cardiol 2007;49(4):403–14.

52. Galassi A, Reynolds K, He J. Metabolic syndrome and risk of cardiovascular disease: a meta-analysis. Am J Med 2006;119(10):812–9.

53. McNeill AM, Rosamond WD, Girman CJ, et al. The metabolic syndrome and 11-year risk of incident cardiovascular disease in the Atherosclerosis Risk in Communities study. Diabetes Care 2005;28(2):385–90.

54. Monami M, Lambertucci L, Ungar A, et al. Is the third component of metabolic syndrome really predictive of outcomes in type 2 diabetic patients? Diabetes Care 2006;29(11):2515–7.

55. Sundstrom J, Riserus U, Byberg L, et al. Clinical value of the metabolic syndrome for long-term prediction of total and cardiovascular mortality: prospective, population-based cohort study. BMJ 2006;332(7546):878–82.

56. Kahn R, Buse J, Ferrannini E, et al. The metabolic syndrome: time for a critical appraisal: joint statement from the American Diabetes Association and the European Association for the Study of Diabetes. Diabetes Care 2005;28:2289–304.

57. Iribarren C, Go AS, Husson G, et al. Metabolic syndrome and early-onset coronary artery disease: is the whole greater than its parts? J Am Coll Cardiol 2006; 48(9):1800–7.

58. Smith DO, LeRoith D. Insulin resistance syndrome, pre-diabetes, and the prevention of type 2 diabetes mellitus. Clin Cornerstone 2004;6(2):7–16.

59. LeRoith D. Beta-cell dysfunction and insulin resistance in type 2 diabetes: role of metabolic and genetic abnormalities. Am J Med 2002;113(Suppl 6A):3S–11S.

60. Armoni M, Harel C, Karnieli E. Transcriptional regulation of the GLUT4 gene: from PPAR-gamma and FOXO1 to FFA and inflammation. Trends Endocrinol Metab 2007;18(3):100–7.

61. Taniguchi CM, Emanuelli B, Kahn CR. Critical nodes in signalling pathways: insights into insulin action. Nat Rev Mol Cell Biol 2006;7(2):85–96.

62. Nisoli E, Clementi E, Carruba MO, et al. Defective mitochondrial biogenesis: a hallmark of the high cardiovascular risk in the metabolic syndrome? Circ Res 2007;100(6):795–806.

63. Larance M, Ramm G, James DE. The GLUT4 code. Mol Endocrinol 2008;22: 226–33.

64. Karnieli E, Armoni M. Transcriptional regulation of the insulin-responsive glucose transporter GLUT4 gene: from physiology to pathology. Am J Physiol Endocrinol Metab 2008;295(1):E38–45.

65. Charron MJ, Katz EB. Metabolic and therapeutic lessons from genetic manipulation of GLUT4. Mol Cell Biochem 1998;182(1–2):143–52.

66. Kahn BB, Flier JS. Obesity and insulin resistance. J Clin Invest 2000;106(4): 473–81.

67. Del Prato S. Loss of early insulin secretion leads to postprandial hyperglycaemia. Diabetologia 2003;46(Suppl 1):M2–8.

68. Minokoshi Y, Kahn CR, Kahn BB. Tissue-specific ablation of the glut4 glucose transporter or the insulin receptor challenges assumptions about insulin action and glucose homeostasis. J Biol Chem 2003;278(36):33609–12.

69. Liang CP, Han S, Senokuchi T, et al. The macrophage at the crossroads of insulin resistance and atherosclerosis. Circ Res 2007;100(11):1546–55.

70. Paz K, Hemi R, LeRoith D, et al. A molecular basis for insulin resistance. Elevated serine/threonine phosphorylation of IRS-1 and IRS-2 inhibits their binding to the juxtamembrane region of the insulin receptor and impairs their ability to undergo insulin-induced tyrosine phosphorylation. J Biol Chem 1997; 272(47):29911–8.

71. Armoni M, Harel C, Karni S, et al. FOXO1 represses peroxisome proliferator-activated receptor-{gamma}1 and -{gamma}2 gene promoters in primary adipocytes: a novel paradigm to increase insulin sensitivity. J Biol Chem 2006; 281(29):19881–91.

72. Nakae J, Biggs WH III, Kitamura T, et al. Regulation of insulin action and pancreatic beta-cell function by mutated alleles of the gene encoding forkhead transcription factor FOXO1. Nat Genet 2002;32(2):245–53.

73. Puigserver P, Rhee J, Donovan J, et al. Insulin-regulated hepatic gluconeogenesis through FOXO1-PGC-1alpha interaction. Nature 2003;423(6939):550–5.

74. Armoni M, Kritz N, Harel C, et al. Peroxisome proliferator-activated receptor-gamma represses GLUT4 promoter activity in primary adipocytes, and rosiglitazone alleviates this effect. J Biol Chem 2003;278(33):30614–23.
75. Yki-Jarvinen H. Thiazolidinediones. N Engl J Med 2004;351(11):1106–18.
76. Guan H-P, Ishizuka T, Chui PC, et al. Corepressors selectively control the transcriptional activity of PPAR{gamma} in adipocytes. Genes Dev 2005;19(4): 453–61.
77. George S, Rochford JJ, Wolfrum C, et al. A family with severe insulin resistance and diabetes due to a mutation in AKT2. Science 2004;304(5675):1325–8.
78. Pegorier JP, Le May C, Girard J. Control of gene expression by fatty acids. J Nutr 2004;134(9):2444S–9S.
79. Poirier P, Giles TD, Bray GA, et al. Obesity and cardiovascular disease: pathophysiology, evaluation, and effect of weight loss: an update of the 1997 American Heart Association scientific statement on obesity and heart disease from the Obesity Committee of the Council on Nutrition, Physical Activity, and Metabolism. Circulation 2006;113(6):898–918.
80. Hutley L, Prins JB. Fat as an endocrine organ: relationship to the metabolic syndrome. Am J Med Sci 2005;330(6):280–9.
81. Kloting N, Graham TE, Berndt J, et al. Serum retinol-binding protein is more highly expressed in visceral than in subcutaneous adipose tissue and is a marker of intra-abdominal fat mass. Cell Metab 2007;6(1):79–87.
82. Khayat ZA, Patel N, Klip A. Exercise- and insulin-stimulated muscle glucose transport: distinct mechanisms of regulation. Can J Appl Physiol 2002;27(2):129–51.
83. Yang Q, Graham TE, Mody N, et al. Serum retinol binding protein 4 contributes to insulin resistance in obesity and type 2 diabetes. Nature 2005;436(7049): 356–62.
84. Abel ED, Peroni O, Kim JK, et al. Adipose-selective targeting of the GLUT4 gene impairs insulin action in muscle and liver. Nature 2001;409(6821):729–33.
85. Graham TE, Yang Q, Bluher M, et al. Retinol-binding protein 4 and insulin resistance in lean, obese, and diabetic subjects. N Engl J Med 2006;354(24): 2552–63.
86. Brown CD, Higgins M, Donato KA, et al. Body mass index and the prevalence of hypertension and dyslipidemia. Obes Res 2000;8(9):605–19.
87. Sharma AM, Staels B. Review: peroxisome proliferator-activated receptor gamma and adipose tissue—understanding obesity-related changes in regulation of lipid and glucose metabolism. J Clin Endocrinol Metab 2007;92(2): 386–95.
88. Zhang Y, Proenca R, Maffei M, et al. Positional cloning of the mouse obese gene and its human homologue. Nature 1994;372(6505):425–32.
89. Farooqi IS, Jebb SA, Langmack G, et al. Effects of recombinant leptin therapy in a child with congenital leptin deficiency. N Engl J Med 1999;341(12):879–84.
90. Maffei M, Fei H, Lee GH, et al. Increased expression in adipocytes of ob RNA in mice with lesions of the hypothalamus and with mutations at the db locus. Proc Natl Acad Sci U S A 1995;92(15):6957–60.
91. Kim C-H, Pennisi P, Zhao H, et al. MKR mice are resistant to the metabolic actions of both insulin and adiponectin: discordance between insulin resistance and adiponectin responsiveness. Am J Physiol Endocrinol Metab 2006;291(2): E298–305.
92. Tsatsanis C, Zacharioudaki V, Androulidaki A, et al. Peripheral factors in the metabolic syndrome: the pivotal role of adiponectin. Ann N Y Acad Sci 2006; 1083:185–95.

93. Tuncman G, Erbay E, Hom X, et al. A genetic variant at the fatty acid-binding protein aP2 locus reduces the risk for hypertriglyceridemia, type 2 diabetes, and cardiovascular disease. Proc Natl Acad Sci USA 2006;103:6970–5.

94. Xu A, Tso AW, Cheung BM, et al. Circulating adipocyte-fatty acid binding protein levels predict the development of the metabolic syndrome: a 5-year prospective study. Circulation 2007;115(12):1537–43.

95. Matias I, Vergoni AV, Petrosino S, et al. Regulation of hypothalamic endocannabinoid levels by neuropeptides and hormones involved in food intake and metabolism: insulin and melanocortins. Neuropharmacology 2008;54(1): 206–12.

96. Cota D. CB1 receptors: emerging evidence for central and peripheral mechanisms that regulate energy balance, metabolism, and cardiovascular health. Diabetes Metab Res Rev 2007;23(7):507–17.

97. Woods SC. The endocannabinoid system: mechanisms behind metabolic homeostasis and imbalance. Am J Med 2007;120(2 Suppl 1):S9–17 [discussion S29–32].

98. Kakafika AI, Mikhailidis DP, Karagiannis A, et al. The role of endocannabinoid system blockade in the treatment of the metabolic syndrome. J Clin Pharmacol 2007;47(5):642–52.

99. Walker BR, Andrew R. Tissue production of cortisol by 11beta-hydroxysteroid dehydrogenase type 1 and metabolic disease. Ann N Y Acad Sci 2006;1083: 165–84.

100. van der Klaauw AA, Biermasz NR, Feskens EJ, et al. The prevalence of the metabolic syndrome is increased in patients with GH deficiency, irrespective of long-term substitution with recombinant human GH. Eur J Endocrinol 2007; 156(4):455–62.

101. Wilson PW, D'Agostino RB, Levy D, et al. Prediction of coronary heart disease using risk factor categories. Circulation 1998;97(18):1837–47.

102. Orchard TJ, Temprosa M, Goldberg R, et al. The effect of metformin and intensive lifestyle intervention on the metabolic syndrome: the diabetes prevention program randomized trial. Ann Intern Med 2005;142(8):611–9.

103. Expert Panel on the Identification, Evaluation and Treatment of Overweight in Adults. Clinical guidelines on the identification, evaluation, and treatment of overweight and obesity in adults: executive summary. Am J Clin Nutr 1998; 68(4):899–917.

104. Knowler W, Barrett-Connor E, Fowler S, et al. Reduction in the incidence of type 2 diabetes with lifestyle intervention or metformin. N Engl J Med 2002;346(6): 393–403.

105. Tuomilehto J, Lindstrom J, Eriksson JG, et al. Prevention of type 2 diabetes mellitus by changes in lifestyle among subjects with impaired glucose tolerance. N Engl J Med 2001;344(18):1343–50.

106. Kraus WE, Houmard JA, Duscha BD, et al. Effects of the amount and intensity of exercise on plasma lipoproteins. N Engl J Med 2002;347(19):1483–92.

107. Kim HJ, Lee JS, Kim CK. Effect of exercise training on muscle glucose transporter 4 protein and intramuscular lipid content in elderly men with impaired glucose tolerance. Eur J Appl Physiol 2004;93(3):353–8.

108. Goodyear LJ, Kahn BB. Exercise, glucose transport, and insulin sensitivity. Annu Rev Med 1998;49(1):235–61.

109. Pi-Sunyer FX. Use of lifestyle changes, treatment plans, and drug therapy in controlling cardiovascular and metabolic risk factors. Obesity 2006; 14(Suppl 3):135S–42S.

110. Elder KA, Wolfe BM. Bariatric surgery: a review of procedures and outcomes. Gastroenterology 2007;132(6):2253–71.
111. National Cholesterol Education Program (NCEP) Expert Panel on Detection, Evaluation, and Treatment of High Blood Cholesterol in Adults (Adult Treatment Panel III). Third report of the National Cholesterol Education Program (NCEP) Expert Panel on Detection, Evaluation, and Treatment of High Blood Cholesterol in Adults (Adult Treatment Panel III) final report. Circulation 2002;106(25): 3143–421.
112. Bottorff MB. Statin safety and drug interactions: clinical implications. The American Journal of Cardiology 2006;97(8 Suppl 1):S27–31.
113. Chobanian AV, Bakris GL, Black HR, et al. Seventh report of the Joint National Committee on Prevention, Detection, Evaluation, and Treatment of High Blood Pressure. Hypertension 2003;42(6):1206–52.
114. DREAM Trial Investigators, Gerstein HC, Yusuf S, et al. Effect of rosiglitazone on the frequency of diabetes in patients with impaired glucose tolerance or impaired fasting glucose: a randomised controlled trial. Lancet 2006;368(9541):1096–105.
115. Nissen SE, Wolski K. Effect of rosiglitazone on the risk of myocardial infarction and death from cardiovascular causes. N Engl J Med 2007;356(24):2457–71.

Insulin Resistance: the Link Between Obesity and Cardiovascular Disease

Gerald M. Reaven, MD

KEYWORDS

- Insulin resistance • Obesity • Cardiovascular disease
- Insulin-mediated glucose uptake • Body mass index
- Waist circumference

One need not be an epidemiologist to recognize the fact that the prevalence of over-weight/obesity is increasing rapidly in the United States, and by simply strolling down the streets of any city, going to the movies, attending a ballgame, and so forth, the magnitude of this problem (no pun intended) is identified. The impact of the "obesity epidemic" has also been chronicled in probably every magazine published in this country, and hardly a month goes by without this dilemma occupying prominent space in some newspaper.

The fact that more and more Americans are overweight has been well documented in the medical literature,[1,2] as has the association between overweight/obesity and mortality.[3–7] The relationship between obesity and excess mortality is consistent with evidence that these individuals are at increased risk of essential hypertension, type 2 diabetes mellitus (2DM), and cardiovascular disease (CVD).[8–10] In light of these findings, it is not surprising that a "call to action" has been issued to health care professionals to begin addressing the harmful effects of the increase in adiposity and the decrease in physical activity that seem to characterize the United States population.[11]

In view of the apparent consensus over the adverse impact of obesity on important clinical syndromes and overall morality, a recent study's conclusion that the magnitude of the impact of the increase in prevalence of overweight/obesity on excess death may not be as great as is feared was unexpected.[12] In this report, moderately obese participants (body mass index [BMI] 30.0 kg/m^2 to <35.0 kg/m^2) in the National

A version of this article appeared in the 37:3 issue of the *Endocrinology and Metabolism Clinics of North America*.

Division of Cardiovascular Medicine, Stanford University School of Medicine, Falk CVRC, Stanford Medical Center, 300 Pasteur Drive, Stanford, CA 94305, USA

E-mail address: greaven@cvmed.stanford.edu

Med Clin N Am 95 (2011) 875–892

doi:10.1016/j.mcna.2011.06.002

Health and Nutrition Examination Survey (NHANES) demonstrated only modestly increased mortality compared with individuals whose BMI was 18.5 kg/m² to <25.0 kg/m², with increased relative risk statistically significant in NHANES I but not in NHANES II or III.[12] The investigators did not contest the view that being obese increases the likelihood of developing a number of serious clinical syndromes but suggested that the association between obesity and mortality may have decreased over time because of improvements in public health or medical care for obesity-related conditions. Indeed, analysis of trends in CVD risk factors shows decreases in the prevalence of hypercholesterolemia and high blood pressure and a stable prevalence of diabetes despite increasing prevalence of obesity.[13]

There is no simple way to reconcile these conflicting views of the impact that obesity has on mortality, and doing so is not the goal of this article. Such conflicting views, however, open the door to propose a somewhat different approach to the relationship between obesity and disease, and in particular, the relationship between excess adiposity and CVD. Specifically, it is argued that (1) resistance to insulin action (and associated abnormalities) is the link between obesity and CVD; and (2) overweight/obese individuals differ in terms of their degree of insulin resistance and, therefore, their risk of CVD.

FITNESS VERSUS FATNESS

Although there is general agreement that overweight/obese individuals tend to be sedentary, relatively little attention is paid to the impact that variations in physical activity might have on the putative relationships among obesity, metabolic abnormalities, and disease. The result is that the adverse health-related consequences of being overweight are exaggerated and the deleterious effects of decreases in physical activity receive much less attention.

Relationship Between Insulin-mediated Glucose Uptake and Fitness

Rosenthal and colleagues[14] quantified insulin-mediated glucose uptake (IMGU) by using the hyperinsulinemic, euglycemic clamp technique and physical fitness by measuring maximal aerobic capacity ($\dot{V}o_2$max) in 33 apparently healthy individuals of Caucasian ancestry and found the two variables to be highly correlated ($r = 0.63$, $P<.001$). This relationship was independent of age and obesity; it was also noted that the higher the $\dot{V}o_2$max, the lower the plasma glucose and insulin responses during an oral glucose tolerance test ($P<.05$).

Essentially similar findings were noted in a study of 55 nondiabetic, apparently healthy Pima Indians.[15] The values of IMGU varied considerably in these subjects, and it was estimated that differences in maximal oxygen uptake appeared to make an independent contribution of approximately 20% to the variations in IMGU seen in this population. The results of a subsequent study of 55 Pima Indians and 35 Caucasians also indicated that differences in $\dot{V}o_2$max were significantly related to IMGU and pointed out that differences in $\dot{V}o_2$max and estimates of adiposity, taken together, could account for approximately 50% of the variation in measures of IMGU, with each making independent contributions of approximately 25%.[16]

The existence of a positive relationship between degree of physical fitness and insulin sensitivity in cross-sectional studies of apparently healthy individuals is not surprising in view of the substantial evidence of the beneficial effects of training on improving insulin sensitivity.[17–19]

The convergence of the facts that overweight/obese individuals tend to be less physically active and that decreased activity is associated with insulin resistance supports the notion that the adverse impact of obesity may, at least partly, be due to obesity-related sedentary lifestyle, rather than obesity, per se. This distinction may be scientifically the case, but it could also be argued that this issue is somewhat irrelevant, and the relative importance of the untoward effects of obesity versus those of fitness is beside the point; pragmatically, both are bad. It could also be well argued that not truly understanding the problem makes devising solutions infinitely more difficult.

Impact of Variations in Adiposity Versus Activity Level on Clinical Outcome

Efforts have been made to evaluate the relative importance of obesity and inactivity to increasing risk of CVD and 2DM.[20–24] In some cases, measures of obesity appeared to incur greater risk,[21,24] and in other cases, level of activity seemed to be the more important risk factor,[20] whereas in some instances, the contribution seemed to be approximately the same.[22,23] A good example of this last finding is the study by Sullivan and colleagues[23] that evaluated data collected from 2000 to 2002 by the Medical Expenditure Panel Survey on 68,500 adults. These investigators found that the likelihood of developing diabetes, diabetes plus heart disease, diabetes plus hypertension, and diabetes plus hyperlipidemia was lowest in those who had a normal BMI and increased progressively with degree of obesity. Within each specific obesity category, however, the likelihood of developing all of these morbidities was higher in those individuals classified as being inactive. For example, in individuals who had a normal BMI (<25.0 kg/m^2), the odds ratio for developing 2DM was 1.52 (1.25–1.86) when inactive to active individuals were compared; the odds ratio of 1.65 (1.40–1.96) for active overweight individuals (BMI = 25.0–29.9 kg/m^2) did not increase compared with inactive individuals who had normal weight (BMI <25.0 kg/m^2). As a result of their analysis, Sullivan and colleagues[23] concluded, "both physical inactivity and obesity seem to be strongly and independently associated with diabetes and diabetes-related comorbidities."

OBESITY AND INSULIN RESISTANCE
Relationship Between Obesity and Insulin-mediated Glucose Uptake

It has been known for more than 30 years that obesity is associated with a decrease in IMGU.[25] Despite this long history, however, the relationship between obesity and insulin resistance remains controversial at several levels. Indeed, it is frequently assumed that obesity is essentially synonymous with insulin resistance and associated metabolic abnormalities. If this were not the case, it would be difficult to understand the genesis of the concept of a metabolically obese, normal-weight individual.[26] This notion is obviously based on the belief that the natural state of the obese individual is to be insulin resistant and metabolically abnormal and that these findings rarely occur in nonobese persons. Perhaps the strongest evidence that insulin resistance is not a simple function of overweight/obesity comes from the report from the European Group for the Study of Insulin Resistance[27]: the results of euglycemic, hyperinsulinemic clamp studies in 1146 nondiabetic, normotensive volunteers showed that only approximately 25% of the obese volunteers were classified as being insulin resistant with the criteria used.

Although not the major focus of their study, these investigators also pointed out that waist circumference (WC) and ratio of waist-to-hip girth were not related to insulin sensitivity after adjustments for age, sex, and BMI.[27] This observation seems to have been overlooked in the emphasis on the importance of the role played by abdominal obesity in the development of insulin resistance and CVD. For example, the criteria published by the Adult Treatment Panel III (ATP III)[28] for the diagnosis of the metabolic syndrome included obesity as one of the components, but an individual could not be considered obese unless he or she exceeded an arbitrary value of WC. The importance of abdominal obesity reached its apotheosis with the publication of the International Diabetes Federation definition of the metabolic syndrome.[29] Not only is an abnormal WC the only criterion with which to define obesity but an abnormal WC is also the one essential ingredient that must be present to make a diagnosis of the metabolic syndrome.

Relationship Between Overall (Body Mass Index) or Abdominal Obesity (Waist Circumference) and Insulin Resistance

The apparent hegemony of abdominal (WC) compared with overall (BMI) obesity in the association with insulin resistance seemed somewhat surprising in light of the fact that BMI and WC are so closely related. For example, measurements obtained from approximately 15,000 participants in the NHANES indicated that the correlation coefficient between BMI and WC was greater than 0.9, irrespective of the age, sex, and ethnicity of the groups evaluated.[30]

Given these data, we have made an effort to evaluate the magnitude of the relationship between BMI and WC to a specific measure of IMGU. For this purpose, IMGU was quantified with the insulin suppression test (IST). The IST was introduced and validated some years ago[31,32] and, in its current form, involves the continuous infusion for 180 minutes of octreotide, insulin, and glucose.[33] Under these conditions, endogenous insulin secretion is inhibited, as is the secretion of all other hormones that modulate glucose uptake. Steady-state plasma insulin (SSPI) and steady-state plasma glucose (SSPG) concentrations are reached 90 to 120 minutes after the start of the infusion, and blood is drawn for measurement of plasma insulin and glucose concentrations every 10 minutes during the last 30 minutes of the continuous infusion. These four values are averaged and used to determine the SSPI and SSPG concentrations observed during that study. Because the SSPI concentrations at the end of the infusion are similar in all individuals and because the glucose infusion rate during the infusion is also identical, the SSPG concentrations provide a direct estimate of the ability of the same amount of insulin to promote glucose disposal in the person being studied: the higher the SSPG concentration, the more insulin resistant the individual. It should be emphasized that quantification of insulin action with the IST and the hyperinsulinemic, euglycemic clamp technique yields results that are highly correlated ($r > 0.9$) in normal subjects and in patients who have 2DM, both obese and nonobese.[32]

The relationship between BMI or WC and SSPG concentration was examined in 330 apparently healthy individuals[34]; the results of this analysis are shown in **Fig. 1**. It is clear from these data that there was no difference in the magnitude of the correlation coefficient between BMI and SSPG ($r = 0.58$, $P<.001$) compared with that between WC and SSPG ($r = 0.57$, $P<.001$). Furthermore, the best-fit lines describing the relationship between the specific adiposity measures and SSPG concentrations were also not different ($P = .90$). It is also clear that there are many obese individuals, whether defined by an abnormal BMI or by WC, who are insulin sensitive (low SSPG concentrations).

The fact that BMI and WC are significantly related to measures of IMGU has been shown by other groups, but the putative superiority of WC is based on the argument that the relationship between WC and insulin sensitivity remains significant when adjusted for differences in BMI; however, and for unclear reasons, the converse is rarely attempted—that is, determining whether the relationship between BMI and insulin sensitivity remains significant when adjusted for differences in WC. Our attempt to address this issue is illustrated in **Figs. 2** and **3**.[34] **Fig. 2** displays the impact of

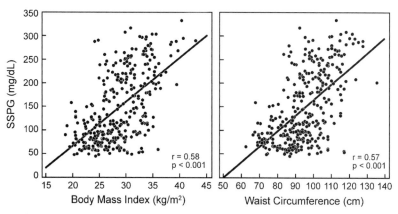

Fig. 1. Relationship between SSPG concentration and BMI (*left panel*) and WC (*right panel*). (*From* Farin HMF, Abbasi F, Reaven GM. Body mass index and waist circumference both contribute to differences in insulin-mediated glucose disposal in nondiabetic adults. Am J Clin Nutr 2006;83:47–51; with permission.)

differences in WC classification on SSPG concentration when participants are subdivided based on BMI category. These data show that 96% of individuals who had a normal BMI also had a normal WC, and that 93% of those within the obese BMI category were abdominally obese. Thus, a valid comparison of the impact of differences in WC on IMGU within a given BMI category was limited to those who had a BMI between 25 kg/m^2 and 29.9 kg/m^2, and the results show that abdominally obese individuals had significantly higher ($P<.05$) SSPG concentrations than those who had a normal WC.

The data in **Fig. 3** illustrate the alternative analysis, that is, the impact of differences in BMI category when the same population is subdivided on the basis of being

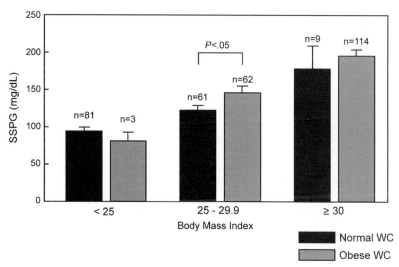

Fig. 2. Comparison of SSPG concentrations as a function of WC classification in subjects stratified by BMI category. (*From* Farin HMF, Abbasi F, Reaven GM. Body mass index and waist circumference both contribute to differences in insulin-mediated glucose disposal in nondiabetic adults. Am J Clin Nutr 2006;83:47–51; with permission.)

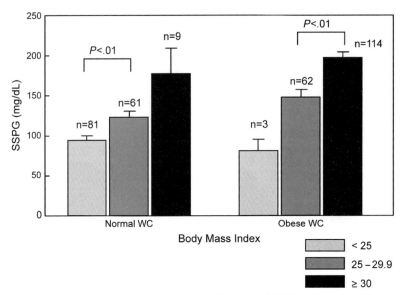

Fig. 3. Comparison of SSPG concentrations as a function of BMI category in subjects stratified by WC classification. (*From* Farin HMF, Abbasi F, Reaven GM. Body mass index and waist circumference both contribute to differences in insulin-mediated glucose disposal in nondiabetic adults. Am J Clin Nutr 2006;83:47–51; with permission.)

abdominally obese (abnormal WC) or not (normal WC). Similar to the results in, **Fig. 2** only 6% of those in the normal WC group were obese by BMI criteria, and only 2% of the 179 persons classified as abdominally obese had a normal BMI. Consequently, within the normal WC group, we could only compare the SSPG concentrations of individuals who were normal or overweight by BMI criteria. Likewise, in the abdominally obese group, the comparison was limited to those whose BMI classified them as being overweight or obese. These comparisons show that irrespective of WC classification, the greater the BMI, the higher the SSPG concentration. Thus, among those who had a normal WC, the mean SSPG concentration of overweight subjects (123 ± 7 mg/dL) was significantly greater (*P*<.01) than that of normal-weight individuals (94 ± 5 mg/dL). The magnitude of the effect on IMGU due to differences in BMI was even greater in abdominally obese participants, with significantly higher (*P*<.01) SSPG concentrations in those who had an obese BMI (197 ± 7 mg/dL) compared with individuals whose BMI classified them as being overweight (147 ± 9 mg/dL).

The results in **Figs. 1–3** are based on measurements made in 330 apparently healthy individuals and provide evidence at the simplest level that there is an extremely close relationship between the two indices of obesity: it is rare for an individual classified as being obese to have a normal WC and rare for someone who is of normal weight to have abdominal adiposity (an abnormal WC). Furthermore, the relationship to a quantitative measure of IMGU is essentially identical, irrespective of which index of adiposity is used (WC or BMI), and that in either instance, there are substantial numbers of individuals who have excess adiposity who are not insulin resistant, just as there are persons who have a normal WC or BMI who are insulin resistant.

Relationship Between Visceral Obesity and Insulin-mediated Glucose Uptake

The evidence presented to this point has demonstrated that measurements of BMI and WC are closely related and are associated with a specific measure of IMGU to an identical degree. These conclusions are at odds with the conventional wisdom that overweight/obesity is synonymous with insulin resistance and the notion, codified by the ATP III[28] and the International Diabetes Federation,[29] that abdominal obesity is the source of all metabolic evil. One possible explanation for this discrepant view of the central role (pun intended) of abdominal obesity in the genesis of insulin resistance and its consequences is the failure to take into consideration the importance of visceral obesity.

The results of 21 studies attempting to define the relative magnitude of the relationship between IMGU and various estimates of adiposity in nondiabetic subjects are provided in **Table 1**.[35–55] The studies are listed in chronologic order, and the following inclusion criteria were used to construct the table: imaging techniques had to be used to determine the magnitude of the various fat depots; IMGU had to be quantified with a reasonably specific method (studies using surrogate estimates of IMGU were not included); and the experimental data had to be available before the use of arbitrary "adjustments" or multiple regression analysis. **Table 1** provides a comprehensive list of studies that meet these criteria; the omission of any published study that would have been appropriately included was inadvertent. In-depth analysis of the possible impact of differences in the experimental populations, the imaging techniques used in each study, and the specific methods used to quantify IMGU are not possible within the context of this presentation.

The results of this analysis are presented in **Table 1**, and it should be noted that the correlation coefficients (r values) between visceral fat (VF) and IMGU are certainly no better than the r values between IMGU and BMI or WC seen in **Fig. 1**. Indeed, r values between IMGU and VF varied from 0.33 to 0.6 in 20 of the 25 measurements in **Table 1**, with differences in VF accounting for approximately 25% of the variability in IMGU in most instances.

Although total fat (TF) was not quantified as often as VF, the magnitude of the relationship between IMGU and TF seemed to be comparable to that between IMGU and VF.

The emphasis in the analysis of these studies was a comparison of the relationship between IMGU and subcutaneous abdominal fat (SF) with that between IMGU and VF. Although the magnitude of the relationship with IMGU was reasonably comparable with VF or SF, there were two examples in which the values were discrepant.[42,48] In the remaining 20 available comparisons, the r values between IMGU and VF or SF did not vary a great deal, being somewhat higher with VF in nine studies, higher with SF in nine studies, and identical on two occasions.

Given the information in **Figs. 1–3** and **Table 1**, the basis for the "conventional wisdom" that abdominal obesity, and in particular visceral obesity, has a uniquely adverse effect on IMGU is not self-evident. Most likely, it is the widespread use of multiple regression analysis to decide which variable is an "independent" predictor of IMGU that is responsible for this belief. Although this approach may provide useful information, it is understood that it presents problems when closely related variables are entered into the model being used. Because all measures of adiposity are highly correlated, it is not clear what the biologic significance is of the results of multivariate analysis that indicate that only one measure is an "independent" predictor of IMGU. In any event, the data presented to this point make it legitimate to at least question the notion of a uniquely close relationship between IMGU and WC or VF, in contrast to the relationship between IMGU and BMI, SF, or TF. Indeed, this conclusion should not be too surprising in view of the results of a study showing that "independent of age and sex, the combination of BMI and WC explained a greater variance in nonabdominal, abdominal, subcutaneous and visceral fat than either BMI or WC alone."[56]

Table 1
Correlation coefficients (r values) between insulin-mediated glucose uptake and body fat distribution in nondiabetic subjects

Study	Population	Visceral Fat	Subcutaneous Abdominal Fat	Total Fat
Abate et al, 1995[35]	39 men	-0.51	-0.62	-0.61
Cefalu et al, 1995[36]	60 subjects	-0.50	-0.50	-0.57
Macor et al, 1997[37]	26 obese subjects	-0.56	—	-0.54
Goodpaster et al, 1997[38]	54 subjects	-0.52	-0.61	-0.58
Banerji et al, 1999[39]	20 Southeast Asian men	-0.59	-0.54	-0.56
Kelley et al, 2000[40]	47 men	-0.61	-0.53	—
Sites et al, 2000[41]	27 postmenopausal women	-0.39	-0.43	-0.30
Brochu et al, 2001[42]	44 obese postmenopausal women	-0.40	-0.17	—
Goran et al, 2001[43]	68 Caucasian children	-0.59	-0.70	-0.68
	51 African American children	-0.43	-0.47	-0.52
Rendell et al, 2001[44]	55 postmenopausal women	-0.49	0.43	—
Purnell et al, 2001[45]	48 subjects	-0.58	-0.41	—
Raji et al, 2001[46]	24 subjects	-0.55	-0.47	-0.61
Ross et al, 2002[47]	89 obese men	-0.41	—	—
Ross et al, 2002[48]	40 obese premenopausal women	-0.34	-0.06	—
Cnop et al, 2002[49]	174 subjects	-0.69	-0.57	—
Cruz et al, 2002[50]	32 Hispanic children	-0.44	-0.46	-0.46
Gan et al, 2003[51]	39 men	-0.71	—	—
Tulloch-Reid et al, 2004[52]	44 African American men	-0.57	-0.57	—
	35 African American women	-0.50	-0.67	—
Rattarasarn et al, 2004[53]	11 Thai women	-0.60	-0.47	-0.38
	11 Thai men	-0.54	-0.45	-0.80
Raji et al, 2004[54]	40 Southeast Asian/Caucasian subjects	-0.33	-0.45	-0.46
	25 Southeast Asian subjects	-0.55	-0.46	-0.54
Bush et al, 2005[55]	150 African American/Caucasian children	-0.33	-0.38	-0.54

OBESITY, INSULIN RESISTANCE, AND CARDIOVASCULAR DISEASE RISK
Body Mass Index and Waist Circumference As Predictors of Cardiovascular Disease Risk

The discussion to this point has focused on the relationship between adiposity and insulin resistance. Although this issue is clearly important, it is necessary to also consider how these variables interact in increasing the risk of adverse clinical outcomes. More specifically, what are the relationships among obesity, insulin resistance, and CVD risk? For example, WC and BMI may be related to insulin resistance to a similar degree, but what is their impact on the abnormalities related to insulin resistance that are more closely related to the risk of clinical disease? We recently addressed this latter question in 261 apparently healthy adults who were divided into two groups based on having a normal or abnormal WC using ATP III criteria[28] or into three groups based on their BMI: normal weight (<25.0 kg/m^2), overweight (25.0 to <30.0 kg/m^2), or obese (≥30.0 kg/m^2). **Table 2** compares the SSPG, plasma glucose, triglyceride (TG), and total cholesterol, low-density lipoprotein cholesterol (LDL-C), and high-density lipoprotein cholesterol (HDL-C) concentrations of the non-obese (normal WC) and abdominally obese (obese WC) subgroups. These data show that abdominally obese individuals had significantly higher SSPG, glucose, and TG concentrations than their normal WC counterparts; however, there were no significant differences in the total cholesterol, LDL-C, or HDL-C concentrations between the non-obese and abdominally obese groups.

Changes in insulin sensitivity and CVD risk factors as a function of differences in BMI are presented in **Table 3**. By one-way analysis of variance it can be seen that every variable measured differed as a function of BMI group. Furthermore, all of the CVD risk factors were significantly different when normal-weight individuals (BMI <25.0 kg/m^2) were compared with obese subjects (BMI 30.0–35.0 kg/m^2). It should also be noted that SSPG concentrations of all three BMI groups were different from each other.

Results in **Tables 2** and **3** show that insulin sensitivity and related metabolic CVD risk factors worsened as a function of increased obesity whether BMI or WC was used as the index of excess adiposity. To further asses the clinical relevance of using BMI or WC to identify individuals at increased CVD risk, we compared all of the experimental variables in individuals classified as being overweight/obese by BMI criteria or abdominally obese on the basis of their WC values. The metabolic characteristics of

Table 2
Metabolic variables in 261 apparently healthy individuals classified by waist circumference

	WC		
Variables	Normal (n = 128)	Obese (n = 133)	P
SSPG (mg/dL)	107 ± 5	174 ± 6	<.001
Glucose (mg/dL)	92 ± 1	98 ± 1	<.001
Triglyceride (mg/dL)	128 ± 10	163 ± 9	.01
Total cholesterol (mg/dL)	193 ± 3	201 ± 3	.09
LDL-C (mg/dL)	118 ± 3	124 ± 3	.14
HDL-C (mg/dL)	52 ± 1	49 ± 1	.13

Data are expressed as mean ± SEM; statistical significance by Student *t* test.
Abbreviations: HDL-C = high-density lipoprotein cholesterol; LDL-C = low-density lipoprotein cholesterol.
Data from Farin HFM, Abbasi F, Reaven GM. Comparison of body mass index versus waist circumference with the metabolic changes that increase the risk of cardiovascular disease in insulin-resistant individuals. Am J Cardiol 2006;98:1053–6.

Table 3
Metabolic variables in the 261 apparently healthy individuals classified by body mass index

| Variables | BMI (kg/m²) | | | P |
	<25 (n = 68)	25–29.9 (n = 106)	≥30 (n = 87)	
SSPG (mg/dL)*	91 ± 5	132 ± 6	192 ± 8	<.001
Glucose (mg/dL)**	91 ± 1	95 ± 1	98 ± 1	<.001
TG (mg/dL)**	98 ± 7	154 ± 12	173 ± 12	<.001
Total cholesterol (mg/dL)**	186 ± 4	201 ± 4	201 ± 4	.03
LDL-C (mg/dL)**	111 ± 3	124 ± 3	126 ± 4	.01
HDL-C (mg/dL)**	56 ± 2	50 ± 1	47 ± 1	<.001

Data are expressed as mean ± SEM; statistical significance by analysis of variance.

* $P<.001$ for pairwise comparisons of BMI groups <25 versus 25–29.9, <25 versus ≥30, and 25–29.9 versus ≥30; ** $P<.05$ for pairwise comparisons of BMI groups <25 versus 25–29.9 and <25 versus ≥30.

Data from Farin HFM, Abbasi F, Reaven GM. Comparison of body mass index versus waist circumference with the metabolic changes that increase the risk of cardiovascular disease in insulin-resistant individuals. Am J Cardiol 2006;98:1053–6.

the subjects identified by the two different obesity criteria were then compared. Comparison of the two groups in **Table 4** shows that more individuals met criteria for being overweight/obese (n = 193) than were classified as abdominally obese (n = 133). It can also be seen that the values for all of the CVD risk factors measured were comparable, irrespective of whether BMI or WC was used to classify the groups. Thus, if the goal is to have normal and abnormal values for classifying individuals as being obese and therefore at increased risk to develop adverse outcomes, it seems that applying criteria for an abnormal BMI or an abnormal WC identifies populations at comparable CVD risk.

Variability of Cardiovascular Disease Risk in Equally Obese, Apparently Healthy Individuals

Because it is apparent that not all overweight/obese individuals are insulin resistant, the question then becomes what proportion of this population displays the metabolic abnormalities associated with the defect in insulin action.[57,58] In several relatively

Table 4
Metabolic variables in 261 apparently healthy individuals classified as overweight/obese or abdominally obese

Variables	Overweight/Obese[a] (n = 193)	Abdominally Obese[b] (n = 133)
SSPG (mg/dL)	159 ± 5	174 ± 6
Glucose (mg/dL)	96 ± 1	98 ± 1
TG (mg/dL)	163 ± 8	163 ± 9
Total cholesterol (mg/dL)	200 ± 3	201 ± 3
LDL-C (mg/dL)	123 ± 3	124 ± 3
HDL-C (mg/dL)	49 ± 1	49 ± 1

[a] BMI ≥25.0 kg/m².
[b] WC >88 cm for women, >102 cm for men.

Data from Farin HFM, Abbasi F, Reaven GM. Comparison of body mass index versus waist circumference with the metabolic changes that increase the risk of cardiovascular disease in insulin-resistant individuals. Am J Cardiol 2006;98:1053–6.

small studies, we presented evidence that a significant proportion of obese individuals are insulin sensitive and do not demonstrate the panoply of CVD risk factors that equally obese insulin-resistant individuals do.[59-65] More recently, we compared a number of CVD risk factors in 211 obese individuals[64] who were divided into three groups based on their SSPG concentration (ie, their degree of insulin resistance). SSPG concentrations (mean ± SD) increased progressively from 81 ± 26 mg/dL, to 166 ± 25 mg/dL, and to 247 ± 29 mg/dL, going from the most insulin-sensitive to the most insulin-resistant tertile. BMI values also tended to increase in parallel with the higher SSPG concentrations, with values of 31.7 kg/m^2, 32.0 kg/m^2, and 32.5 kg/m^2 in SSPG tertiles 1, 2, and 3, respectively.

Table 5 presents the comparison of multiple metabolic variables in the three SSPG tertiles, adjusted for any differences in age, sex, and BMI. For the purposes of this analysis, impaired fasting glucose and impaired glucose tolerance were as defined by the American Diabetes Association.[66] In the most general sense, it is apparent that the values of every risk factor measured were accentuated as a function of the degree of insulin resistance, with the exception of LDL-C concentration. Regarding every other variable, the comparison of the three SSPG groups showed that they were all worse when comparing tertile 3 (the most insulin-resistant group) to tertile 1 (the most insulin-sensitive group), and most of the values in tertile 3 were also significantly different from those in tertile 2 (the intermediate group).

There are many clinical implications of these findings, but at least two points are worth emphasizing. All of the values of the subjects in SSPG tertile 1 indicate that the risk for

Table 5
Comparison of cardiovascular and diabetes risk factors in obese individuals as a function of steady-state plasma glucose tertile

Risk Factor	Tertile 1 (n = 70)	Tertile 2 (n = 70)	Tertile 3 (n = 71)	P[d]	P for Trend[e]
Systolic blood pressure (mm Hg)	123 (18)	130 (17)	139 (20)[a,b]	<.001	<.001
Diastolic blood pressure (mm Hg)	75 (10)	78 (12)	83 (3)[a]	<.001	<.001
TG (mg/dL)	114 (51)	156 (66)[c]	198 (105)[a,b]	<.001	<.001
HDL-C (mg/dL)	50 (13)	47 (13)	41 (9)[a,b]	<.001	<.001
LDL-C (mg/dL)	123 (38)	134 (33)	123 (29)	.88	.77
Fasting plasma glucose (mg/dL)	95 (11)	99 (10)	103 (11)[a]	<.001	<.001
2-h plasma glucose during OGTT (mg/dL)	104 (19)	124 (35)[c]	139 (39)[a]	<.001	<.001
% Impaired fasting glucose	29%	46%	68%[a,b]	<.001	<.001
% Impaired glucose tolerance	1%	29%[c]	46%[a,b]	<.001	<.001

Data are expressed as mean (SD).
Abbreviation: OGTT, oral glucose tolerance test.
[a] P < .05 for tertile 3 versus tertile 1.
[b] P < .05 for tertile 3 versus tertile 2.
[c] P < .05 for tertile 2 versus tertile 1.
[d] Analysis of covariance, adjusted for age, BMI, and sex.
[e] P for trend analyzed by way of general linear model for continuous variables and Cochran-Armitage test for categoric variables.

CVD (or 2DM for that matter) in the most insulin-sensitive third of this obese population is markedly attenuated. In dramatic contrast are the findings in the most insulin-resistant third of this obese population, in which the level of risk is clearly greatly magnified. Perhaps the most striking example of the disparity in metabolic abnormalities in obese individuals is a prevalence of impaired glucose tolerance of 1% in the most insulin-sensitive third compared with a 46% in the most insulin-resistant tertile. These findings clearly point out that not all obese individuals are insulin resistant and that approximately one third of them are at reduced risk to develop CVD.

EFFECTS OF WEIGHT LOSS ON CARDIOVASCULAR DISEASE RISK
Insulin Resistance and The Metabolic Benefits of Weight Loss

The biologic implications of the findings in **Table 5** are substantial and require consideration of the clinical approach to weight loss in overweight/obese individuals. At the simplest level, the most insulin-sensitive third of an apparently healthy group of obese individuals was at greatly decreased risk of CVD and 2DM compared with the most insulin-resistant third of this population. Are the metabolic benefits of weight loss similar in these two groups? The answer, not surprisingly, is no, and whereas obese insulin-resistant individuals become more insulin sensitive (lower SSPG concentrations) and have an improvement in all CVD risk factors associated with insulin resistance, there is essentially no change in insulin sensitivity and related CVD risk factors when insulin-sensitive obese individuals lose the same amount of weight.[59–65] Given this information, it seems mandatory to reconsider how health care professionals approach the overweight/obese individual. At the most elementary, it is necessary to cease thinking of overweight/obesity as a cosmetic issue and focus on its importance as increasing the risk of serious clinical syndromes. When that is realized, it also becomes necessary to stop thinking of obese individuals as an undifferentiated group of subjects that is at equal risk for adverse clinical outcomes and to realize that it is the insulin-resistant subset of these individuals who are at greatest health risk. The obvious corollary to this is the necessity to identify those overweight/obese individuals who are insulin resistant and initiate an aggressive weight loss program aimed at improving their insulin sensitivity and associated CVD risk factors.

How to Identify the Overweight/Obese Individual at Greatest Cardiovascular Disease Risk

Based on the data in **Table 5**, it could be argued that the first step in the clinical approach to overweight/obese individuals should be to identify the subset of overweight/obese individuals that is insulin resistant. As simple as this may seem at first glance, it is not clear whether it is necessary or attainable. For example, although being insulin resistant may increase the risk of developing the CVD risk factors listed in **Table 5**, it is not clear whether it is insulin resistance per se or the CVD risk factors associated with the defect in insulin action that are the culprit to be focused on. Therefore, simply measuring fasting plasma glucose, TG, LDL-C, and HDL-C concentrations provides an enormous degree of insight into those individuals who are insulin resistant (and thereby at greatest CVD risk) and who will benefit the most from weight loss.

Parenthetically, and of particular relevance to 2DM, it would be prudent to include a measurement of plasma glucose concentration 120 minutes after a 75-g oral glucose load as part of a health care evaluation in overweight/obese individuals. Conversely, patients who have values for these measurements that resemble those seen in the most insulin-sensitive tertile in **Table 5** are at greatly reduced risk to develop CVD or 2DM and will gain little metabolic benefit from weight loss.

In addition to understanding that insulin resistance, by itself and in the absence of its associated metabolic abnormalities, may not increase risk of CVD, it should also be understood that although insulin-resistant individuals are more likely to be glucose intolerant, dyslipidemic, and hypertensive, these abnormalities do not necessarily always develop. Thus, at a clinical level, it is more important to know whether the potential adverse consequences of being insulin resistant are present, rather than whether or not a given individual can be classified as being insulin resistant. For example, results of studies in 490 apparently healthy individuals[67] showed that values of IMGU vary more than sixfold, without any obvious cut-point in the values of SSPG concentration that provides an objective way to define a person as being insulin resistant or insulin sensitive. In our two relatively small prospective studies, however, we showed that the third of an apparently healthy population that has the highest SSPG concentrations (the most insulin resistant) is at significantly greater risk to develop the adverse clinical outcomes related to the defect in insulin action.[68,69]

Despite the complexity of trying to relate insulin resistance per se to clinical outcome, there seems to be a desire among health care professionals to "know" whether a subject is or is not insulin resistant. Even if it was possible to come up with a clear definition of who is or is not insulin resistant, the techniques necessary to determine this are not possible within the context of the clinical practice of medicine. As a consequence, an effort has been made to use surrogate markers of insulin resistance, with an emphasis on plasma insulin concentrations. Although nondiabetic insulin-resistant individuals tend to be hyperinsulinemic, there are two basic problems with the use of plasma insulin concentrations as a clinical tool to classify an individual as being insulin resistant. At the simplest level, there is no standardized clinical assay to measure plasma insulin concentration, making it essentially impossible to come up with a specific value that can be applied that will have meaning beyond the specific methodology used.

In addition to the technical problem related to the measurement of plasma insulin concentration, there remains the issue of how closely related insulin concentration is to a specific measure of IMGU. The best surrogate estimate of IMGU is the plasma insulin response to a 75-g oral glucose challenge, with a correlation coefficient (r value) of approximately 0.8,[67] accounting for approximately two thirds of the variability in IMGU. The correlation drops to an r value of approximately 0.6 when the fasting plasma insulin concentration is used instead of the response to oral glucose,[67] thereby accounting for no more than one third of the variability in IMGU. Furthermore, surrogate estimates of IMGU based on combining concentrations of fasting plasma glucose with fasting insulin (ie, the homeostasis model assessment of insulin resistance or the quantitative insulin sensitivity check index) provide essentially the same information as the fasting plasma insulin concentration.[67,70,71]

Following hyperinsulinemia, hypertriglyceridemia is the metabolic abnormality most closely related to differences in IMGU.[63] For example, in a recent analysis of 449 apparently healthy individuals, we found that the correlation coefficient between SSPG and TG concentrations was 0.57, which was not that different from the r value of 0.6 between SSPG and fasting plasma insulin concentrations in the same population.[72] There was also an inverse relationship ($r = -0.40$) between SSPG and HDL-C concentrations, and the plasma concentration ratio of TG to HDL-C was as closely related ($r = 0.6$) to SSPG concentration as was fasting plasma insulin concentration. Because a high TG concentration and a low HDL-C concentration are known to increase CVD risk,[73–76] the use of the TG/HDL-C concentration ratio could provide the means to identify insulin-resistant subjects who also display the characteristic dyslipidemia associated with the defect in insulin action. In pursuit of this issue, we applied receiver operating characteristic curves to 258 apparently healthy overweight/obese individuals[63] and found that a plasma TG concentration greater than 130 mg/dL and a TG/HDL-C concentration ratio greater than 3.0 were relatively comparable in their ability to identify overweight/obese individuals classified (based on their SSPG concentration) as being insulin resistant. If BMI were the only criterion to initiate an intensive program of weight loss, then 258 individuals would be started; however, only 129 individuals were identified as insulin resistant and would benefit metabolically in response to weight loss. In contrast, only 125 of the 258 had the increase in TG concentration suggesting that they were insulin resistant, and in this instance, 87 would derive substantial metabolic benefit from weight loss. Essentially similar findings were obtained using the TG/HDL-C concentration ratio. Thus, if the goal is to reserve more aggressive attempts at weight loss for those overweight/ individuals who are insulin resistant and at greater risk for CVD, then the use of these dyslipidemic markers appears to be of some clinical benefit by reducing the number of subjects identified for this purpose and ensuring that the individuals chosen would gain substantial clinical benefit from successful weight loss.

SUMMARY

There seems to be general agreement that the prevalence of obesity is increasing in the United States[1,2] and that we are in the midst of an obesity epidemic.[11] The disease-related implications of this epidemic have received an enormous amount of publicity in the popular media, but public awareness of the untoward effects of excess weight has not led to an effective approach to dealing with the dilemma. The gravity of the problem is accentuated in light of the report that only approximately 50% of physicians polled provided weight loss counseling.[77]

Given the importance of excess adiposity as increasing the risk of CVD, 2DM, and hypertension[8–10] and the combination of an increase in the prevalence of overweight/ obesity and a health care system unprepared to deal with this situation, it is essential that considerable thought be given as to how to best address this dilemma. In this context, it must be emphasized that CVD, 2DM, and hypertension are characterized by resistance to insulin-mediated glucose disposal[57,58] and that insulin resistance and the compensatory hyperinsulinemia associated with insulin resistance have been shown to be independent predictors of all three clinical syndromes.[68,69,78] It has also been apparent for many years that overweight/obese individuals tend to be insulin resistant and become more insulin sensitive with weight loss.[25] In light of these observations, it seems reasonable to suggest that insulin resistance is the link between overweight/obesity and the adverse clinical syndromes related to excess adiposity. The evidence summarized in this review shows that the more overweight an individual, the more likely he or she is insulin resistant and at increased risk to develop all the abnormalities associated with this defect in insulin action. Not all overweight/obese individuals are insulin resistant, however, any more than all insulin-resistant individuals are overweight/obese. More important, there is compelling evidence that CVD risk factors are present to a significantly greater degree in the subset of overweight/obese individuals that is also insulin resistant. Not surprisingly, we have also demonstrated that an improvement in CVD risk factors with weight loss occurs to a significantly greater degree in those overweight/obese individuals who are also insulin resistant at baseline. In view of the ineffectiveness of current clinical approaches to weight loss, it seems necessary to recognize that not all overweight/obese individuals are at equal risk to develop CVD and that it is clinically useful to identify those at highest risk. The simplest way to achieve this task seems to be focusing on the CVD risk factors that are highly associated with insulin resistance/hyperinsulinemia. If this is done, then intense efforts at weight control can be brought to bear on those who not only need it the most but also have the most to gain by losing weight.

REFERENCES

1. Flegal KM, Carroll MD, Ogden CL, et al. Prevalence and trends in obesity among US adults, 1999–2000. JAMA 2002;288:1723–7.
2. Hedley AA, Ogden CL, Johnson CL, et al. Prevalence of overweight and obesity among US children, adolescents, and adults, 1999–2002. JAMA 2004;291:2847–50.
3. Allison DB, Fontaine KR, Manson JE, et al. Annual deaths attributable to obesity in the United States. JAMA 1999;282:1530–8.
4. Fontaine KR, Redden DT, Wang C, et al. Years of life lost due to obesity. JAMA 2003;289:187–93.
5. Hu FB, Willett WC, Li T, et al. Adiposity as compared with physical activity in predicting mortality among women. N Engl J Med 2004;351:2964–703.
6. Calle EE, Thun MJ, Petrelli JM, et al. Body-mass index and mortality in a prospective cohort of US adults. N Engl J Med 1999;341:1097–105.
7. Yan LL, Daviglus ML, Liu K, et al. Midlife body mass index and hospitalization and mortality in older age. JAMA 2006;295:190–8.
8. West KM, Kalbfleisch JM. Influence of nutritional factors on prevalence of diabetes. Diabetes 1971;20:99–108.
9. Havlik RJ, Hubert HB, Fabsitz RR, et al. Weight and hypertension. Ann Intern Med 1983;98:855–9.
10. Wilson PW, D'Agostino RB, Sullivan L, et al. Overweight and obesity as determinants of cardiovascular risk: the Framingham experience. Arch Intern Med 2002; 162:1867–72.
11. Manson JE, Skerrett PJ, Greenland P, et al. The escalating pandemics of obesity and sedentary lifestyle. Arch Intern Med 2004;164:249–58.
12. Flegal KM, Graubard BI, Williamson DF, et al. Excess deaths associated with underweight, overweight, and obesity. JAMA 2005;293:1861–7.
13. Gregg EW, Cheng YJ, Cadwell BL, et al. Secular trends in cardiovascular disease risk factors according to body mass index in US adults. JAMA 2005;293: 1868–74.
14. Rosenthal M, Haskell WL, Solomon R, et al. Demonstration of a relationship between level of physical training and insulin-stimulated glucose utilization in normal humans. Diabetes 1983;32:408–11.
15. Bogardus C, Lillioja S, Mott D, et al. Relationship between obesity and maximal-insulin stimulated glucose uptake in vivo and in vitro in Pima Indians. J Clin Invest 1984;73:800–5.
16. Bogardus C, Lillioja S, Mott DM, et al. Relationship between degree of obesity and in vivo insulin action in man. Am J Physiol 1985;248:E286–91.
17. Soman VR, Koivisto VA, Deibert D, et al. Increased insulin sensitivity and insulin binding to monocytes after physical training. N Engl J Med 1978;301:1200–4.
18. Koivisto VA, Yki-Jarvinen H, DeFronzo RA. Physical training and insulin sensitivity. Diabetes Metab Rev 1986;445–81.
19. Goodyear LJ, Kahn BB. Exercise, glucose transport, and insulin sensitivity. Annu Rev Med 1998;49:235–61.
20. Wessel TR, Arant CB, Olson MB, et al. Relationship of physical fitness vs body mass index with coronary artery disease and cardiovascular events in women. JAMA 2004;292:1179–87.

21. Weinstein AR, Sesso HD, Lee IM, et al. Relationship of physical activity vs body mass index with type 2 diabetes in women. JAMA 2004;292:1188–94.

22. Li TY, Rana JS, Manson JE, et al. Obesity as compared with physical activity in predicting risk of coronary heart disease in women. Circulation 2006;31:499–506.

23. Sullivan PW, Morrato EH, Ghushchyan V, et al. Obesity, inactivity, and the prevalence of diabetes and diabetes-related cardiovascular comorbidities in the U.S., 2000–2002. Diabetes Care 2005;28:1599–603.

24. Rana JS, Li TY, Manson JE, et al. Adiposity compared with physical inactivity and risk of type 2 diabetes in women. Diabetes Care 2007;30:53–8.

25. Olefsky JM, Reaven GM, Farquhar JW. Effects of weight reduction on obesity: studies of carbohydrate and lipid metabolism. J Clin Invest 1974;53:64–76.

26. Ruderman NB, Schneider SH, Berchtold P. The "metabolically-obese," normal weight individual. Am J Clin Nutr 1981;1617–21.

27. Ferrannini E, Natali A, Bell P, et al. Insulin resistance and hypersecretion in obesity. J Clin Invest 1997;100:1166–73.

28. Executive summary of the third report of the National Cholesterol Education Program (NCEP) Expert Panel on Detection, Evaluation, and Treatment of High Blood Cholesterol in Adults (Adult Treatment Panel III). JAMA 2002;285:2486–97.

29. Alberti KG, Zimmet P, Shaw J, for the IDF Epidemiology Task Force Consensus Group. The metastatic syndrome—a new worldwide definition. Lancet 2004;366:1059–61.

30. Ford ES, Mokdad AH, Giles WH. Trends in waist circumference among U.S. adults. Obes Res 2003;11:1223–31.

31. Pei D, Jones CN, Bhargava R, et al. Evaluation of octreotide to assess insulin-mediated glucose disposal by the insulin suppression test. Diabetologia 1994;37:843–5.

32. Shen S-W, Reaven GM, Farquhar JW. Comparison of impedance to insulin mediated glucose uptake in normal and diabetic subjects. J Clin Invest 1970;49:2151–60.

33. Greenfield MS, Doberne L, Kraemer FB, et al. Assessment of insulin resistance with the insulin suppression test and the euglycemic clamp. Diabetes 1981;30:387–92.

34. Farin HM, Abbasi F, Reaven GM. Body mass index and waist circumference both contribute to differences in insulin-mediated glucose disposal in nondiabetic adults. Am J Clin Nutr 2006;83:47–51.

35. Abate N, Garg A, Peshock RM, et al. Relationships of generalized and regional adiposity to insulin sensitivity in man. J Clin Invest 1995;96:88–98.

36. Cefalu WT, Wang ZQ, Werbgel S, et al. Contribution of visceral fat to the insulin resistance of aging. Metabolism 1995;44:954–9.

37. Macor C, Ruggeri A, Mazzonetto P, et al. Visceral adipose tissue impairs insulin secretion and sensitivity, but not energy expenditure in obesity. Metabolism 1997;46:123–9.

38. Goodpaster BH, Thaete JA, Simoneau JA, et al. Subcutaneous abdominal fat and thigh muscle composition predict insulin sensitivity independently of visceral fat. Diabetes 1997;46:1579–85.

39. Banerji MA, Faridi N, Atluri R, et al. Body composition, visceral fat, leptin and insulin resistance in Asian Indian men. J Clin Endocrinol Metab 1999;84:137–44.

40. Kelley DE, Thaete FL, Troost F, et al. Subdivisions of subcutaneous abdominal tissue and insulin resistance. Am J Physiol Endocrinol Metab 2000;278:E941–8.

41. Sites CK, Calles-Escandon J, Brochu M, et al. Relation of regional fat distribution to insulin sensitivity in postmenopausal women. Fertil Steril 2000;73:61–5.

42. Brochu M, Starling RD, Tchernof A, et al. Visceral adipose tissue is an independent correlate of glucose disposal in older postmenopausal women. J Clin Endocrinol Metab 2001;85:2378–84.

43. Goran MI, Bergman RN, Gower BA. Influence of total vs. visceral fat on insulin action and secretion in African American and white children. Obes Res 2001;423–31.

44. Rendell M, Hulthen UL, Tornquist C, et al. Relationship between abdominal fat compartments and glucose and lipid metabolism in early postmenopausal women. J Clin Endocrinol Metab 2001;86:744–9.

45. Purnell JQ, Kahn SE, Schwartz RS, et al. Relationship of insulin sensitivity and apoB levels to intra-abdominal fat in subjects with combined hyperlipidemia. Arterioscler Thromb Vasc Biol 2001;21:567–72.

46. Raji A, Seeley EW, Arky RA, et al. Body fat distribution and insulin resistance in healthy Asian Indians and Caucasians. J Clin Endocrinol Metab 2001;86:5366–71.

47. Ross R, Aru J, Freman J, et al. Abdominal obesity and insulin resistance in obese men. Am J Physiol Endocrinol Metab 2002;282:E657–63.

48. Ross R, Freeman J, Hudson R, et al. Abdominal obesity, muscle composition and insulin resistant in premenopausal women. J Clin Endocrinol Metab 2002;87:5044–51.

49. Cnop M, Landchild MJ, Vidal J, et al. The concurrent accumulation of intra-abdominal and subcutaneous fat explains the association between insulin resistance and plasma leptin concentrations. Diabetes 2002;51:1005–15.

50. Cruz ML, Bergman RN, Goran MI. Unique effect of visceral fat on insulin sensitivity in obese Hispanic children with a family history of type 2 diabetes. Diabetes Care 2002;25:1631–6.

51. Gan SK, Krikeos AD, Poynten AM, et al. Insulin action, regional fat, and myocyte lipid; altered relationships with increased adiposity. Obes Res 2003;11:1295–305.

52. Tulloch-Reid MK, Hanson RL, Sebring NG, et al. Both subcutaneous and visceral adipose tissues correlate highly with insulin resistance in African Americans. Obes Res 2004;1352–9.

53. Rattarasarn C, Leelawattan R, Soonthornpun S, et al. Gender differences of regional abdominal fat distribution and their relationships with insulin sensitivity in healthy and glucose-intolerant Thais. J Clin Endocrinol Metab 2004;89:6266–70.

54. Raji A, Gerhard-Herman MD, Warren M, et al. Insulin resistance and vascular dysfunction in nondiabetic Asian Indians. J Clin Endocrinol Metab 2004;89:3965–72.

55. Bush NC, Darnell BE, Oster RA, et al. Adiponectin is lower among African Americans and is independently related to insulin sensitivity in children and adolescents. Diabetes 2005;54:2772–8.

56. Janssen I, Heymsfield SB, Allison DB, et al. Body mass index and waist circumference independently contribute to the prediction of nonabdominal, abdominal, subcutaneous, and visceral fat. Am J Clin Nutr 2002;75:683–8.

57. Reaven GM. Role of insulin resistance in human disease. Diabetes 1988;37:1595–607.

58. Reaven GM. The insulin resistance syndrome. Curr Atheroscler Rep 2003;5:364–71.

59. McLaughlin T, Abbasi F, Carantoni M, et al. Differences in insulin resistance do not predict weight loss in response to hypocaloric diets in healthy obese women. J Clin Endocrinol Metab 1999;84:578–81.

60. Jones CN, Abbas F, Carantoni M, et al. Roles of insulin resistance and obesity in regulation of plasma insulin concentrations. Am J Physiol Endocrinol Metab 2000; 278:E501–8.
61. McLaughlin T, Abbasi F, Kim H-S, et al. Relationship between insulin resistance, weight loss, and coronary heart disease risk in healthy, obese women. Metabolism 2001;50:795–800.
62. McLaughlin T, Abbasi F, Lamendola C, et al. Differentiation between obesity and insulin resistance in the association with C-reactive protein. Circulation 2002;106: 2908–12.
63. McLaughlin T, Abbasi F, Cheal K, et al. Use of metabolic markers to identify overweight individuals who are insulin resistant. Ann Intern Med 2003;139:802–9.
64. McLaughlin T, Abbasi F, Lamendola C, et al. Heterogeneity in the prevalence of risk factors for cardiovascular disease and type 2 diabetes in obese individuals: effect of differences in insulin sensitivity. Arch Intern Med 2007;167:642–8.
65. McLaughlin T, Stuhlinger M, Lamendola C, et al. Plasma asymmetric dimethylarginine concentrations are elevated in obese insulin resistant women and fall with weight loss. J Clin Endocrinol Metab 2006;91:1896–900.
66. Genuth S, Alberti KG, Bennett P, et al. Follow-up report on the diagnosis of diabetes mellitus. Diabetes Care 2003;26:3160–7.
67. Yeni-Komshian H, Carantoni M, Abbasi F, et al. Relationship between several surrogate estimates of insulin resistance and quantification of insulin-mediated glucose disposal in 490 healthy, nondiabetic volunteers. Diabetes Care 2000; 23:171–5.
68. Yip J, Facchini FS, Reaven GM. Resistance to insulin-mediated glucose disposal as a predictor of cardiovascular disease. J Clin Endocrinol Metab 1998;83:2773–6.
69. Facchini FS, Hua N, Abbasi F, et al. Insulin resistance as a predictor of age-related diseases. J Clin Endocrinol Metab 2001;86:3574–8.
70. Abbasi F, Reaven GM. Evaluation of the quantitative insulin sensitivity check index as an estimate of insulin sensitivity in humans. Metabolism 2002;51:235–7.
71. Kim SH, Abbasi F, Reaven GM. Impact of degree of obesity on surrogate estimates of insulin resistance. Diabetes Care 2004;27:1998–2002.
72. McLaughlin T, Reaven G, Abbasi F, et al. Is there a simple way to identify insulin-resistant individuals at increased risk of cardiovascular disease? Am J Cardiol 2005;96:399–404.
73. Miller GJ, Miller NE. Plasma high-density-lipoprotein concentration and development of ischaemic heart disease. Lancet 1975;1:16–9.
74. Carlson LA, Bottiger LE, Ahfeldt PE. Risk factors for myocardial infarction in the Stockholm prospective study: a 14-year follow-up focusing on the role of plasma triglycerides and cholesterol. Acta Med Scand 1979;206:351–60.
75. Castelli WP, Garrison RJ, Wilson PW, et al. Incidence of coronary heart disease and lipoprotein cholesterol levels: the Framingham Study. JAMA 1986;256: 2385–7.
76. Hokanson JE, Austin MA. Plasma triglyceride level in a risk factor for cardiovascular disease independent of high-density lipoprotein cholesterol level: a meta-analysis of population-based prospective studies. J Cardiovasc Risk 1996;3: 213–9.
77. Galuska DA, Will JC, Serdula MK, et al. Are health care professionals advising obese patients to lose weight? JAMA 1999;282:1576–8.
78. Zavaroni I, Bonini L, Gasparini P, et al. Hyperinsulinemia in a normal population as a predictor of non-insulin-dependent diabetes mellitus, hypertension, and coronary heart disease: the Barilla factory revisited. Metabolism 1999;48:989–94.

Obesity and Dyslipidemia

Remco Franssen, MD, Houshang Monajemi, MD,
Erik S.G. Stroes, MD, PhD, John J.P. Kastelein, MD, PhD*

KEYWORDS

- Obesity • Adipocyte dysfunction • Dyslipidemia
- Hyperlipidemia • Lipid metabolism

Cardiovascular (CV) disease is a major cause of mortality worldwide. Traditional risk factors for cardiovascular disease are smoking, hypertension, dyslipidemia, hyperinsulinemia, and obesity. Because these risk factors tend to cluster and most patients have multiple risk factors, the term "metabolic syndrome" has been introduced. Although the precise cause, definition, and additional CV risk of the metabolic syndrome are still under debate, in 2001 the National Cholesterol Education Program Adult Treatment Panel III defined the metabolic syndrome as an independent risk factor for atherosclerosis.[1] Currently, three different definitions are being used to classify the metabolic syndrome. Recently, the International Diabetes Foundation has added yet another classification to the available options, in which waist circumference can be corrected for ethnicity.[2,3] During the last 2 decades, there has been an unprecedented increase in the prevalence of obesity, as well as the metabolic syndrome, closely associated with an increased CV risk. The prevalence of obesity (body mass index or BMI $\geq$30 kg/m^2) in the United States now exceeds 30%, which makes obesity a leading public health problem.[4] The United States has the highest rates of obesity worldwide. From 1980 to 2002, obesity prevalence has doubled in adults and, even more compelling, overweight prevalence has tripled in children and adolescents.[5] The prevalence of overweight adolescence in 2000 was 16.7% in boys and 15.4% in girls; based on these data it is predicted that by 2020 30% to 37% of adolescent boys and 34% to 44% of adolescent girls will be overweight. Based on the current child obesity numbers in the United States, it is speculated that by 2035 the prevalence of chronic heart disease (CHD) will increase by a range of 5% to 16%.[6] Not only in the United States but also in socioeconomic upcoming countries, such as India and Poland, childhood obesity is already progressing rapidly.[7]

A version of this article appeared in the 37:3 issue of the *Endocrinology and Metabolism Clinics of North America*.

Department of Vascular Medicine, Academic Medical Center, Meibergdreef 9, Room F4-159.2, 1105 AZ, Amsterdam, The Netherlands

* Corresponding author.

E-mail address: j.j.kastelein@amc.uva.nl

Med Clin N Am 95 (2011) 893–902

doi:10.1016/j.mcna.2011.06.003

medical.theclinics.com

The dyslipidemia associated with obesity predicts the majority of the increased CV risk seen in obese subjects. The dyslipidemic phenotype, commonly associated with obesity, is characterized by increased triglyceride (TG) levels, decreased high-density lipoproteins (HDL) levels, and a shift in low-density lipoproteins (LDL) to a more pro-atherogenic composition (small dense LDL). Whereas all components of the obesity-associated dyslipidemia have been linked with increased CV risk, low HDL has emerged as one of the most potent risk factors. The strong inverse relationship between HDL-cholesteral (HDL-c) levels and the incidence of CV disease has been substantiated in numerous large observational studies. Even if LDL-c levels are lowered to levels below 70 mg-dl, low HDL-c is still associated with a clearly increased CV disease risk.[8] This potent atheroprotective effect of HDL is traditionally attributed to the role of HDL-c in the reverse cholesterol transport (RCT) pathway, resulting in cholesterol transport from peripheral tissues to the liver followed by excretion in the feces. In the last decade, a wide variety of additional protective effects have been attributed to HDL, comprising inhibition of thrombosis, oxidation, and inflammation.[9] However, low HDL-c is not the only important lipid disorder associated with obesity. High-fasting TGs have also been shown to have independent predictive value for CV risk.[10–12] Although it has proven difficult to dissect the effects mediated by high TGs per se from those conveyed by the concomitant low HDL-c, TGs are shown to convey increased CV risk even after adjusting for HDL-c levels. In a meta-analysis of 21 population-based prospective studies involving a total of 65,863 men and 11,089 women,[13] investigators found that each 1-mmol/L (89-mg/dL) TG increase was associated with a 32% increase in CHD risk in men (relative risk or RR = 1.30; 95% confidence interval or CI, 1.25–1.35) and a 76% increase in women (RR = 1.69; 95% CI, 1.45–1.97). After adjustment for total cholesterol, LDL-c, HDL-c, BMI, blood pressure, and diabetes, the increase in CHD risk associated with each 1-mmol/L increase in TG remained statistically significant: 12% in men (RR = 1.12; 95% CI, 1.06–1.19) and 37% in women (RR = 1.37; 95% CI, 1.13–1.66). Of note, subjects with high TG are invariably characterized by a shift toward small dense LDL. Numerous studies have pointed toward a particular proatherogenic impact of these small dense LDLs. These particles are more likely to be glycosylated and oxidized and, therefore, important in the initiating process of atherosclerosis.[14]

This article focuses on the mechanisms involved in the development of the pro-atherogenic lipid changes associated with obesity. Therefore, it is necessary to first briefly describe normal lipid metabolism before focusing on the obesity associated abnormalities.

NORMAL LIPID METABOLISM

Cholesterol and TGs are both essential for membrane integrity and structure, but also serve as an energy source as well as signaling molecules. Because they are water-insoluble, cholesterol and TGs have to be transported in special water-soluble particles, such as lipoproteins. Triglyceride-rich lipoproteins are secreted in the circulation either by the gut (as chylomicrons) or by the liver (as very low-density lipoprotein [VLDL]) (**Fig. 1**). After a meal, dietary TGs are first digested by pancreatic lipase before they can be absorbed by the intestine and transported into the circulation as chylomicrons. These particles transport the TGs to target tissues, adipose tissue and muscle, where they can be hydrolyzed by the enzyme lipoprotein lipase (LPL) located on the endothelial surface. Upon hydrolysis of TGs, nonesterified fatty acids (NEFA) are formed, which can be taken up by adipose tissue for storage or by skeletal muscle for use as an energy source. The LPL involved in this process is mainly produced

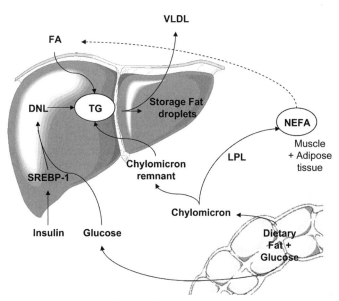

Fig. 1. Schematic representation of normal triglyceride metabolism. DNL, de novo lipogenesis; FA, fatty acids; LPL, lipoprotein lipase; NEFA, nonesterified fatty acids; SREBP1, sterol regulatory element binding protein.

by adipose tissue and muscle itself, and its synthesis and function are under strict control of insulin. This control mechanism through insulin results in activation of LPL in adipose tissue, with a concomitant decrease in LPL activity in muscle during the fed state.[15,16] During the fasted state, when the body relies on fatty acids as an energy source, the hormone glucagon signals the breakdown of TGs by hormone-sensitive lipase (HSL) to release NEFA.

The liver itself is also able to produce TGs from fatty acids and glycerol, also under the influence of insulin. These TGs are then secreted into the blood as VLDL. The fatty acids used by the liver for TG formation are either derived from the plasma or newly formed within the liver by a process called de novo lipogenesis (DNL). In DNL, glucose serves as a substrate for fatty acid synthesis. The uptake of fatty acids in the liver from the plasma is uncontrolled and driven by free fatty acid (FFA) plasma levels. If the liver is taking up more fatty acids than it can use in the VLDL formation and excretion, these surplus fatty acids will be stored in the liver in the form of fat droplets. Through the study of these processes, part of the problem with surplus dietary intake becomes immediately clear: more dietary TGs (chylomicrons), fatty acids, and glucose (source for VLDL) intake can promote liver fat accumulation. Besides up-regulating LPL and stimulation of gene expression of multiple intracellular lipogenic enzymes, insulin controls the uptake and processing of NEFA in adipose tissue and muscle during the fed state. Insulin also acts in the liver on the sterol regulatory element binding protein (SREBP) 1-c, a protein located on hepatocyte cell membranes which transcriptionally activates most genes involved in DNL.[17]

OBESITY-ASSOCIATED DYSLIPIDEMIA

The unraveling of the metabolic mechanisms underlying these proatherogenic lipid changes has made large strides in the last decade. In fact, the lipid changes associated with obesity are similar to those seen in patients with type-2 diabetes or insulin resistance (IR).[18] Insulin resistance itself is a hallmark of the metabolic syndrome, and has a profound impact on the lipid profiles seen in patients suffering from the syndrome.[19] The presence of IR has also been shown to precede the onset of dyslipidemia in most obese individuals.

In the IR state, a reduced efficiency of insulin to inhibit hepatic glucose production and stimulate glucose use in skeletal muscle and adipose tissue leads to hyperglycemia and a subsequent compensatory hyperinsulinemia.[19] In IR, insulin is also no longer capable of inhibiting TG-lipolysis by HSL in fat stores.[20,21] As a consequence, the flux of FFAs to the liver increases profoundly, and this will contribute to increased fat accumulation within the liver. Unfortunately, the IR also results in impaired activation of LPL within the vasculature, contributing to a further increase in circulating TG levels. Thus, in the IR state the responses of both LPL and HSL are blunted and the resulting inefficient trapping of dietary energy will produce a postprandial lipemia and an increase in NEFA, as is seen in both obesity and hyperinsulinemia. This increase in NEFA will result in an increased NEFA flux to tissues, like the liver and muscle, during the fed state. The liver will be the major recipient of this increased flux because of the uncontrolled plasma level-driven uptake. To maintain TG homeostasis, VLDL production is increased in the liver, particularly large VLDL1 particles,[22] as is also observed in obese- and IR patients.[23] When plasma NEFA are raised in normal individuals, VLDL secretion will increase.[24] The formation and excretion of VLDL is then the consequential rate-limiting step and the newly synthesized, but not excreted surplus TGs, will therefore be stored as lipid droplets in the liver that ultimately might lead to nonalcoholic fatty liver disease (NAFLD).[25] NAFLD has numerous causes, but is often encountered in patients with obesity or other components of the metabolic syndrome. The prevalence of NAFLD increases to 74% in obese and up to 90% in morbidly obese individuals.[26,27]

Even when these changes in peripheral energy metabolism caused by IR are not sufficient to disturb lipid profiles and increase liver fat content, hyperinsulinemia per se is also capable of stimulating DNL in the liver through activation of the previously described SREBP-1 pathway. And the hyperglycemia resulting from the IR can also stimulate lipogenesis directly by activation of the carbohydrate response element-binding protein, which in its turn activates the transcription of numerous genes also involved in DNL.[28]

LIPID COMPOSITION IN OBESITY

These changes will also have a dramatic impact on the lipid composition and levels of, for instance, HDL-c particles, that are (besides hypertriglyceridemia) commonly low in both obesity and hyperinsulinemia. The increased assembly, secretion, and decreased clearance of VLDL, and the resulting hypertriglyceridemia, all contribute to lower HDL-c levels. This results partly from the decreased flux of apolipoproteins and phospholipids from chylomicrons and VLDL particles, which are normally used in HDL-c maturation.[15] The enzyme cholesteryl ester transfer protein (CETP), the mass of which and activity are found to be increased in obese patients, also contributes to the decreased HDL-c levels through facilitating transfer of cholesteryl esters from HDL to TG-rich lipoproteins (chylomicrons, VLDL).[29] CETP is also secreted by adipose tissue, which is thought of as an important source of plasma CETP in human beings.[30,31] This cholesteryl ester transfer decreases HDL-c levels but also creates a TG-rich HDL that serves as a better substrate for clearance by hepatic lipase.[32–34] Increased CETP mass and activity also cause the shift that is observed in the LDL composition in obesity. Because of the increased VLDL pool size and delayed particle clearance, an induction of cholesteryl ester exchange in LDL takes place for TGs in VLDL. These LDL particles enriched with TGs are similarly like HDL-c, a better substrate for lipolysis by hepatic lipase.

Besides the decrease of HDL-c levels, there is also evidence that the changes in HDL composition result in a less antiatherogenic function of HDL.[35] HDL isolated from patients with metabolic syndrome was shown to be less capable of attenuating anti-apoptotic activities, indicating defective protection of endothelial cells from oxLDL-induced apoptosis. This antiapopototic function was inversely correlated with abdominal obesity, atherogenic dyslipidemia, and systemic oxidative stress.

ADIPOCYTE DYSFUNCTION AND OBESITY

During the last decade, it has become widely accepted that adipose tissue is not only a storage organ, but also an active endocrine organ with key regulatory functions in both inflammation and metabolism, capable of excreting a wide array of cytokines called adipokines.[36,37] These molecules have been shown to exert significant effects on total body glucose metabolism, insulin sensitivity, and satiety. During obesity an expansion of adipose tissue is associated with an increased influx of mononuclear white blood cells,[38] resulting in the generation of "dysfunctional" fat, characterized by disturbances in the excretion of these adipokines. Defective insulin signaling is also thought to play a role in this expansion of adipose tissue. When the insulin receptor is selectively knocked out in adipose tissue in mice, these mice become resistant to obesity, suggesting that a defect in insulin signaling in adipocytes is important for developing obesity.[39]

Some of the more extensively researched adipokines, such as leptin, adiponectin, resistin, and interleukin (IL)-6 exhibit interactions with lipid metabolism and IR. Leptin was one of the first adipokines discovered, and underlined the impact of adipokines on human energy and fat metabolism.[40] Leptin is the protein, encoded by the ob gene which, when deficient, is responsible for the obesity in the ob/ob mouse and plays a major role in the food intake and energy homeostasis. Absence of leptin drives hunger and suppresses energy expenditure. Notably, leptin has both central as well as peripheral actions. Central administration of leptin increases resting metabolic rates, resulting in reduced TG content in tissues with a concomitant decrease in plasma TG levels.[37,41] In contrast, peripheral leptin stimulates lipolysis of TGs. The complete absence of leptin in both animal models and human patients is associated with a lipotoxicity that can be reversed by administration of leptin itself.[42,43] Patients with lipoatrophy, who have no fat tissue at all or who experienced a loss of fat tissue, suffer from IR, diabetes, and leptin deficiency. When these patients are treated with recombinant leptin the IR can be reversed.[44] Although leptin administration can reverse metabolic disturbances in these patients, this is not a potential cure for obesity because many obese individuals already have high plasma leptin levels and are somewhat leptin resistant.[45]

Whereas attention has now shifted from leptin to novel adipokines, the metabolic consequences of these adipokines are less clear. Adiponectin is a unique adipokine in the sense that as far as we know, it is the only adipokine with antiatherothrombotic effects. In line, plasma levels are reduced in obese, insulin resistant, diabetic, and dyslipidemic patients. Adiponectin-deficient mice develop IR on a high fat diet. When recombinant adiponectin is administrated in obese mouse models, this results in multiple beneficial effects, including a reduction of glucose and lipid levels, increased lipid oxidation, and reduced vascular thickening.[46,47] Adiponectin levels are inversely related to plasma TG and positively correlated with HDL-c levels in human beings.[48] The correlation between HDL-c levels and adiponectin is independent of BMI and IR; however, whether adiponectin directly influences HDL-c metabolism has as of yet to be proven.[49,50]

The gene encoding for another adipokine involved in obesity, resistin, was found to be suppressed by treatment with antidiabetic thiazoladinediones, and therefore also thought to play a role in IR and obesity. However, the precise mechanism of action of this molecule remains unclear. Resistin levels are elevated in diet-induced or genetic mouse models of obesity; however, in human beings data are conflicting.[51] IL-6 is an immune modulating cytokine and its expression in adipose tissue is increased in obesity. IL-6 deficient mice develop late onset obesity that can be prevented by low-dose IL-6 infusion into the brain. Obviously, IL-6 is not really an adipokine. Whereas fat cells have the capacity to produce IL-6, the majority of this cytokine is likely to derive from macrophages located within the fat tissue, actively recruited by local expression of monocyte chemotactic protein 1 (MCP-1).[38]

CENTRAL REGULATION OF LIPID METABOLISM AND OBESITY

Certain parts of the brain are devoted to the control of energy homeostasis and food intake. Foremost, the hypothalamus is known to play a major role in the regulation of satiety and energy expenditure.[45] There are now numerous hormonal mechanisms shown to participate in the regulation of appetite and food intake, relative size of lean and fat mass, and the development of IR. For instance leptin and ghrelin, which are both produced peripherally, are able to exert their effect on appetite through the central nervous system via the hypothalamus. Ghrelin is produced by the stomach and was first found to stimulate growth hormone release from the pituary gland, but is now seen as a short-term appetite controller that is released in response to stretch of the stomach with a function complementary to leptin.[52] The arcuate nucleus has several circuits linking it to different parts of the hypothalamus: the lateral hypothalamus, which is important in feeding, and the ventromedial hypothalamus, which is important in satiety.[53] The arcuate nucleus contains two distinct groups of neurons to exert its effects. The first group coexpresses neuropeptide Y (NPY) and agouti-related peptide (AgRP) and has stimulatory inputs to the lateral hypothalamus and inhibitory inputs to the ventromedial hypothalamus.[54,55] The second group coexpresses pro-opiomelanocortin (POMC) and cocaine- and amphetamine-regulated transcript (CART), and has stimulatory inputs to the ventromedial hypothalamus and inhibitory inputs to the lateral hypothalamus. Consequently, the NPY/AgRP neurons will stimulate feeding and inhibit satiety, while the POMC/CART neurons stimulate satiety and inhibit feeding. Leptin exerts its action to both groups of these arcuate nucleus neurons by inhibiting the NPY/AgRP group while stimulating the POMC/CART group.[56] Besides neuropetides and neurocytokines coming from the adipose tissue, metabolic substrates can influence these hypothalamic regions as well. Glucose and fatty acids also have a central influence on satiety feeling and the metabolic pathways. When an inhibitor of fatty acid synthesis is given centrally, both food intake and body weight are decreased.[57] More recently, central glucose levels were also shown to play a pivotal role in the obesity-associated dyslipidemia. A selective increase in hypothalamic glucose is able to inhibit VLDL secretion by the liver and, therefore, to decrease TG levels in rats. These effects are lost during diet-induced obesity, indicating a role for defective brain glucose signaling in the etiology of the dyslipidemia associated with the metabolic syndrome.[58]

SUMMARY

Dyslipidemia associated with obesity and the metabolic syndrome is one of the central features contributing to the increased CV risk in these patients. In view of the pandemic of the metabolic syndrome, it is imperative to fully understand the mechanisms leading to the metabolic lipid phenotype before embarking upon optimal treatment strategies. The traditional concept that insulin resistance causes increased FFA flux via increased TG hydrolysis in adipose tissue is still of a central theme in the general hypothesis. The combination of increased hepatic VLDL secretion with impaired LPL-mediated TG clearance explains the hypertriglyceridemia phenotype of the metabolic syndrome. Hence, central IR may be an important factor contributing to peripheral hypertriglyceridemia. Recently recognized regulatory systems include the profound impact of the hypothalamus on TG secretion and glucose control. In addition, dysfunctional (or inflamed) intra abdominal adipose tissue has emerged as a potent regulator of dyslipidemia and IR. It will be a challenge to design novel treatment modalities that target "dysfunctional" fat or central IR to attempt to prevent the epidemic of CV disease secondary to the metabolic syndrome.

REFERENCES

1. Third report of the National Cholesterol Education Program (NCEP) Expert Panel on detection, evaluation, and treatment of high blood cholesterol in adults (Adult Treatment Panel III) final report. Circulation 2002;106:3143–421.
2. Alberti KG, Zimmet P, Shaw J. The metabolic syndrome—a new worldwide definition. Lancet 2005;366:1059–62.
3. Alberti KG, Zimmet PZ. Definition, diagnosis and classification of diabetes mellitus and its complications. Part 1: diagnosis and classification of diabetes mellitus provisional report of a WHO consultation. Diabet Med 1998;15:539–53.
4. Mokdad AH, Ford ES, Bowman BA, et al. Prevalence of obesity, diabetes, and obesity-related health risk factors, 2001. JAMA 2003;289:76–9.
5. Ford ES. Prevalence of the metabolic syndrome defined by the International Diabetes Federation among adults in the U.S. Diabetes Care 2005;28:2745–9.
6. Bibbins-Domingo K, Coxson P, Pletcher MJ, et al. Adolescent overweight and future adult coronary heart disease. N Engl J Med 2007;357:2371–9.
7. Kelishadi R. Childhood overweight, obesity, and the metabolic syndrome in developing countries. Epidemiol Rev 2007;29:62–76.
8. Castelli W. Lipoproteins and cardiovascular disease: biological basis and epidemiological studies. Value Health 1998;1:105–9.
9. Ansell BJ, Watson KE, Fogelman AM, et al. High-density lipoprotein function: recent advances. J Am Coll Cardiol 2005;46:1792–8.
10. Onat A, Sari I, Yazici M, et al. Plasma triglycerides, an independent predictor of cardiovascular disease in men: a prospective study based on a population with prevalent metabolic syndrome. Int J Cardiol 2006;108:89–95.
11. Bansal S, Buring JE, Rifai N, et al. Fasting compared with nonfasting triglycerides and risk of cardiovascular events in women. JAMA 2007;298:309–16.
12. Jacobson TA, Miller M, Schaefer EJ. Hypertriglyceridemia and cardiovascular risk reduction. Clin Ther 2007;29:763–77.
13. Abdel-Maksoud MF, Hokanson JE. The complex role of triglycerides in cardiovascular disease. Semin Vasc Med 2002;2:325–33.
14. Sobenin IA, Tertov VV, Orekhov AN. Atherogenic modified LDL in diabetes. Diabetes 1996;45(Suppl 3):S35–9.

15. Goldberg IJ. Lipoprotein lipase and lipolysis: central roles in lipoprotein metabolism and atherogenesis. J Lipid Res 1996;37:693–707.

16. Merkel M, Eckel RH, Goldberg IJ. Lipoprotein lipase: genetics, lipid uptake, and regulation. J Lipid Res 2002;43:1997–2006.

17. Horton JD, Goldstein JL, Brown MS. SREBPs: activators of the complete program of cholesterol and fatty acid synthesis in the liver. J Clin Invest 2002;109:1125–31.

18. Taskinen MR. Diabetic dyslipidaemia: from basic research to clinical practice. Diabetologia 2003;46:733–49.

19. Ginsberg HN. Insulin resistance and cardiovascular disease. J Clin Invest 2000; 106:453–8.

20. Arner P. Human fat cell lipolysis: biochemistry, regulation and clinical role. Best Pract Res Clin Endocrinol Metab 2005;19:471–82.

21. Kraemer FB, Shen WJ. Hormone-sensitive lipase: control of intracellular tri-(di-)acylglycerol and cholesteryl ester hydrolysis. J Lipid Res 2002;43:1585–94.

22. Adiels M, Boren J, Caslake MJ, et al. Overproduction of VLDL1 driven by hyperglycemia is a dominant feature of diabetic dyslipidemia. Arterioscler Thromb Vasc Biol 2005;25:1697–703.

23. Ginsberg HN, Zhang YL, Hernandez-Ono A. Metabolic syndrome: focus on dyslipidemia. Obes Res 2006;14:S41–9.

24. Lewis GF. Fatty acid regulation of very low density lipoprotein production. Curr Opin Lipidol 1997;8:146–53.

25. Qureshi K, Abrams GA. Metabolic liver disease of obesity and role of adipose tissue in the pathogenesis of nonalcoholic fatty liver disease. World J Gastroenterol 2007;13:3540–53.

26. Angulo P, Lindor KD. Treatment of nonalcoholic fatty liver: present and emerging therapies. Semin Liver Dis 2001;21:81–8.

27. Abrams GA, Kunde SS, Lazenby AJ, et al. Portal fibrosis and hepatic steatosis in morbidly obese subjects: a spectrum of nonalcoholic fatty liver disease. Hepatology 2004;40:475–83.

28. Yamashita H, Takenoshita M, Sakurai M, et al. A glucose-responsive transcription factor that regulates carbohydrate metabolism in the liver. Proc Natl Acad Sci U S A 2001;98:9116–21.

29. Arai T, Yamashita S, Hirano K, et al. Increased plasma cholesteryl ester transfer protein in obese subjects. A possible mechanism for the reduction of serum HDL cholesterol levels in obesity. Arterioscler Thromb 1994;14:1129–36.

30. Radeau T, Lau P, Robb M, et al. Cholesteryl ester transfer protein (CETP) mRNA abundance in human adipose tissue: relationship to cell size and membrane cholesterol content. J Lipid Res 1995;36:2552–61.

31. Dullaart RP, Sluiter WJ, Dikkeschei LD, et al. Effect of adiposity on plasma lipid transfer protein activities: a possible link between insulin resistance and high density lipoprotein metabolism. Eur J Clin Invest 1994;24:188–94.

32. Lewis GF, Lamarche B, Uffelman KD, et al. Clearance of postprandial and lipolytically modified human HDL in rabbits and rats. J Lipid Res 1997;38:1771–8.

33. Rashid S, Uffelman KD, Lewis GF. The mechanism of HDL lowering in hypertriglyceridemic, insulin-resistant states. J Diabet Complications 2002;16:24–8.

34. Horowitz BS, Goldberg IJ, Merab J, et al. Increased plasma and renal clearance of an exchangeable pool of apolipoprotein A-I in subjects with low levels of high density lipoprotein cholesterol. J Clin Invest 1993;91:1743–52.

35. de Souza JA, Vindis C, Hansel B, et al. Metabolic syndrome features small, apolipoprotein A-l-poor, triglyceride-rich HDL3 particles with defective anti-apoptotic activity. Atherosclerosis 2008;197(1):84–94.

36. Yu YH, Ginsberg HN. Adipocyte signaling and lipid homeostasis: sequelae of insulin-resistant adipose tissue. Circ Res 2005;96:1042–52.

37. Ahima RS. Adipose tissue as an endocrine organ. Obes Res 2006;14:242S–9S.

38. Wellen KE, Hotamisligil GS. Obesity-induced inflammatory changes in adipose tissue. J Clin Invest 2003;112:1785–8.

39. Bluher M, Michael MD, Peroni OD, et al. Adipose tissue selective insulin receptor knockout protects against obesity and obesity-related glucose intolerance. Dev Cell 2002;3:25–38.

40. Zhang F, Basinski MB, Beals JM, et al. Crystal structure of the obese protein leptin-E100. Nature 1997;387:206–9.

41. Ahima RS, Saper CB, Flier JS, et al. Leptin regulation of neuroendocrine systems. Front Neuroendocrinol 2000;21:263–307.

42. Farooqi IS, Jebb SA, Langmack G, et al. Effects of recombinant leptin therapy in a child with congenital leptin deficiency. N Engl J Med 1999;341:879–84.

43. Halaas JL, Gajiwala KS, Maffei M, et al. Weight-reducing effects of the plasma protein encoded by the obese gene. Science 1995;269:543–6.

44. Oral EA, Ruiz E, Andewelt A, et al. Effect of leptin replacement on pituitary hormone regulation in patients with severe lipodystrophy. J Clin Endocrinol Metab 2002;87:3110–7.

45. Flier JS. Obesity wars: molecular progress confronts an expanding epidemic. Cell 2004;116:337–50.

46. Pajvani UB, Scherer PE. Adiponectin: systemic contributor to insulin sensitivity. Curr Diab Rep 2003;3:207–13.

47. Berg AH, Combs TP, Scherer PE. ACRP30/adiponectin: an adipokine regulating glucose and lipid metabolism. Trends Endocrinol Metab 2002;13:84–9.

48. Yamamoto Y, Hirose H, Saito I, et al. Correlation of the adipocyte-derived protein adiponectin with insulin resistance index and serum high-density lipoprotein-cholesterol, independent of body mass index, in the Japanese population. Clin Sci 2002;103:137–42.

49. Cote M, Mauriege P, Bergeron J, et al. Adiponectinemia in visceral obesity: impact on glucose tolerance and plasma lipoprotein and lipid levels in men. J Clin Endocrinol Metab 2005;90:1434–9.

50. Martin LJ, Woo JG, Daniels SR, et al. The relationships of adiponectin with insulin and lipids are strengthened with increasing adiposity. J Clin Endocrinol Metab 2005;90:4255–9.

51. Steppan CM, Bailey ST, Bhat S, et al. The hormone resistin links obesity to diabetes. Nature 2001;409:307–12.

52. Kojima M, Hosoda H, Date Y, et al. Ghrelin is a growth-hormone-releasing acylated peptide from stomach. Nature 1999;402:656–60.

53. Fan W, Boston BA, Kesterson RA, et al. Role of melanocortinergic neurons in feeding and the agouti obesity syndrome. Nature 1997;385:165–8.

54. Batterham RL, Cowley MA, Small CJ, et al. Physiology: does gut hormone PYY3-36 decrease food intake in rodents? [reply]. Nature 2004;430:3–4.

55. Ollmann MM, Wilson BD, Yang YK, et al. Antagonism of central melanocortin receptors in vitro and in vivo by agouti-related protein. Science 1997;278:135–8.

56. Cowley MA, Smith RG, Diano S, et al. The distribution and mechanism of action of ghrelin in the CNS demonstrates a novel hypothalamic circuit regulating energy homeostasis. Neuron 2003;37:649–61.

57. Loftus TM, Jaworsky DE, Frehywot GL, et al. Reduced food intake and body weight in mice treated with fatty acid synthase inhibitors. Science 2000;288: 2379–81.

58. Lam TK, Gutierrez-Juarez R, Pocai A, et al. Brain glucose metabolism controls the hepatic secretion of triglyceride-rich lipoproteins. Nat Med 2007;13:171–80.

Hypertension in Obesity

L. Romayne Kurukulasuriya, MD[a,b,]*, Sameer Stas, MD[a,b],
Guido Lastra, MD[a,b], Camila Manrique, MD[a,b],
James R. Sowers, MD[a,c,d,e]

KEYWORDS

- Obesity • Hypertension • Cardiovascular disease
- Insulin resistance • Chronic kidney disease • Adipocyte

There have been significant increases in hypertension (HTN), obesity, and diabetes in the last several years. The increase in these comorbid conditions will contribute to an increased incidence of cardiovascular disease (CVD) and chronic kidney disease (CKD). Central or visceral obesity is much more closely related to metabolic risk factors, CVD, and CKD, than peripheral or lower-body obesity. Furthermore, the European Prospective Investigation into Cancer Norfolk (EPIC) study of 22,090 men and women showed that systolic blood pressure (SBP) and diastolic blood pressure (DBP) increased linearly across the whole range of waist-to-hip ratio in both men and women.[1] As per National Health and Nutrition Examination Survey (NHANES) data, in 1999 to 2000 only 68.9% of people with HTN were aware of their high blood pressure (BP), only 58.4% were treated, and HTN was controlled in only 31%. Women,

---

A version of this article appeared in the 37:3 issue of the *Endocrinology and Metabolism Clinics of North America*.

Dr Sowers's research is supported by grants from the National Institutes of Health (R01 HL73101-01A1 NIH/NHLBI) and from the Veterans Affairs Research Service (VA Merit Review). Dr Sowers is a member of the Speakers' Bureau and has received grant funding from Novaritis Pharmaceutical Company. Dr Sowers is also a member of the Speakers' Bureau for Merck Pharmaceutical Company and has received grant funding from Forest Research Institute and is on their Advisory Board.

[a] Department of Internal Medicine, University of Missouri-Columbia School of Medicine, Columbia, MO 65212, USA

[b] Cosmopolitan International Diabetes and Endocrinology Center, University of Missouri-Columbia, Columbia, MO 65212, USA

[c] Department of Medical Pharmacology and Physiology, University of Missouri-Columbia School of Medicine, Columbia, MO 65212, USA

[d] Thomas W. Burns Center of Diabetes and Cardiovascular Research, University of Missouri-Columbia School of Medicine, Colmbia, MO 65212, USA

[e] Harry S. Truman VA Medical Center, University of Missouri-Columbia School of Medicine, Columbia, Columbia, MO 65212, USA

* Corresponding author. Division of Internal Medicine, University of Missouri-Columbia, Columbia, MO 65212.

E-mail address: romaynel@health.missouri.edu

Med Clin N Am 95 (2011) 903–917
doi:10.1016/j.mcna.2011.06.004

Mexican Americans, and those aged 60 years or older had significantly lower rates of control when compared with men, younger individuals, and non-Hispanic whites.[2] In the United States population with HTN, inadequate BP control was estimated to result in 39,702 cardiovascular events, 8,374 CVD deaths, and $964 million in direct medical expenditures. In the medicated population with CVD, the incremental costs of failure to attain BP goals reached approximately $467 million. These results reflect the importance of adequate BP control (in particular, SBP control) in reducing CVD morbidity, mortality, and overall health care expenditures among patients with HTN.[3] Based on the NHANES III sample, approximately 63% of men and 55% of women aged 25 years or older in the United States population, were overweight or obese.[4] Obesity is becoming recognized as one of the most important risk factors for the development of HTN in both males and females.[5] Several genetic and environmental factors play a role in the pathogenesis of obesity, HTN, and CVD (**Fig. 1**). This article discusses the underlying mechanisms of obesity-related HTN and their clinical implications.

MECHANISMS OF HYPERTENSION IN OBESITY

The mechanisms involved in obesity-related HTN are complex and involve derangements in multiple systems. They include increased activation of the renin-angiotensin-aldosterone system (RAAS), increased sympathetic nervous system (SNS) activity, and insulin resistance. In addition, obesity is associated with increased renal sodium reabsorption, impaired pressure natriuresis, and volume expansion. Furthermore, obesity may also cause marked structural changes in the kidneys that will eventually lead to CKD and further increases in BP.[6] In addition, alterations in

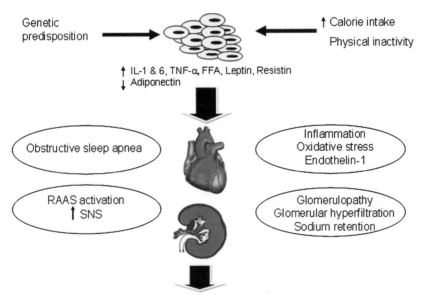

Fig. 1. Pathophysiologic events implicated in the relationship between obesity and development of hypertension and cardiovascular disease. FFA, free fatty acids; IL, interleukin; RAAS, renin-angiotensin-aldosterone syste; SNS, sympathetic nervous system; TNFα, tumor necrosis factor alpha.

adipokines, free fatty acids (FFA), endothelial dysfunction, systemic inflammation, and sleep apnea promote hypertension and CVD (**Box 1**).

RENIN ANGIOTENSIN ALDOSTERONE SYSTEM

There is evidence to suggest that the activation of the RAAS plays an important role in obesity-related HTN. This system has a crucial role in regulating fluid volume and vascular tone. In a study of 449 individuals from Jamaica, serum angiotensin converting enzyme (ACE) and circulating angiotensinogen levels were significantly higher in individuals with a body mass index (BMI) over 31.[6] A study of postmenopausal women showed that obese women had higher circulating angiotensinogen, renin, aldosterone, and ACE levels than lean women. Weight reduction by 5% reduced plasma angiotensinogen by 27%, renin by 43%, aldosterone by 31%, ACE activity by 12%, and angiotensinogen expression by 20% in adipose tissue (all $P<.05$). The decrease in plasma angiotensinogen levels was highly correlated with the waist circumference decline ($r = 0.74$; $P<.001$).[7] Studies on animal models have demonstrated that angiotensinogen produced by adipose tissue plays a role in local adipose tissue differentiation. In addition, angiotensinogen produced in the adipose tissue can be released into the blood stream (an endocrine effect). This suggests that high blood angiotensinogen levels and associated HTN seen in obese patients may be because of the increased fat mass.[8] Furthermore, activation of systemic and tissue RAAS can cause increased renal sodium reabsorption and a hypertensive shift of pressure natriuresis.[9]

Box 1
Factors involved in obesity-related hypertension

Insulin resistance

RAAS activation

SNS activation

Endothelial dysfunction and oxidative stress

Endothelin-1

Adiposity

    Leptin resistance

    Resistin

    Low adiponectin

    FFAs

    Hydroxysteroid dehydrogenase type 1 enzyme

    Increased abdominal pressure

    Local RAAS and SNS activiation

Renal derangement

    Sodium retention

    Obesity-related glomerulopathy

    Perirenal fat accumulation

    Renal RAAS and SNS activation

Obstructive sleep apnea

Plasma aldosterone levels are higher in obese subjects. This cannot be explained by the impact of increased plasma renin activity or other factors promoting aldosterone production. Some predictors of plasma aldosterone include abdominal obesity, measured as waist/hip ratio or by CT scan, and insulin resistance measured by glucose tolerance tests or euglycemic clamp techniques. These studies suggest that aldosterone participates in HTN associated with insulin resistance, both components of the cardiometabolic syndrome (CMS).[10] Aldosterone increases BP in obesity by its action on both mineralocorticoid and glucocorticoid receptors located in different tissues, including brain, heart, kidney, and vasculature.[11]

In a study of 223 obese patients, lisinopril was shown to be as effective as hydrochlorothiazide in treating obese subjects with HTN. This study also showed that ACE inhibitors may show greater efficacy as monotherapy at lower doses (compared with thiazide diuretics), may have a more rapid rate of response, and may offer advantages in patients at high risk of metabolic disorders.[12]

Aldosterone antagonist eplerenone markedly attenuated glomerular hyperfiltration, sodium retention, and HTN associated with chronic dietary-induced obesity in dogs fed a high fat diet. Collectively, these data indicate that aldosterone plays an important role in the pathogenesis of obesity HTN.[13]

SYMPATHETIC NERVOUS SYSTEM

The SNS plays an important role in the regulation of cardiovascular homeostasis. There are several proposed mechanisms linking obesity with SNS activation. These include baroreflex dysfunction, hypothalamic-pituitary axis dysfunction, hyperinsulinemia/insulin resistance, hyperleptinemia, and elevated circulating angiotensin II concentrations.[14,15] Muscle sympathetic nervous system activity (MSNA) in men is more closely associated with the level of abdominal visceral fat than total fat mass or abdominal subcutaneous fat. MSNA does not differ in subcutaneous obese and nonobese men with similar levels of abdominal visceral fat.[16] Furthermore, these findings may have important implications in understanding the increased risk of developing CVD in individuals with visceral obesity. Men with higher visceral adiposity seem to be at higher risk for CVD than their total body fat-matched peers.[15] The increase in renal sympathetic activity in obesity may possibly be necessary for the development of HTN in obese individuals, but not a sufficient cause, being present in both normotensive and hypertensive obese individuals. The discriminating feature of obesity-related HTN has been shown to be an absence of the suppression of the cardiac sympathetic outflow seen in normotensive obese individuals.[17] Interestingly, the lack of increase in SNS activity with increasing adiposity and insulinemia in Pima Indians may contribute to the low prevalence of HTN in this population.[18] Nevertheless, increased renal sodium absorption associated with increased renal SNS activity appears to contribute to obesity-related HTN in many individuals. A study of both lean and obese hypertensives has shown that BP is more sensitive to alpha and beta adrenergic blockade in obese than in lean hypertensive patients, and suggests that increased sympathetic activity may be an important factor in the development and maintenance of HTN in obesity.[19]

INSULIN RESISTANCE

Diabetes mellitus is commonly associated with HTN. One link between diabetes and essential HTN may be hyperinsulinemia. When hypertensive patients, whether obese or of normal body weight, are compared with age- and weight-matched normotensive control subjects, a heightened plasma insulin response to a glucose challenge is consistently found. Insulin resistance predisposes an individual to hyperinsulinism.[20] Most glucose uptake under control of insulin occurs in skeletal muscle tissue. Interestingly, the insulin resistance in skeletal muscle accompanying essential HTN is limited to nonoxidative pathways of glucose disposal (glycogen synthesis). This resistance correlates directly with the severity of HTN. Mechanisms involved in the association of insulin resistance and essential HTN include renal sodium retention, SNS overactivity, disturbed membrane cation transport, and proliferation of vascular smooth muscle cells.[20] The conclusion of a study of 2,475 subjects was that insulin resistance or hyperinsulinemia is present in the majority of hypertensives, and constitutes a common pathophysiologic feature linking obesity, glucose intolerance, and HTN. Insulin resistance is associated with decreased metabolic signaling, which normally modulates intracellular calcium levels. With insulin resistance there is increased intracellular calcium and calcium sensitization, resulting in increased peripheral vascular resistance.[21]

Despite this evidence, the direct role of insulin resistance or hyperinsulinemia in the pathophysiology of HTN is not well understood. In a study of obese dogs, chronic hyperinsulinemia did not raise BP, even though they were resistant to the metabolic and vasodilator effects of insulin.[22] A study of 14 normotensive subjects infused with high and low doses of insulin showed that the acute increases in plasma insulin within the physiologic range elevate sympathetic neural outflow but do not elevate arterial pressure in normal human beings.[23] Insulinoma patients have inappropriately high plasma concentrations of insulin and proinsulin, but their BP levels do not typically differ from those of normal control subjects, and surgical removal of the insulinomas does not reduce their BP. These findings argue against the hypothesis that hyperinsulinemia is an independent causal factor in the development of essential hypertension in humans.[24] Studies with spontaneously hypertensive rats support the view that HTN does not lead to insulin resistance, hyperinsulinemia, and hypertriglyceridemia.[25] Interestingly, the relationship between plasma insulin levels and HTN seen in essential HTN does not occur with secondary forms of HTN.[26] Therefore, insulin resistance and hyperinsulinemia are not consequences of HTN; instead, a genetic predisposition may exist that contributes to both disorders.[27] This concept is supported by the occurrence of hyperinsulinemia and insulin resistance in normotensive offspring of hypertensive adults.[28,29] Even though hyperinsulinemia may not be a major cause of obesity-related HTN, insulin resistance may contribute to HTN by other mechanisms involving inflammation and oxidative stress superimposed on abnormalities in glucose and lipid metabolism. Mechanisms for the development of HTN in insulin resistance/hyperinsulinemia include activation of the SNS, renal sodium retention, altered membrane cation transport, vascular smooth muscle growth and remodeling, and vasoconstriction.[27]

RENAL STRUCTURAL AND FUNCTIONAL CHANGES

There is substantial evidence that abnormal kidney function plays a key role in obesity-related HTN. Obesity increases tubular sodium reabsorption and shifts pressure natriuresis toward higher BP. Increased tubular sodium reabsorption is closely linked to activation of the SNS and RAAS, and possible changes in intrarenal physical forces. For example, medullary compression because of accumulation of adipose tissue around the kidney and increased extracellular matrix within the kidney can result in enhanced tubular reabsorption and altered pressure natriuresis. Obesity is also associated with marked afferent renal artery vasodilatation and increased glomerular filtration rate, which are compensatory responses that help overcome the increased tubular sodium reabsorption and maintain sodium balance. However, chronic renal vasodilation causes increased hydrostatic pressure and wall stress in the glomeruli that, along with increased lipids and glucose, may cause glomerulosclerosis and loss of nephron function in obese patients. Obesity is increasingly a primary cause of essential HTN as well as type 2 diabetes, and consequently is an increasingly frequent cause of end-stage renal disease.[30] Kambham and colleagues[31] have defined obesity related glomerulopathy (ORG) as a focal segmental glomerulosclerosis (FSG) and glomerulomegaly in patients with a BMI of over 30 kg/m². They showed that ORG is distinct from idiopathic FSGS, with a lower incidence of nephrotic syndrome, a more indolent course, consistent presence of glomerulomegaly, and milder foot process fusion. The 10-fold increase in incidence over the past 15 years suggests a newly emerging epidemic. Increased intra abdominal pressure (IAP) produced by progressively inflating an intra-abdominal balloon in dogs caused significant increases in SBP and DBP that resolved with balloon deflation. This has lead to the concept that increased IAP and accompanying changes in renal dynamics may be a cause for systemic HTN in those with central obesity.[32]

In summary, persistent obesity causes renal injury and functional nephron loss, contributing to an elevated BP. This in turn leads to further renal injury, thereby setting off a vicious cycle of events leading to further BP elevation and renal injury. It is difficult to dissociate the cause from the effect in this nexus, as the overall burden of obesity on renal injury and BP may be strongly time dependent.[33]

ROLE OF ADIPOCYTES

Excess energy-intake leads to an expansion of adipose tissue, which is a hallmark of obesity, but the location and adipocyte morphology of the expanded adipose tissue differs among individuals. The presence of large adipocytes is associated with functional and structural abnormalities of adipose tissue. These include: (1) the increased production of bioactive molecules, such as leptin, resistin, angiotensinogen, proinflammatory cytokines, and reactive oxygen species (ROS); (2) an insufficient capacity to accommodate excess energy-intake related increases in serum lipids, leading to ectopic fat storage in tissues such as skeletal muscle and liver, which, in turn, enhances insulin resistance and hyperinsulinemia; (3) augmented macrophage infiltration of the adipose tissue enhancing the production of proinflammatory cytokines and ROS. This "dysfunctional" adipose tissue may, in turn, induce activation of the SNS and RAAS, and enhance systemic oxidative stress, all of which promote the development of obesity-associated HTN.[34] It has been shown that weight reduction is associated with a marked decrease in fat cell volume, leptin secretion, and serum leptin concentration. Fat cell volume, but not percent body fat or BMI, was directly proportional to leptin secretion and serum leptin concentrations.[35]

It has been shown that secretory products from human adipocytes stimulated steroidogenesis in human adrenocortical cells with a predominant effect on mineralocorticoid secretion, suggesting a direct link between obesity, RAAS activation, and HTN.[36]

Resistin

Resistin (named for resistance to insulin) is a recently discovered polypeptide that antagonizes insulin action and may play a part in the pathogenesis of insulin resistance. Resistin is increased in diet-induced and genetic forms of obesity.[37] A Chinese study with 1,102 subjects has shown resistin gene polymorphism to be an independent factor associated with elevated SBP and DBP in patients with type 2 diabetes.

These findings suggest that resistin may play a part in the pathogenesis of type 2 diabetes and insulin resistance-related HTN.[38] Another study from China, with 71 subjects, showed that resistin was not related to systolic or diastolic HTN.[39]

Endothelin

Some hypertensive patients have increased endothelin-1 (ET-1) dependent vasoconstrictor tone. It has been shown in subjects with a BMI of over 25 kg/m^2, that DBP is significantly associated with G/T polymorphism of ET-1.[40] In human HTN, increased BMI may be associated with enhanced ET$_A$ receptor-dependent vasoconstrictor activity, suggesting that this abnormality may play a role in the pathophysiology of obesity-related HTN. Therefore, targeting the ET-1 system may be useful in the treatment of these patients.[41] In addition, BP increases in relation to BMI in carriers of the T allele of ET-1/C198 polymorphism when compared with GG homozygotes. As a consequence of this interaction, the T allele was associated with a significant increase of SBP and DBP levels in overweight subjects with a BMI over 26 kg/m^2, whereas no significant effect was observed in lean subjects (BMI <26 kg/m^2).[42] Endothelin antagonism unmasks or augments nitric oxide synthesis capacity in obese patients. Thus, in addition to direct vasoconstrictor effects of endothelin, impaired nitric oxide bioavailability as a result of elevated endogenous endothelin may also contribute to endothelial dysfunction in obesity.[43]

Free Fatty Acids

It has been shown that increases in portal venous delivery of FFA (ie, oleic acid- a cis unsaturated nonesterified fatty acid or NEFA) to the liver, stimulates a neurally mediated reflex that results in an increase in vascular sympathetic tone and an increase in BP.[44] In vivo data from both animal and human studies support the notion that acute plasma NEFA elevation leads to an increase in BP levels. Epidemiologic evidence suggests a link between increased NEFA levels and HTN. Accumulating evidence indicates the existence of several pathways through which NEFA could promote BP elevation. These include alpha (1)-adrenergic stimulation, endothelial dysfunction, increases in oxidant stress, and stimulation of vascular smooth muscle cell growth and remodeling. Collectively, these data support a possibly important role of NEFA in the development of HTN in patients with obesity and CMS.[45]

Glucocorticoid Excess

Glucocorticoids play an essential role in adaptation to stress, regulation of metabolism, and inflammatory responses. Patients with Cushing's Syndrome develop insulin resistance, dyslipidemia, and HTN. Adipose stromal cells from omental fat, but not subcutaneous fat, can generate active cortisol from inactive cortisone mediated via 11 beta- hydroxysteroid dehydrogenase type 1 (11beta-HSD1) enzyme activity. In vivo, such a mechanism would ensure a constant exposure of glucocorticoid specifically to omental adipose tissue, suggesting that central obesity may reflect "Cushing's disease of the omentum".[46] Type 1 enzyme (11beta-HSD1) in vitro is an NADP(H)-dependent bidirectional enzyme; it promotes conversion of cortisone to active cortisol. In contrast, 11beta HSD type 2 enzyme, residing in the distal tubule and collecting duct of the kidney, converts cortisol to cortisone, thus protecting the mineralocorticoid receptor from occupation by cortisol. HSD1 amplifies glucocorticoid receptor activation and promotes preadipocyte differentiation and adipocyte hypertrophy. Although initial studies in transgenic mice and human beings support this concept, more data is required to conclusively demonstrate that the adipose-tissue specific overexpression of HSD1 and increases in adipose tissue cortisol lead to obesity, insulin resistance, high BP, and CMS.[47] Patients with essential HTN usually do not have overt signs of mineralocorticoid excess, but nevertheless can show a positive correlation between BP and increased serum sodium levels, or a negative correlation with potassium concentrations, suggesting a mineralocorticoid influence. Recent studies revealed a prolonged half-life of cortisol and an increased ratio of urinary cortisol to cortisone metabolites in some patients with essential HTN. These abnormalities may be genetically determined.[48] For example, the P2-HSD1 mouse with over expression of HSD1 is hypertensive with apparent activation of the circulating RAAS and features of the CMS.[49] These mice highlight the potential role of adipose glucocorticoid activation in the pathophysiology of HTN seen in the CMS. They develop visceral obesity, salt-sensitive HTN, insulin resistance, dyslipidemia, and increased plasma levels of angiotensinogen, angiotensin II, and aldosterone.[49]

Leptin

Leptin is important in regulating appetite, body weight, and energy balance. It plays a vital role in the cross-talk between the brain and adipose tissue. Moreover, leptin has a wide range of biologic actions, including effects on the SNS, glucose and insulin metabolism, lipolysis, vascular tone, the hypothalamic-pituitary-adrenal axis, and reproduction.[50] Normally, leptin alters energy intake by decreasing appetite and increasing energy expenditure via SNS stimulation.[50] Leptin deficiency, or disruption of leptin signaling in the hypothalamus, can lead to obesity.[51] Plasma leptin levels are typically elevated in obese people and are positively correlated with the amount of adipose tissue. In fact, hyperleptinemia is an independent risk factor for coronary artery disease.[52] The failure of high levels of leptin in most obese individuals to promote weight loss is thought to be because of hypothalamic insensitivity to leptin action. It was proposed that hypothalamic leptin resistance in obesity is selective; the appetite-controlling and weight-reducing effects of leptin are disrupted while the excitatory effects on SNS are maintained.[53]

The cardiovascular effects of leptin have recently been reviewed.[54,55] The mechanisms of leptin's vascular effects are complex. Despite the experimental reports of beneficial vascular effects, including improved nitric oxide production and endothelium-dependent vasodilatation,[56] the predominant vascular effect of chronic hyperleptinemia is a pressor effect mediated by increased SNS activity. Leptin infusion in animal models causes increases in arterial BP, heart rate, and sympathetic nerve signals in several tissues.[50,57,58] Finally, leptin has been found to increase ROS and ET-1, which might contribute to HTN.[59,60]

Adiponectin

Adiponectin has insulin-sensitizing, antiatherogenic, and anti-inflammatory effects.[61] Plasma levels of adiponectin are inversely related to obesity. Cross-sectional studies have shown that hypoadiponectinemia is an independent risk factor for HTN.[62–64] Recently, in a prospective 5-year nested study in a nondiabetic Chinese cohort, hypoadiponectinemia predicted the development of HTN in normotensive subjects, independent of sex, age, C-reactive protein, waist circumference, or BMI.[65]

Several mechanisms might be involved in the association between hypoadiponectinemia and HTN.[61,65,66] Reduced adiponectin levels can be caused by interactions of genetic factors and environmental factors, such as lifestyle changes that cause obesity. Hypoadeponectinemia, in turn, appears to play an important causal role in the development of insulin resistance and HTN.[67] Studies of overexpression or knock-down of adiponectin receptors suggest that adiponectin increases adenosine monophosphate kinase and peroxisome proliferaltor-activator receptor (PPAR) ligand activity.[61] Adiponectin replenishment reduces BP in the hypertensive obese KKAy mice (a model of obesity-related HTN). Independent of obesity and insulin resistance, salt-fed adiponectin knockout mice develop HTN and adiponectin delivery improves HTN.[68] Furthermore, adiponectin induces nitric oxide production and increases nitric oxide bioavailability by up-regulating eNOS expression and reducing ROS production in endothelial cells.[69,70] It was shown both in human beings and in adiponectin-deficient mice that hypoadiponectinemia is associated with endothelial dysfunction and impaired endothelium-dependent vasodilatation.[71] It is likely that angiotensin receptor blocker induced adiponectin production is mediated by way of PPARγ activation.[72]

OBSTRUCTIVE SLEEP APNEA

Obesity, especially upper body obesity, is a major risk factor for obstructive sleep apnea (OSA). OSA frequently coexists with HTN. Approximately 5% to 10% of the general population and 50% to 60% of hypertensive patients have OSA.[73] The association between sleep-disordered breathing and the risk of developing HTN were studied prospectively in the Wisconsin Sleep Cohort Study. After adjustment for base-line HTN status, BMI, neck and waist circumference, age, sex, and weekly use of alcohol and cigarettes, there was a dose-response association between sleep-disordered breathing at base line and the presence of HTN 4 years later.[74] Despite its common prevalence, OSA is largely undetected and undertreated.

OSA results from a partial or complete collapse of the upper respiratory airways because of physiologic or anatomic causes. There is a wide spectrum of the manifestations of OSA, ranging from intermittent simple snoring to frequent episodes of apneas (absence of airflow), hypoxia, and hypercapnia with frequent arousals. The arousals from sleep, which are usually unrecognized by the patient, are associated with acute spikes in SBP.[75] People with OSA lose the physiologic nocturnal drop in arterial BP and have an average mean pressure that is higher during OSA episodes than it is during wakefulness. Symptoms of OSA include frequent snoring, nocturnal apnea and choking, diurnal hypersomnolence despite getting 8 hours of sleep, dyspnea, and nocturia.

Mechanisms of Hypertension in Obstructive Sleep Apnea

Patients with untreated OSA have increased SNS activity. Plasma and urine norepinephrine levels and baseline MSNA are also elevated in individuals with OSA.[76–78] Intermittent hypoxia in an animal model of sleep apnea results in prolonged high BP. Surgical denervation of peripheral chemoreceptors, adrenal demedullation, and chemical denervation of the peripheral SNS prevented such increases in arterial BP.[79] Moreover, in OSA hypoxia-induced autonomic and ventilatory responses in the peripheral chemoreceptor activation are exaggerated, with a blunted response to hypotensive stimulation.[77] There is evidence that patients with OSA have attenuated baroreflex control.[80] Finally, continuous positive airway pressure (CPAP) administered during the night, the most widely used treatment for OSA, decreases sympathetic activity and improves baroreflex control of heart rate, thus improving HTN.[73]

There is accumulating evidence of endothelial dysfunction in OSA. For instance, endothelium-dependent vasodilatation of resistance vessels is impaired in patients with OSA.[81] This effect is subsequently reversed with CPAP treatment.[82] ET-1 seems to be a pathogenic factor in provoking HTN in OSA. A recent study, in patients with OSA, showed that they had higher plasma levels of ET-1 than did healthy controls.

In this study, the mean nocturnal level of ET-1 was related significantly to the severity of OSA. This correlation remained statistically significant after correction for confounders.[83] In a study of 22 patients who had OSA, CPAP treatment reduced plasma ET-1 and the changes in ET-1 levels were correlated with changes in mean arterial blood pressure and oxygen saturation.[84]

Plasma Ang II and aldosterone are both elevated in OSA patients compared with control subjects. In addition, long-term CPAP therapy resulted in correlated decreases in BP, plasma renin activity, and plasma Ang II concentrations.[85] Activation of the SNS seems to play a role in RAAS activation in OSA. In an animal model of episodic hypoxia, both renal-artery denervated and angiotensin receptor blocker-treated animals did not develop high BP in response to hypoxia, while control rats had progressive and sustained elevation in arterial BP.[86] This finding implicates the role of an activated RAAS and the kidney in OSA-related HTN.

Recent work suggests that hypoadiponectemia is independently associated with OSA.[87–89] Moreover, 14 days of CPAP treatment in overweight people with moderate to severe OSA decreased mean arterial pressure and increased adiponectin levels.[90] In summary, the etiology of HTN in OSA is complex. SNS hyperactivity plays a major role, while other factors include abnormalities in baroreflex control, the RAAS system, adipokines, and renal function.

SUMMARY

Obesity and HTN are on the rise in the world. HTN seems to be the most common obesity-related health problem and visceral obesity seems to be the major culprit. Unfortunately, only 31% of hypertensives are treated to goal. This translates into an increased incidence of CVD and related morbidity and mortality. Several mechanisms have been postulated as the causes of obesity-related HTN. Activation of the RAAS, SNS, insulin resistance, leptin, adiponectin, dysfunctional fat, FFA, resistin, 11 Beta dehydrogenase, renal structural and hemodynamic changes, and OSA are some of the abnormalities in obesity-related HTN. Many of these factors are interrelated. Treatment of obesity should begin with weight loss via lifestyle modifications, medications, or bariatric surgery. According to the mechanisms of obesity-related HTN, it seems that drugs that blockade the RAAS and target the SNS should be ideal for treatment. There is not much evidence in the literature that one drug is better than another in controlling obesity-related HTN. There have only been a few studies specifically targeting the obese hypertensive patient, but recent trials that emphasize the importance of BP control have enrolled both overweight and obese subjects.

Until we have further studies with more in-depth information about the mechanisms of obesity-related HTN and what the targeted treatment should be, the most important factor necessary to control the obesity-related HTN pandemic and its CVD and CKD consequences is to prevent and treat obesity and to treat HTN to goal.

REFERENCES

1. Canoy D, Luben R, Welch A, et al. Fat distribution, body mass index and blood pressure in 22,090 men and women in the Norfolk cohort of the European Prospective Investigation into Cancer and Nutrition (EPIC-Norfolk) study. J Hypertens 2004;22(11):2067–74.
2. Hajjar I, Kotchen TA. Trends in prevalence, awareness, treatment, and control of hypertension in the United States, 1988–2000. JAMA 2003;290(2):199–206.
3. Flack JM, Casciano R, Casciano J, et al. Cardiovascular disease costs associated with uncontrolled hypertension. Manag Care Interface 2002;15(11):28–36.

4. Must A, Spadano J, Coakley EH, et al. The disease burden associated with overweight and obesity. JAMA 1999;282(16):1523–9.

5. Narkiewicz K. Diagnosis and management of hypertension in obesity. Obes Rev 2006;7(2):155–62.

6. Cooper R, McFarlane-Anderson N, Bennett FI, et al. ACE, angiotensinogen and obesity: a potential pathway leading to hypertension. J Hum Hypertens 1997; 11(2):107–11.

7. Engeli S, Böhnke J, Gorzelniak K, et al. Weight loss and the renin-angiotensin-aldosterone system. Hypertension 2005;45(3):356–62.

8. Massiera F, Bloch-Faure M, Ceiler D, et al. Adipose angiotensinogen is involved in adipose tissue growth and blood pressure regulation. FASEB J 2001;15(14): 2727–9.

9. Hall JE, Brands MW, Henegar JR. Mechanisms of hypertension and kidney disease in obesity. Ann N Y Acad Sci 1999;892:91–107.

10. Goodfriend TL, Egan BM, Kelley DE. Aldosterone in obesity. Endocr Res 1998; 24(3/4):789–96.

11. Rahmouni K, Correia ML, Haynes WG, et al. Obesity induced hypertension: new insights into mechanism. Hypertension 2005;45(1):9–14.

12. Reisin E, Weir MR, Falkner B, et al. Lisinopril versus hydrochlorothiazide in obese hypertensive patients: a multicenter placebo-controlled trial. Treatment in obese patients with hypertension (TROPHY) study group. Hypertension 1997;30(1 Pt 1): 140–5.

13. De Paula RB, Da Silva AA, Hall JE. Aldosterone antagonism attenuates obesity-induced hypertension and glomerular hyperfiltration. Hypertension 2004;43(1): 41–7.

14. Davy KP, Hall JE. Obesity and hypertension: two epidemics or one? Am J Physiol Regul Integr Comp Physiol 2004;286(5):R803–13.

15. Alvarez GE, Beske SD, Ballard TP, et al. Sympathetic neural activation in visceral obesity. Circulation 2002;106(20):2533–6.

16. Alvarez G, Ballard T, Beske S, et al. Subcutaneous obesity is not associated with sympathetic neural activation. Am J Physiol Heart Circ Physiol 2004;287(1): H14–8.

17. Rumantir MS, Vaz M, Jennings GL, et al. Neural mechanisms in human obesity-related hypertension. J Hypertens 1999;17(8):1125–33.

18. Weyer C, Pratley RE, Snitker S, et al. Ethnic differences in insulinemia and sympathetic tone as links between obesity and hypertension. Hypertension 2000;36(4): 531–7.

19. Wofford MR, Anderson DC Jr, Brown CA, et al. Antihypertensive effect of alpha- and beta-adrenergic blockade in obese and lean hypertensive subjects. Am J Hypertens 2001;14(7 Pt 1):694–8.

20. DeFronzo RA, Ferrannini E. Insulin resistance. A multifaceted syndrome responsible for NIDDM, obesity, hypertension, dyslipidemia, and atherosclerotic cardiovascular disease. Diabetes Care 1991;14(3):173–94.

21. Modan M, Halkin H, Almog S, et al. Hyperinsulinemia. A link between hypertension obesity and glucose intolerance. J Clin Invest 1985;75(3):809–17.

22. Hall JE, Brands MW, Zappe DH, et al. Hemodynamic and renal responses to chronic hyperinsulinemia in obese, insulin resistant dogs. Hypertension 1995; 25(5):994–1002.

23. Anderson EA, Hoffman RP, Balon TW, et al. Hyperinsulinemia produces both sympathetic neural activation and vasodilation in normal humans. J Clin Invest 1991;87(6):2246–52.

24. Sawicki PT, Baba T, Berger M, et al. Normal blood pressure in patients with insulinoma despite hyperinsulinemia and insulin resistance. J Am Soc Nephrol 1992; 3(Suppl 4):S64–8.

25. Reaven GM, Chang H. Relationship between blood pressure, plasma insulin and triglyceride concentration, and insulin action in spontaneous hypertensive and Wistar-Kyoto rats. Am J Hypertens 1991;4(1 Pt 1):34–8.

26. Sechi LA, Melis A, Tedde R. Insulin hypersecretion: a distinctive feature between essential and secondary hypertension. Metabolism 1992;41(11):1261–6.

27. McFarlane SI, Banerji M, Sowers JR. Insulin resistance and cardiovascular disease. J Clin Endocrinol Metab 2001;86(2):713–8.

28. Grunfeld B, Balzareti H, Romo H, et al. Hyperinsulinemia in normotensive offspring of hypertensive parents. Hypertension 1994;23(Suppl 1):I12–5.

29. Beatty OL, Harper R, Sheridan B, et al. Insulin resistance in offspring of hypertensive parents. BMJ 1993;307(6896):92–6.

30. Hall JE, Brands MW, Henegar JR, et al. Abnormal kidney function as a cause and a consequence of obesity hypertension. Clin Exp Pharmacol Physiol 1998;25(1): 58–64.

31. Kambham N, Markowitz GS, Valeri AM, et al. Obesity related glomerulopathy: an emerging epidemic. Kidney Int 2001;59(4):1498–509.

32. Bloomfield GL, Sugerman HJ, Blocher CR, et al. Chronically increased intra-abdominal pressure produces systemic hypertension in dogs. Int J Obes Relat Metab Disord 2000;24(7):819–24.

33. Aneja A, El-Atat F, McFarlane S, et al. Hypertension and obesity. Recent Prog Horm Res 2004;59:169–205.

34. Pausova Z. From big fat cells to high blood pressure: a pathway to obesity-associated hypertension. Curr Opin Nephrol Hypertens 2006;15(2):173–8.

35. Lofgren P, Andersson I, Adolfsson B, et al. Long-term prospective and controlled studies demonstrate adipose tissue hypercellularity and relative leptin deficiency in the postobese state. J Clin Endocrinol Metab 2005;90(11):6207–13.

36. Ehrhart-Bornstein M, Lamounier-Zepter V, Schraven A, et al. Human adipocytes secrete mineralocorticoid-releasing factors. Proc Natl Acad Sci U S A 2003; 100(24):14211–6.

37. Steppan CM, Bailey ST, Bhat S, et al. The hormone resistin links obesity to diabetes. Nature 2001;409(6818):307–12.

38. Tan MS, Chang SY, Chang DM, et al. Association of resistin gene 3'-untranslated region +62G→A polymorphism with type 2 diabetes and hypertension in a Chinese population. J Clin Endocrinol Metab 2003;88(3):1258–63.

39. Zhang J, Qin Y, Zheng X, et al. [The relationship between human serum resistin level and body fat content, plasma glucose as well as blood pressure]. Chung-Hua i Hsueh Tsa Chih. [Chinese Medical Journal] 2002;82(23):1609–12 [in Chinese].

40. Asai T, Ohkubo T, Katsuya T, et al. Endothelin-1 gene variant associates with blood pressure in obese Japanese subjects. Hypertension 2001;38(6):1321–4.

41. Cardillo C, Campia U, Iantorno M, et al. Enhanced vascular activity of endogenous endothelin-1 in obese hypertensive patients. Hypertension 2004;43(1):36–40.

42. Tiret L, Poirier O, Hallet V, et al. The Lys198Asn polymorphism in the endothelin-1 gene is associated with blood pressure in overweight people. Hypertension 1999; 33(5):1169–74.

43. Mather KJ, Lteif A, Steinberg H, et al. Interactions between endothelin and nitric oxide in the regulation of vascular tone in obesity and diabetes. Diabetes 2004; 53(8):2060–6.

44. Grekin RJ, Vollmer AP, Sider RS. Pressor effects of portal venous oleate infusion. A proposed mechanism for obesity hypertension. Hypertension 1995;26(1):193–8.
45. Sarafidis PA, Bakris GL. Non-esterified fatty acids and blood pressure elevation: a mechanism for hypertension in subjects with obesity/insulin resistance? J Hum Hypertens 2007;21(1):12–9.
46. Bujalska IJ, Kumar S, Stewart PM. Does central obesity reflect "Cushing's disease of the omentum"? Lancet 1997;349(9060):1210–3.
47. Sukhija R, Kakar P, Mehta V, et al. Enhanced 11beta-hydroxysteroid dehydrogenase activity, the metabolic syndrome, and systemic hypertension. Am J Cardiol 2006;98(4):544–8.
48. Ferrari P, Lovati E, Frey FJ. The role of the 11beta-hydroxysteroid dehydrogenase type 2 in human hypertension. J Hypertens 2000;18(3):241–8.
49. Masuzaki H, Yamamoto H, Kenyon CJ, et al. Transgenic amplification of glucocorticoid action in adipose tissue causes high blood pressure in mice. J Clin Invest 2003;112(1):83–90.
50. Haynes WG, Morgan DA, Walsh SA, et al. Receptor mediated regional sympathetic nerve activation by leptin. J Clin Invest 1997;100(2):270–8.
51. Münzberg H, Björnholm M, Bates SH, et al. Leptin receptor action and mechanisms of leptin resistance. Cell Mol Life Sci 2005;62(6):642–52.
52. Wallace AM, McMahon AD, Packard CJ, et al. Plasma leptin and the risk of cardiovascular disease in the West of Scotland Cornary Prevention Study (WOSCOPS). Circulation 2001;104(25):3052–6.
53. Mark AL, Correia ML, Rahmouni K, et al. Selective leptin resistance: a new concept in leptin physiology with cardiovascular implications. J Hypertens 2002;20(7):1245–50.
54. Yang R, Barouch LA. Leptin signaling and obesity: cardiovascular consequences. Circ Res 2007;101(6):545–59.
55. Katagiri H, Yamada T, Oka Y. Adiposity and cardiovascular disorders: disturbance of the regulatory system consisting of humoral and neuronal signals. Circ Res 2007;101(1):27–39.
56. Vecchione C, Aretini A, Maffei A, et al. Cooperation between insulin and leptin in the modulation of vascular tone. Hypertension 2003;42(2):166–70.
57. Dunbar JC, Hu Y, Lu H. Intracerebroventricular leptin increases lumbarand renal sympathetic nerve activity and blood pressure in normal rats. Diabetes 1997; 46(12):2040–3.
58. Shek EW, Brands MW, Hall JE. Chronic leptin infusion increases arterial pressure. Hypertension 1998;31(1 Pt 2):409–14.
59. Quehenberger P, Exner M, Sunder-Plassmann R, et al. Leptin induces endothelin-1 in endothelial cells in vitro. Circ Res 2002;90(6):711–8.
60. Bouloumie A, Marumo T, Lafontan M, et al. Leptin induces oxidative stress in human endothelial cells. FASEB J 1999;13(10):1231–8.
61. Kadowaki T, Yamauchi T. Adiponectin and adiponectin receptors. Endocr Rev 2005;26(3):439–51.
62. Adamczak M, Wiecek A, Funahashi T, et al. Decreased plasma adiponectin concentration in patients with essential hypertension. Am J Hypertens 2003; 16(1):72–5.
63. Francischetti EA, Celoria BM, Duarte SF, et al. Hypoadiponectinemia is associated with blood pressure increase in obese insulin-resistant individuals. Metabolism 2007;56(11):1464–9.
64. Iwashima Y, Katsuya T, Ishikawa K, et al. Hypoadiponectinemia is an independent risk factor for hypertension. Hypertension 2004;43(6):1318–23.

65. Chow WS, Cheung BM, Tso AW, et al. Hypoadiponectinemia as a predictor for the development of hypertension: a 5-year prospective study. Hypertension 2007; 49(6):1455–61.
66. Schillaci G, Pirro M. Hypoadiponectinemia: a novel link between obesity and hypertension? Hypertension 2007;49(6):1217–9.
67. Kadowaki T, Yamauchi T, Kubota N, et al. Adiponectin and adiponectin receptors in insulin resistance, diabetes, and the metabolic syndrome. J Clin Invest 2006; 116(7):1784–92.
68. Ohashi K, Kihara S, Ouchi N, et al. Adiponectin replenishment ameliorates obesity-related hypertension. Hypertension 2006;47(6):1108–16.
69. Chen H, Montagnani M, Funahashi T, et al. Adiponectin stimulates production of nitric oxide in vascular endothelial cells. J Biol Chem 2003;278(45):45021–6.
70. Motoshima H, Wu X, Mahadev K, et al. Adiponectin suppresses proliferation and superoxide generation and enhances eNOS activity in endothelial cells treated with oxidized LDL. Biochem Biophys Res Commun 2004;315(2):264–71.
71. Ouchi N, Ohishi M, Kihara S, et al. Association of hypoadiponectinemia with impaired vasoreactivity. Hypertension 2003;42(3):231–4.
72. Clasen R, Schupp M, Foryst-Ludwig A, et al. PPARgamma-activating angiotensin type-1 receptor blockers induce adiponectin. Hypertension 2005;46(1):137–43.
73. Baguet JP, Narkiewicz K, Mallion JM. Update on hypertension management: obstructive sleep apnea and hypertension. J Hypertens 2006;24(1):205–8.
74. Peppard PE, Young T, Palta M, et al. Prospective study of the association between sleep-disordered breathing and hypertension. N Engl J Med 2000; 342(19):1378–84.
75. Davies RJ, Crosby J, Vardi-Visy K, et al. Non-invasive beat to beat arterial blood pressure during non-REM sleep in obstructive sleep apnoea and snoring. Thorax 1994;49(4):335–9.
76. Dimsdale JE, Coy T, Ziegler MG, et al. The effect of sleep apnea on plasma and urinary catecholamines. Sleep 1995;18(5):377–81.
77. Narkiewicz K, Pesek CA, Kato M, et al. Baroreflex control of sympathetic activity and heart rate in obstructive sleep apnea. Hypertension 1998;32(6):1039–43.
78. Robinson GV, Stradling JR, Davies RJ. Sleep 6: obstructive sleep apnea/hypopnea syndrome and hypertension. Thorax 2004;59(12):1089–94.
79. Lesske J, Fletcher EC, Bao G, et al. Hypertension caused by chronic intermittent hypoxia–influence of chemoreceptors and sympathetic nervous system. J Hypertens 1997;15(12 Pt 2):1593–603.
80. Carlson JT, Hedner JA, Sellgren J, et al. Depressed baroreflex sensitivity in patients with obstructive sleep apnea. Am J Respir Crit Care Med 1996;154(5): 1490–6.
81. Kato M, Roberts-Thomson P, Phillips BG, et al. Impairment of endothelium-dependent vasodilation of resistance vessels in patients with obstructive sleep apnea. Circulation 2000;102(21):2607–10.
82. Duchna HW, Stoohs R, Guilleminault C, et al. Vascular endothelial dysfunction in patients with mild obstructive sleep apnea syndrome. Wien Med Wochenschr 2006;156(21/22):596–604.
83. Gjorup PH, Sadauskiene L, Wessels J, et al. Abnormally increased endothelin-1 in plasma during the night in obstructive sleep apnea: relation to blood pressure and severity of disease. Am J Hypertens 2007;20(1):44–52.
84. Phillipps BG, Narkiewicz K, Pesek CA, et al. Effects of obstructive sleep apnea on endothelin-1 and blood pressure. J Hypertens 1999;17(1):61–6.

85. Moller DS, Lind P, Strunge B, et al. Abnormal vasoactive hormones and 24-hour blood pressure in obstructive sleep apnea. Am J Hypertens 2003;16(4):274–80.

86. Fletcher EC, Bao G, Li R. Renin activity and blood pressure in response to chronic episodic hypoxia. Hypertension 1999;34(2):309–14.

87. Zhang XL, Yin KS, Wang H, et al. Serum adiponectin levels in adult male patients with obstructive sleep apnea hypopnea syndrome. Respiration 2006;73(1):73–7.

88. Makino S, Handa H, Suzukawa K, et al. Obstructive sleep apnoea syndrome, plasma adiponectin levels, and insulin resistance. Clin Endocrinol (Oxf) 2006; 64(1):12–9.

89. Masserini B, Morpurgo PS, Donadio F, et al. Reduced levels of adiponectin in sleep apnea syndrome. J Endocrinol Invest 2006;29(8):700–5.

90. Zhang XL, Yin KS, Li C, et al. Effect of continuous positive airway pressure treatment on serum adiponectin level and mean arterial pressure in male patients with obstructive sleep apnea syndrome. Chin Med J (Engl) 2007;120(17):1477–81.

Impact of Obesity on Cardiovascular Disease

Kerstyn C. Zalesin, MD[a],*, Barry A. Franklin, PhD[b],
Wendy M. Miller, MD[c], Eric D. Peterson, MD, MPH[d],
Peter A. McCullough, MD, MPH[e]

KEYWORDS

- Obesity • Cardiovascular disease • Coronary heart disease
- Cardiac risk factors • Body mass index • Visceral obesity

The growing prevalence of obesity has created a global public health threat. Two thirds of the American population is overweight or obese[1]; moreover, the prevalence of obesity is rising in developing countries and now is reaching many impoverished nations.[2] Overweight and obesity portends metabolic and cardiovascular consequences, placing individuals at higher risk for premature coronary heart disease (CHD) morbidity and mortality (**Fig. 1**). The cascade of obesity-related conditions accrues at the upper end of normal body mass index (BMI), highlighting the curious relationship that overweight and obesity share with CHD and metabolic risks.[3] In the United States, it is estimated that obesity causes an excess of 300,000 deaths annually,[4] and potentially reduces lifespan by as much as 5 to 20 years in the morbidly obese.[5] The spread of the obesity epidemic will likely inversely impact life expectancy trends. Accordingly, today's generation of youth may be the first in the United States to not outlive their parents.[6]

In past years, the role of obesity as an independent modulator of coronary risk has been controversial. Recent evidence, however, directly links obesity to intrinsic cardiac conditions including coronary artery disease (CAD), heart failure (HF), cardiomyopathy,

A version of this article appeared in the 37:3 issue of the *Endocrinology and Metabolism Clinics of North America*.

[a] Division of Nutrition and Preventative Medicine, Department of Medicine, William Beaumont Hospital, 4949 Coolidge Highway, Royal Oak, MI 48073, USA

[b] Cardiac Rehabilitation and Exercise Laboratories, William Beaumont Hospital, 4949 Coolidge Highway, Royal Oak, MI 48073, USA

[c] Weight Control Center, Division of Nutrition and Preventative Medicine, William Beaumont Hospital, 4949 Coolidge Highway, Royal Oak, MI 48073, USA

[d] Duke Clinical Research Institute, Duke University School of Medicine, 2400 Pratt Street, Durham, NC 22705, USA

[e] Providence Park Heart Institute, 47601 Grand River Avenue, Suite B-125, Novi, MI 48374, USA

* Corresponding author.

E-mail address: kzalesin@beaumont.edu

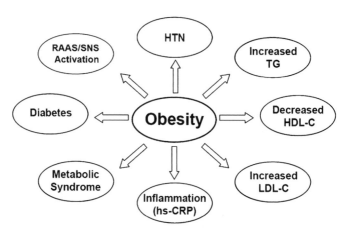

Fig. 1. Obesity is positioned as the only central and reversible cardiovascular risk factor that favorably influences all the other associated factors. HDL-C, high-density lipoprotein cholesterol; hs-CRP, high-sensitivity C-reactive protein; HTN, hypertension; LDL-C, low-density lipoprotein cholesterol; RAAS/SNS, renin-angiotensin-aldosterone system/sympathetic nervous system; TG, triglycerides.

and atrial fibrillation (AF), which collectively carry important health implications. In addition, excess adiposity appears to amplify Framingham CHD risk in patients who are followed over time for actual CHD events (**Fig. 2**). Potentially, many of the obesity-associated risks are partially remediable or preventable with treatment, education, and lifestyle modification. This article explores the impact of obesity on cardiovascular disease.

OBESITY AND CORONARY HEART DISEASE RISK FACTORS IN THE PEDIATRIC POPULATION

For youth, the prevalence of obesity—defined as a BMI (weight in kilograms divided by height in meters squared) at or above the 95th percentile for age and sex—is 10% for children aged 2 to 5 years and 15% for 6- to 19-year-olds.[7] This prevalence represents

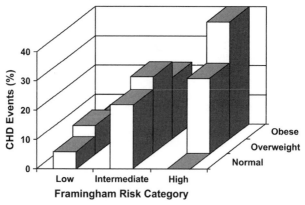

Fig. 2. Amplification of Framingham CHD risk by excess adiposity in 827 apparently healthy siblings (mean age, 46 years) over a mean follow-up of 8.7 years. (*From* Mora S, Yanek LR, Moy TF, et al. Interaction of body mass index and Framingham risk score in predicting incident coronary disease in families. Circulation 2005;111(15):1871–6; with permission.)

a doubling in children and a near tripling among adolescents over the last 2 decades.[8] Childhood obesity significantly increases morbidity and mortality from cardiovascular disease and has great prognostic significance.[9] The presence of cardiovascular risk factors among the pediatric population has become a modern phenomenon. Using the Bogalusa Heart Study database, Freedman and colleagues[10] studied 5- to 10-year-old obese children and reported significant odds ratios (ORs) for systolic blood pressure (OR 4.5, defined as >95th percentile), diastolic blood pressure (OR 2.4, defined as >95th percentile), low-density lipoprotein cholesterol (LDL-C; OR 3.0, defined as >130 mg/dL), triglycerides (OR 7.1, defined as >130 mg/dL), insulin concentration (OR 12.1, defined as >95th percentile), and low levels of high-density lipoprotein cholesterol (HDL-C; OR 3.4, defined as <35 mg/dL). The investigators noted that 58% of the study population had at least one of these cardiovascular risk factors and that 25% had two or more. Similar to the adult population, the presence of atherosclerotic lesions can be predicted by the number of coronary risk factors.[11] Childhood obesity substantially raises the risk of obesity in adulthood, which augments CHD morbidity and mortality risks for future generations.

DEFINITION OF OBESITY AND ABDOMINAL OBESITY

The conventional measurements that define overweight and obesity (ie, BMI, weight, waist circumference, and waist-to-hip ratio) are not sensitive to body composition and merely represent surrogate markers for adiposity. Waist circumference, which is measured halfway between the last rib and the iliac crest, has independently been correlated with visceral obesity and abdominal fat.[12] Abdominal obesity, which is defined as a waist circumference of 103 cm (40 in) or more in men or 88 cm (35 in) or more in women, is associated with several metabolic risks including insulin resistance, type 2 diabetes mellitus (DM), the metabolic syndrome, and CHD. These metabolic alterations are excessively inflammatory in nature and are likely involved in the development of atherosclerosis. Waist circumference measurements among the American population have increased in the last several decades, perhaps even more so than BMI levels, which may be a surrogate marker of greater CHD risks, even among the nonobese.

LEADING RISKS FOR CARDIOVASCULAR DISEASE: THE OBESITY LINK

Cardiovascular disease continues to be a leading cause of morbidity and mortality throughout the world. In 2008 alone, 770,000 Americans will experience an acute myocardial infarction (AMI) and an additional 430,000 will have a recurrent event.[13] There are strong associations between cardiovascular disease risks and obesity. In a prospective study of over a million people followed for 14 years, obesity was strongly associated with an increased risk of all-cause and cardiovascular mortality. This study directly correlated CHD mortality risk with increasing BMI, reporting a twofold to threefold greater risk in individuals who had a BMI of 35 kg/m^2 or higher compared with leaner persons (BMI 18.5–24.9 kg/m^2). An increased risk of cardiovascular mortality was apparent at BMIs greater than 26.5 kg/m^2 and 25.0 kg/m^2 for men and women, respectively (**Fig. 3**).[14]

Data from the INTERHEART study, which evaluated a large controlled population and represented many diverse ethnic groups, confirmed that higher waist-to-hip ratios are associated with greater risks of cardiovascular disease and identified this measurement as a more discriminating risk factor than BMI in men and women of all ages.[15] A recent meta-analysis involving more than 258,000 subjects reported a progressive increase in cardiovascular risk with increasing waist circumference and waist-to-hip ratios.[16] In this study, every 1-cm increase in waist circumference

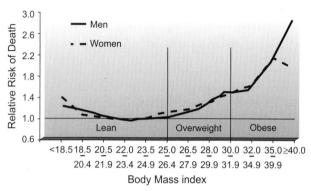

Fig. 3. Mortality risks across the BMI spectrum. (*Data from* Calle EE, Thun MJ, Petrelli JM, et al. Body-mass index and mortality in a prospective cohort of US adults. N Eng J Med 1999;341: 1097–105.)

was associated with a 2% increased relative risk of a cardiovascular event (95% confidence interval [CI]: 1%–3%) for men and women. These findings emphasize the importance of using this simple screening measure as a potential tool in assessing and predicting cardiometabolic risk.

Whether obesity is an independent mediator of CHD risk, apart from its comorbid associations, remains unclear. The Munster Heart Study,[17] which followed more than 23,000 patients over a 7-year span, noted an association of increasing BMI with CHD mortality. After multivariate analysis, however, the increase in death was attributed to confounding medical conditions including hypertension and hypercholesterolemia, negating obesity as an independent mediator of risk. Others studies suggest that obesity augments CHD risk through a codependent mechanism. A recent meta-analysis of more than 300,000 healthy patients identified a 45% increased risk of CHD with overweight and obesity, partially owing to the association with hypertension and hypercholesterolemia. Obesity and overweight, however, were confirmed as significant risk factors warranting treatment.[18] The Framingham Heart Study 26-year follow-up identified obesity as an independent risk factor associated with CHD, stroke, HF, and death from cardiovascular disease.[19] These studies highlight the controversies in the literature with regard to the influence of obesity on cardiovascular risk.

Obesity appears to accelerate established CAD. Obese patients who have acute coronary syndromes tend to be younger at the time of their first cardiovascular event than their normal-weight counterparts and tend to suffer worse outcomes.[20] Based on strong current supportive evidence, the American Heart Association has identified obesity as a major modifiable risk factor for CHD.[21] Despite contemporary guidelines and improved technology for diagnosis, cardiovascular disease remains the leading cause of morbidity and mortality in America.[13] Moreover, the disease often presents without warning, that is, the first clinical manifestation is often an AMI.[22] Heart disease rates are escalating, making primary prevention of cardiovascular disease a major public health objective. Screening for those at elevated risk in the general population is crucial. Arguably, for much of the obese population, excess adiposity serves as a metabolic barometer, which can be highly indicative of excess risk.

OBESITY AND HEART FAILURE

Obesity is gaining support as an independent risk factor for HF, as verified in small population-based studies.[23,24] This hypothesis was strengthened in a prospective population study of approximately 6000 subjects followed for over 14 years that reported a twofold increase in the risk of developing HF among those individuals who had a BMI greater than 30 kg/m^2, even after adjusting for CAD, hypertension, and left ventricular hypertrophy. This study detailed increased HF rates of 5% and 7% for men and women, respectively, with each incremental unit increase in BMI.[25] Furthermore, the risk increased with escalating BMI categories for men and for women and was associated with both diastolic and systolic HF.[25]

Although the mechanisms by which obesity causes HF remains unclear, the relationship may be attributed, at least in part, to the stress of an enlarged body habitus in conjunction with obesity-specific comorbid processes. Obesity is associated with several compensatory structural cardiovascular alterations that result from the increased demands of an excessive body mass and a hyperdynamic circulation. These pathologic changes may stem from the associated increases in blood volume, cardiac output, stroke volume, and filling pressures, culminating in left ventricular hypertrophy and dilation that may induce diastolic dysfunction through impairment in diastolic relaxation.[26]

The established metabolic consequences of obesity also impact HF. There is frequent overlap of obstructive sleep apnea (OSA) with increased vascular tone through activation of the renin-angiotensin and sympathetic systems, resulting in hypertension that can exacerbate left ventricular hypertrophy and diastolic dysfunction and contribute to HF.[27–29] The atherogenic, prothrombotic, and proinflammatory states noted in overweight and obesity enhance atherogenesis and CAD as precursors to HF.[24] It has been suggested that the likelihood of left ventricular dysfunction may be increased by the metabolic syndrome because the components of this medical condition have now been correlated to the degree of myocardial dysfunction.[30]

An emerging hypothesis describes a direct influence of obesity on the myocardium through an accumulation of lipids in the muscle and vasculature, which increases with the extent of adiposity.[31] This association was first described in 1933 from autopsy findings that suggested fatty degeneration of the myocardial tissues as a direct consequence of obesity.[32] The theory suggests that when excessive body fat accumulates, visceral storage sites fill to capacity, promoting a release of triglycerides and free fatty acids into the circulation that then accumulate within the myocardium itself. There is also an abnormal aggregation of epicardial and paracardial adipose tissue, which are forms of visceral fatty accumulation.[33] These pathologic fatty depots secrete hormones, inflammatory cytokines, and proteins that apply a direct and continued exposure of the myocardium to an inflammatory milieu through a paracrine influence. This proximal association may intensify the progression of atherosclerosis and serve as a unique marker for cardiovascular disease risk.[33] The accumulation of lipid metabolism by-products within the myocardium promotes lipotoxicity through a pathologic activation of adverse signaling cascades, which can culminate in cellular death.[34] Animal research has also established the relationship of steatosis and interstitial dysfunction in other organ systems.[35] Collectively, these consequences induce left ventricular remodeling and diastolic dysfunction that in some cases may culminate in an obesity-specific dilated nonischemic cardiomyopathy. The term *obesity-specific lipotoxic cardiomyopathy* has been used to describe the relationship between obesity and HF and includes pathologic changes that may be arrhythmogenic.[36]

OBESITY AND ATRIAL FIBRILLATION

Incidence rates of AF have increased dramatically over the last several decades. Approximately 2.5 million Americans now have AF, and these numbers are expected to soar with the aging of the population and the obesity epidemic.[37] The obese population demonstrates a twofold to fivefold increased risk of stroke and a twofold increase in early mortality as a consequence of its excessive adiposity.[38] Although previous reports regarding the link between obesity and AF have been inconsistent, a recent large community-based observational long-term follow-up (mean 13.7 years) of Framingham subjects delineated a close association between these two syndromes.[39] In this multivariate model adjusted for cardiovascular diseases (including a history of myocardial infarction and HF), a 4% increase in AF risk per 1-unit increase in BMI among men ($P = .02$) and women ($P = .009$) was reported. Adjusted hazard ratios for AF associated with obesity were 1.52 (95% CI: 1.09–2.13; $P = .02$) for men and 1.46 (95% CI: 1.03–2.07; $P = .03$) for women compared with normal-weight participants. In this study, left atrial diameter enlargement emerged as the strongest echocardiographic predictor of AF and has been directly correlated with increasing BMI levels.[40] These associations have been substantiated in another large population-based prospective cohort study, further strengthening the connection between obesity and AF.[41] Using many of the same hypotheses that explain the association of obesity and HF, researchers have now described common modulators that promote left atrial enlargement and AF, including elevated plasma volume, hypertension, left ventricular hypertrophy, diastolic dysfunction, stimulation of sympathetic tone, and OSA.[30,42] A theoretic direct influence of lipotoxicity promoting atrial enlargement has also been offered as a potential mechanism.[36]

THE OBESITY OUTCOME PARADOX: FINDINGS AFTER DISEASE MANIFESTATION AND TREATMENT

Despite the fact that obesity is tightly linked to earlier CHD presentation, there has been a frequently reported "survival paradox" associated with overweight and obesity in patients who experience acute coronary events and in those who undergo emergent or elective coronary revascularization procedures.[43,44] A large population-based cohort study found that although there was a higher prevalence of overweight and obesity and related comorbidities among patients who had previous myocardial infarction, there were no adverse outcomes associated with obesity.[45] Recently, Uretsky and colleagues[46] noted this paradox among hypertensive patients who had known cardiovascular disease. This study evaluated 22,576 obese and overweight patients and found a decreased risk of primary end points (defined as death, nonfatal myocardial infarction, or nonfatal stroke) compared with a normal-weight control group. The results from the Arterial Revascularization Therapy Study trial (ARTS), a multicenter randomized trial comparing normal, overweight, and stage 1 obese patients who underwent coronary artery bypass grafting (CABG) or coronary stenting, reported a significant decrease in repeat revascularizations in the stage 1 obese subgroup ($P = .03$). At the 3-year end point, obese subjects who underwent CABG demonstrated a superior outcome with regard to survival and had a significantly decreased rate of major cardiac and cerebrovascular events ($P = .008$).[47]

The obesity survival benefit has been substantiated in similar multicenter randomized trials, whereby lower mortality rates after coronary angioplasty among hospitalized patients, at 30 days, and at 1-year intervals compared with patients who had normal BMI levels were noted.[48] Similar findings highlighting the existence of an obesity paradox have been noted in HF patients. Curtis and colleagues[49] reported that overweight and obesity provided a relative risk reduction of 12% and 19%, respectively, for all-cause mortality compared with a normal-weight group in patients who had established HF.

A meta-analysis[50] of 40 different studies with over 250,000 subjects who had known coronary disease followed for over a mean of 3.8 years revealed an inverse relationship with increasing BMI and CHD mortality rates that persisted through class II obesity. In this study, a BMI of less than 20 kg/m^2 was associated with an increased relative risk for CHD mortality of 1.45 (1.16–1.81). In the overweight group (BMI 25–29.9 kg/m^2), CHD mortality was lowest, with a relative risk of 0.88 (0.75–1.02), whereas class I obesity (BMI 30–35 kg/m^2) had a relative risk of 0.97 (0.82–1.15). Among patients who had class II obesity and above (BMI $\geq$35 kg/m^2), the cardiac mortality was significantly elevated and corresponded to a relative risk of 1.88 (1.05–3.34). Similarly, Kaplan and colleagues[51] correlated obesity with a higher mortality after AMI, reporting a U-shaped mortality curve by BMI levels, highlighting the complex association of mortality risks at BMI extremes (see **Fig. 2**).

Although this U-shaped association has been found in most studies, a few have reported decreased survival with increasing BMI levels after coronary revascularization. In the Bypass Angioplasty Revascularization Investigation (BARI) trial,[52] there was a strikingly worse long-term prognosis after CABG as BMI increased, described as an 11% higher adjusted 5-year cardiac mortality rate among CABG-treated subjects with each incremental unit of BMI. These cumulative findings describe the controversy that surrounds the obesity paradox.

The mechanism underlying higher survival rates among obese CHD individuals is not fully clear. Some of these observed differences are due to the fact that the disease is manifest in patients at an earlier age.[53] It is also possible that obese cardiac patients tolerate the catabolic stress of myocardial ischemia or HF better than their normal-weight counterparts.[53] Conversely, weight loss due to chronic disease and cachexia may serve as a confounding variable, worsening outcomes in lower-weight individuals.

OBESITY AND DIABETES MELLITUS

The worldwide prevalence of DM is rapidly increasing and is projected to increase to roughly 300 million by the year 2025. At least 95% of the new cases are a result of type 2 DM.[54] Obesity is strongly associated with the development of type 2 DM, and nearly 90% of individuals who have this metabolic condition are overweight or obese.[55] A recent study reported a reduction of 8 years in life expectancy in an individual who is diagnosed with DM by the age of 40 years compared with an individual who is not diagnosed with DM.[56] Approximately 65% of patients who have type 2 DM die from a cardiovascular event,[57] and 7-year outcomes of patients who have CHD are similar to those of patients who have DM without known coronary disease. In a meta-analysis of 27 studies that evaluated mortality from CHD in the presence of diabetes, the risk of a fatal coronary event was three times higher in those affected with type 2 DM.[58] These sobering statistics support diabetes as risk equivalent to known cardiovascular disease.[59]

Hyperglycemia with insulin resistance in conjunction with dyslipidemia, chronic inflammation, and procoagulability all contribute to endothelial dysfunction and macrovascular disease, leading to the development of CHD. Aggressive strategies to improve these metabolic markers are useful to prevent initial and recurrent cardiovascular events. The United Kingdom Prospective Diabetes Study found that poor diabetic control (hemoglobin A_{1c} >7.9%) was associated with a greater cardiovascular mortality rate when compared with tight glycemic control (hemoglobin A_{1c} <6%). In patients who have type 1 DM, intensive control of blood glucose involving three or more injections of insulin per day with appropriate adjustments has been shown to reduce the incidence of cardiovascular disease. Among the intensively treated group, there was a 42% reduction in the risk of cardiovascular events and a 57% decrease in the risk for nonfatal myocardial infarction, cerebrovascular accidents, and death from cardiovascular disease.[60]

To achieve comprehensive cardiovascular risk reduction in a diabetic patient, optimization of risk factors is required from a multifactorial approach, including sustaining blood glucose levels (hemoglobin A_{1c} around 7%), appropriate blood pressure levels (<130/80 mm Hg), and targeted lipid levels (triglycerides <150 mg/dL, LDL-C <100 mg/dL, and HDL-C >40 mg/dL and >50 mg/dL in men and women, respectively). Gaede and colleagues[61] compared conventional treatment with intensive behavioral modification in patients who had type 2 DM that was aimed at achieving these goals and reported that the latter was superior, with behavioral modification resulting in a 53% cardiovascular risk reduction over 7-year period.

The reduction of cardiovascular risk factors has been repeatedly documented with therapeutic lifestyle intervention. Three separate large randomized controlled studies have concluded that lifestyle modification in an at-risk population is a successful method of diabetes prevention and is superior to pharmacologic intervention alone.[62–64] These strategies, however, employ behavior modification, which is labor-intensive and subject to recidivism.

OBESITY AND HYPERTENSION

Obesity is strongly associated with hypertension, which is a major risk factor for the development of CHD. The Framingham Heart Study reported that 79% of the hypertension in men and 65% in women was a direct result of excess weight.[65] Data from the Third National Health and Nutritional Examination Survey indicate a linear relationship between BMI and systolic and diastolic blood pressure.[66] In age-adjusted regression models, an increase in BMI of 1.25 kg/m^2 and 1.70 kg/m^2 and an increase in waist circumference of 2.5 cm and 4.5 cm among women and men, respectively, was associated with a 1-mm Hg increase in systolic blood pressure.[67] Uncontrolled hypertension increases CHD risks and exacerbates vascular complications including CAD, chronic kidney disease, stroke, peripheral vascular disease, and retinopathy.[68] The risk of developing CHD and of coronary death is increased in a progressive manner, with higher systolic and diastolic blood pressure levels seen among all age categories including the elderly.[69,70]

The etiologic mediators of these increased risks are likely multifactorial. The consequence of obesity combined with hypertension promotes hemodynamic cardiac compensations from increased preload, stroke work, and blood volume, producing an eccentric cardiac hypertrophy[71] These alterations are clinically meaningful because they are mediators of HF, ventricular arrhythmias, and sudden cardiac death. Obesity is associated with sympathetic stimulation and renin-angiotensin-aldosterone activation, exacerbating these hemodynamic alterations and increasing the likelihood of hypertension.[72] Collectively, these changes may heighten the risk of chronic kidney disease, which by way of a viscous feedback mechanism may accelerate the development of CHD.

Blood pressure lowering has been shown to be a successful strategy to reduce cardiovascular events. A meta-analysis of 10 randomized trials revealed that a 12- to 13-mm Hg lowering in systolic blood pressure over a 4-year follow-up was associated with a 21% reduction in CHD, a 37% reduction in stroke, and a 25% decrease in total cardiovascular mortality.[73] To minimize the likelihood of cardiovascular events, lowering blood pressure to normal ranges, especially in patients who have known cardiovascular disease, is of utmost importance. The last Joint National Committee guidelines recommended a blood pressure goal of less than 130/85 mm Hg and acknowledged that higher-risk patients who have known chronic kidney disease and proteinuria (>1 g) may benefit from even lower pressures (125/75 mm Hg).[74] Concomitant diet/lifestyle intervention and pharmacotherapy are recommended strategies to achieve these goals. Currently, there is no evidence-based approach to direct obesity-related hypertension treatment other than empiric experience. Angiotensin-converting enzyme inhibitors or angiotensin-receptor blockers, however, may produce benefits beyond blood pressure lowering by improving modulators in DM, HF, and microalbuminuria, delaying the onset of DM and potentially reducing the risk of death, MI, and stroke.[75,76] β-blockers are routinely prescribed for patients who have known coronary disease and are an attractive treatment option for inhibition of the adrenergic response [77,78]; however, these agents may promote weight gain and potentially worsen glycemic control, limiting their appeal.

OBESITY AND DYSLIPIDEMIA

Cholesterol is one of the greatest mediators for cardiovascular risk in visceral obesity. Indeed, approximately 70% of patients who have premature CHD also have dyslipidemia.[79] Increasing BMI levels mediate a common pattern of dyslipidemia characterized by higher triglycerides, lower HDL-C, and increased small, dense LDL particles, which are all independent risk factors for coronary disease.[80,81] This abnormal pattern of cholesterol is typically compounded in obesity by secondary associations to type 2 DM, the metabolic syndrome, and dietary influences from high fat and high sugar intakes. The small, dense LDL particles are excessively atherogenic due to their tendency for oxidation and their ability to penetrate the endothelial barrier of vessel walls, impairing nitric oxide production, blunting endothelial-mediated vasodilation, and augmenting inflammation, smooth muscle proliferation, and platelet aggregation.[82–84]

The National Cholesterol Education Program Expert Panel on Detection, Evaluation, and Treatment of High Blood Cholesterol in Adults (Adult Treatment Panel III) guidelines provide evidence-based recommendations on the management of LDL-C using the Framingham Score, a 10-year prognostic assessment for identifying those at risk of developing cardiovascular disease. This score is derived from a formula using age, sex, tobacco use, HDL-C, LDL-C, blood pressure, and presence of diabetes. Modifying LDL-C is the major treatment goal for risk reduction within this model that incorporates lifestyle modifications and pharmacologic intervention, when appropriate. This validated model has the power to predict greater than 90% of all cardiac events, identifying those individuals at greatest risk.[59] A significant limitation of this common risk assessment tool is the absence of the variables obesity, physical inactivity, and insulin resistance—the metabolic syndrome parameters that are uniquely associated with cardiovascular disease and that are highly modifiable. If these variables were included in traditional risk assessments, then a significantly higher proportion of the population would meet criteria for treatment.

Treatment of these lipid/lipoprotein markers may decrease systemic inflammation, improve endothelial dysfunction, and stabilize and promote regression of atherosclerotic plaques, which all serve to reduce cardiovascular event rates and total mortality.[85] Statin therapy is highly effective for treating elevated LDL-C and triglycerides and reduced HDL-C. Certain patients who have elevated triglycerides and low HDL-C may benefit from the addition of a fibrate, which also has anti-inflammatory and antiatherosclerotic properties.[86] The Veterans Affairs HDL Intervention trial[87] found that the benefits of fibrate therapy depended on insulin resistance and, to a lesser extent, triglyceride or HDL-C abnormalities, supporting their potential use in the patient who has DM or the metabolic syndrome. Fibrate therapy was evaluated in the treatment of diabetic dyslipidemia in the Fenofibrate Interventions and Event-Lowering in Diabetes study,[88] which found a significant benefit in secondary treatment outcomes among the intervention group; however, there was no significant benefit with respect to primary prevention. The Action to Control Cardiovascular risk in Diabetes study is currently investigating the use of statins and fibrate therapy in diabetics to determine the value of combined treatments with regard to cardiovascular and all-cause mortality outcomes.[89]

OBESITY AND THE METABOLIC SYNDROME

The association of visceral obesity and cardiovascular risks stems from the clustering of metabolic conditions (including hypertension, dyslipidemia, and type 2 DM) that are mediated through insulin resistance, leading to the metabolic syndrome. The purpose of this unique designation was to identify those at higher metabolic risk for cardiovascular disease and the development of diabetes and to respond with more aggressive strategies for prevention. The metabolic syndrome, as defined by the guidelines from the National Cholesterol Education Program Adult Treatment Panel III, is characterized by three or more of the criteria listed in **Box 1**. The metabolic syndrome is present in 24% of all adults in the United States and in more than 40% of men and women over the age of 65 years.[90] Each component of the metabolic syndrome is associated with a heightened risk for developing cardiovascular disease and diabetes.[91] Patients who have the metabolic syndrome have a 1.5- to 3-fold increased risk for developing CHD or stroke.[92] In the primary prevention arm of the San Antonio Heart Study (mean follow-up, 12.7 years), the metabolic syndrome was associated with a twofold higher risk for developing cardiovascular disease,[93] which distinguishes the metabolic syndrome as a unique marker for increased cardiovascular risk and highlights the need for aggressive risk-factor reduction in this population.

LINKS WITH NONTRADITIONAL RISK FACTORS

Recent studies suggest that traditional risk factors do not fully encompass global cardiovascular risks. A new set of nontraditional risk factors are emerging (**Box 2**).[85,94] Insulin resistance is the primary mediator in the development of diabetes (along with visceral obesity) and is a significant and independent risk factor for cardiovascular disease.[95] This condition adversely impacts insulin action and glucose disposal. β cells of the pancreas secrete higher levels of insulin to maintain

---

Box 1
National Cholesterol Education Program Adult Treatment Panel III guidelines for diagnosing the metabolic syndrome

- Abdominal obesity defined as a waist circumference of 102 cm (40 in) in men and 88 cm (35 in) in women
- TG levels of 150 mg/dL or more (1.7 mmol/L)
- HDL-C levels of less than 40 mg/dL (1 mmol/L) in men and less than 50 mg/dL (1.3 mmol/L) in women
- Blood pressure levels of 130/85 mm Hg or higher
- Fasting glucose levels of 100 mg/dL or greater (5.5 mmol/L)

Box 2
Emerging risk factors for cardiovascular risk

- Insulin resistance
- Abnormal fibrinolysis
- Endothelial dysfunction
- Microalbuminuria
- Inflammation
- Procoagulation
- Obstructive sleep apnea

Data from Grundy SM, Cleeman JI, Mez CNB, et al. Implications of recent clinical trials for the National Cholesterol Education Program Adult Treatment Panel III Guidelines. Circulation 2004;110:227–39.

---

blood glucose concentrations, which leads to hyperinsulinemia. These changes promote an impairment of lipolysis and the release of free fatty acids, leading to hypertriglyceridemia and the accumulation of fatty acids in the muscle and liver, which exacerbates insulin resistance and dyslipidemia.[96]

Visceral obesity also promotes an inflammatory environment and increased levels of resistin, free fatty acids, and interleukin-6, which are the primary mediators of insulin resistance that accelerate atherogenic dyslipidemia and the likelihood of the metabolic syndrome and type 2 DM.[97] Obesity and insulin resistance contribute to vascular dysfunction by inhibiting the release of nitric oxide, a natural promoter of endothelial integrity and a mediator of vascular homeostasis. A recent study noted that increasing BMI was paralleled by abnormal vascular reactivity, increased vasoconstriction, and procoagulant influences.[98] Hyperinsulinemia with insulin resistance promotes multiple other metabolic derangements and is proportional to the risk of cardiovascular mortality.[99]

Numerous studies have demonstrated beneficial effects of insulin sensitizers in modifying cardiovascular risk factors. Insulin sensitivity can be moderated by up-regulating peroxisome proliferator–activated receptors within adipose tissue, which favorably alters lipid and carbohydrate metabolism. Thiazolidinediones are peroxisome proliferator–activating receptor gamma agonists that are used in the treatment of type 2 DM. These agents improve lipid/lipoprotein profiles and emerging vascular risk factors by enhancing vascular reactivity and inhibiting markers of thrombosis and inflammation, distinguishing this class of medications as an attractive intervention.[100] The carotid intima-media thickness is highly correlated with the risk of developing cardiovascular disease. In the Carotid Intima-Media Thickness in Atherosclerosis Using Pioglitazone trial, diabetic subjects were randomized to pioglitazone or glimepiride. Using carotid intima-media thickness as the criterion measure, investigators reported a significant benefit in the thiazolidinedione group compared with the glimepiride group.[101]

Thiazolidinediones, however, are associated with weight gain and a more resistant adipose mass, which represent potential limitations. In contrast, fibrate therapy used in the treatment of dyslipidemia may up-regulate insulin receptors, facilitating glucose disposal in adipose and muscle tissue, thereby improving insulin sensitivity.[102]

Microalbuminuria is now recognized as an early independent risk factor for chronic kidney disease, cardiovascular disease, insulin resistance, type 2 DM, and hypertension.[103] The exact mechanisms by which microalbuminuria is associated with cardiovascular disease are not known; however, it has been suggested that proteinuria serves as a generalized marker for endothelial dysfunction and, in this manner, signals a greater risk of generalized vascular disease and atherosclerosis.[104]

There is an inverse relationship between microalbuminuria and insulin sensitivity. Conversely, with the reduction of urinary protein concentrations, there are associated metabolic improvements that translate to a markedly diminished cardiovascular risk.[105] DeZeaw and colleagues[106] examined type 2 DM patients who had nephropathy and reported that a decrease in proteinuria of 50% translated to an 18% reduction in cardiovascular risk. Pharmacologic treatment aimed at improving glycemia and hypertension has also proved to be beneficial at lowering microalbuminuria. Adequate blood pressure control is essential in improving the degree of urinary albumin excretion and hence the degree of nephropathy. Angiotensin-converting enzyme inhibitors and angiotensin II–receptor blockers improve albuminuria through their antihypertensive effects and lowering of intraglomerular pressure, reducing the progression of chronic kidney disease risks.[107]

Visceral adipose cells were once considered inert but have now been shown to behave similarly to endocrine tissue, releasing cytokines and adhesion molecules including tumor necrosis factor α, which stimulates high-sensitivity C-reactive protein; P-selectin; and interleukin-6, which limits adiponectin release and is known for its antiatherogenic and insulin sensitivity–promoting properties. Excessive visceral adipose tissue secretions have been confirmed in biopsy studies in obese compared with normal-weight subjects.[108] These inflammatory changes further exacerbate hyperinsulinemia, hyperglycemia, and dyslipidemia in the obese patient, promoting oxidative stress, endothelial dysfunction, and cardiovascular alterations that are compatible with atherosclerotic heart disease. Rosito and colleagues[109] studied over 3230 subjects and found that increasing BMI values and hip-to-waist ratios were independently associated with prothrombotic factors, including impaired fibrinolytic activity, as well as abnormalities with fibrinogen, factor VII, plasminogen activating inhibitor 1, and tPA antigen in men and women ($P<.002$). Accordingly, the investigators found greater thrombotic potential in overweight and obese subjects.

Higher levels of plasminogen activator inhibitor 1, increased platelet aggregation, and elevated levels of fibrinogen promote a thrombotic state that exacerbates atherogenesis and cardiovascular risks.[110] These conditions function in concert with the metabolic syndrome and are highly atherogenic in nature. Presumably, the mechanisms involve an up-regulation of adhesion molecules and the inhibition of endothelial synthesis of nitrous oxide, which promote an increased risk for atherogenesis.

Using the notion that inflammation plays a key role in the development of cardiovascular disease, clinicians have increasingly examined the role of inflammatory markers in predicting risks for CAD. C-reactive protein levels of 2 mg/L or higher may be a powerful predictor for future cardiovascular events.[111] The current American Heart Association/Centers for Disease Control and Prevention Scientific Statement on Markers of Intervention and Cardiovascular Disease recommends that in the patient who has an intermediate Framingham 10-year risk (10%–20%) and an LDL-C level below the cut-off for initiation of pharmacotherapy it may be appropriate to measure C-reactive protein to aid in risk stratification and assessment.[112] The Justification for the Use of Statins in Primary Prevention (JUPITER) trial,[113] which is currently ongoing, will assist in evaluating the utility of this inflammatory marker to help identify patients who may require more aggressive treatment. More recently, lipoprotein-associated phospholipase A_2 has emerged as a promising inflammatory marker associated with cardiovascular risk that may be able to predict atherosclerosis independent from obesity or other nonspecific inflammatory conditions. This ability would distinguish it as a potentially more sensitive screening tool that may further enhance risk assessments.[114]

OSA is characterized by repeated partial or complete cessation of airflow during sleep, causing transient oxygen desaturation. Obesity is also a major determinant in risk for OSA.[115] Approximately 70% of patients diagnosed with OSA are obese, and the risk of OSA increases incrementally with escalating BMI levels.[116] For example, for every 10-kg increase in body weight, the risk of OSA doubles.[117] This condition contributes to the risks of hypertension, fatal and nonfatal cardiovascular events, stroke, HF, and cardiac arrhythmias.[42] Some of the metabolic disruptions associated with OSA stem from the activation of the sympathetic nervous system and the concurrent associations with systemic and pulmonary hypertension, atherosclerotic heart disease, dilated cardiomyopathy with or without HF, and cerebrovascular disease, arrhythmias, and AF.[118–121] Observational studies suggest that OSA is associated with a threefold increased risk for coronary disease apart from these related comorbid conditions.[122] There are also numerous thrombotic parameters that are associated with OSA that may increase cardiovascular events, including the exacerbation of coagulation defects, inflammatory responders, and endothelial dysfunction.[123] Despite these associations, OSA continues to be underdiagnosed and undertreated. In patients who have known coronary disease, OSA bears important prognostic significance, in that those patients who have untreated OSA experience a significantly higher mortality rate (38%) than their counterparts who do not have OSA (9%), which distinguishes OSA as a risk factor in need of diagnosis and of treatment.

SUMMARY

Obesity promotes a cascade of secondary pathologies including diabetes, insulin resistance, dyslipidemia, inflammation, thrombosis, hypertension, the metabolic syndrome, and OSA, which collectively heighten the risk for cardiovascular disease. Obesity may also be an independent moderator of cardiac risk apart from these comorbid conditions. Rates of obesity and cardiac disease continue to rise in a parallel and exponential manner. Because obesity is potentially one of the most modifiable mediators of cardiovascular morbidity and mortality, effective treatment and prevention interventions should have a profound and favorable impact on public health.

REFERENCES

1. Flegal KM, Carroll MD, Ogden CL, et al. Prevalence and trends in obesity among U.S. adults, 1999–2000. JAMA 2002;288:1723–7.
2. Popkin BM. The nutrition transition and its health implications in lower income countries. Public Health Nutr 1998;1:5–21.
3. Willett WC, Manson JE, Stampfer MJ, et al. Weight, weight change and coronary heart disease in women: risk within the "normal" weight range. JAMA 1995; 273(6):461–5.
4. Allison DB, Fontaine KR, Manson JE, et al. Annual deaths attributable to obesity in the United States. JAMA 1999;282:1530–8.
5. Fontaine KR, Redden DT, Wang C, et al. Years lost of life due to obesity. JAMA 2003;289:187–93.
6. Olshansky SJ, Passaro DJ, Hershow RC, et al. A potential decline in life expectancy in the United States in the 21st century. N Eng J Med 2005;352:1138–45.
7. Ogden CL, Flegal KM, Carroll MD, et al. Prevalence and trends in overweight among U.S. children and adolescents, 1999–2000. JAMA 2002;288:1728–32.

8. U.S. Department of Health and Human Services. The Surgeon General's call to action to prevent and decrease overweight and obesity. Rockville (MD): U.S. Department of Health and Human Services, Public Health Service, Office of the Surgeon General; 2001. Available from: U.S. GPO, Washington.

9. Must A, Jacques PF, Dallal GE, et al. Long-term morbidity and mortality of overweight adolescents: a follow-up of the Harvard Growth Study of 1922 to 1935. N Eng J Med 1992;327:1350–5.

10. Freedman DS, Dietz WH, Srinivasan SR, et al. The relation of overweight to cardiovascular risk factors among children and adolescents: the Bogalusa Heart Study. Pediatrics 1999;103:1175–82.

11. Berenson GS, Srinivasan SR, Bao W, et al. Association between multiple cardiovascular risk factors and atherosclerosis in children and young adults. N End J Med 1998;338:1650–6.

12. Pouliot MC, Despres JP, Lemieux S, et al. Waist circumference and abdominal sagittal diameter: best simple anthropometric indices of abdominal visceral adipose tissue accumulation and related cardiovascular risk in men and women. Am J cardiol 1994;73:460–8.

13. Heart disease and stroke statistics–2008 update. A report from the American Heart Association Statistics Committee and Stroke Statistics Subcommittee. Circulation 2008;117:e25–146.

14. Calle EE, Thun MJ, Petrelli JM, et al. Body-mass index and mortality in a prospective cohort of US adults. N Eng J Med 1999;341:1097–105.

15. Yusuf S, Hawken S, Ōunpuu S, et al. Obesity and the risk of myocardial infarction in 27000 participants from 52 countries: a case-control study. Lancet 2005; 366:1640–9.

16. De Koning L, Merchant AT, Pogue J, et al. Waist circumference and waist-to-hip ratio as predictors of cardiovascular events: meta-regression analysis of prospective studies. Eur heart J 2007;28(7):850–6.

17. Schulte H, Cullen P, Assmann G. Obesity, mortality and cardiovascular disease in the Munster Heart Study (PROCAM). Atherosclerosis 1999;144(1):199–209.

18. Bogers RP, Bemelmans WJ, Hoogenveen RT, et al. Association of overweight with increased risk of coronary heart disease partly independent of blood pressure and cholesterol levels. Arch Intern Med 2007;167(16):1720–8.

19. Hubert HB, Feinleib M, McNamara PM, et al. Obesity as an independent risk factor for cardiovascular disease: a 26-year follow-up of participants in the Framingham Heart Study. Circulation 1983;67(5):968–77.

20. Eisenstein E, Shaw L, Nelson C, et al. Obesity and long-term clinical and economic outcomes in coronary artery disease patients. Obes Res 2002;10:83–91.

21. Eckel RH. Obesity and heart disease: a statement for healthcare professionals from the Nutrition Committee, American Heart Association. Circulation 1997; 96(9):3248–50.

22. Levy D, Wilson PW. Atherosclerotic cardiovascular disease: an epidemiologic perspective. In: Topol EJ, editor. Text of cardiovascular medicine. Philadelphia: Lippincott-Raven; 1998. p. 13–30.

23. Chen YT, Vaccarino V, Williams CS, et al. Risk factors for heart failure in the elderly: a prospective community-based study. Am J Med 1999;106:605–12.

24. He J, Ogden LG, Bazzano LA, et al. Risk factors for congestive heart failure in US men and women: NHANES I epidemiologic follow-up study. Arch Intern Med 2001;161:996–1002.

25. Kenchaiah S, Evans JC, Levy D, et al. Obesity and the risk of heart failure. N Engl J Med 2002;347(5):305–13.

26. Alpert MA. Obesity cardiomyopathy: pathophysiology and evolution of the clinical syndrome. Am J Med Sci 2001;321:225–36.

27. Kasper EK, Hruban RH, Baughman KL. Cardiomyopathy of obesity: a clinicopathologic evaluation of 43 obese patients with heart failure. Am J Cardiol 1992;70:921–4.

28. Ku CS, Lin SL, Wang DJ, et al. Left ventricular filling in young normotensive obese adults. Am J Cardiol 1994;73:613–5.

29. Masserli FH. Cardiomyopathy of obesity—a not so Victorian disease. N Engl J Med 1986;314:378–80.

30. Wong CY, O'Moore-Sullican T, Fang ZY, et al. Myocardial and vascular dysfunction and exercise capacity in the metabolic syndrome. Am J Cardiol 2005;96:1686–91.

31. Malavazos AE, Ermetici F, Coman C, et al. Influence of epicardial adipose tissue and adipocytokine levels on cardiac abnormalities in visceral obesity. Int J Cardiol 2007;121(1):132–4.

32. Smith HL, Willius FA. Adiposity of the heart. Arch Intern Med 1933;52:811–31.

33. Iacobellis G, Corradi D, Sharma AM. Epicardial adipose tissue: anatomic, biomolecular and clinical relationship with the heart. Nat clin pract Cardiovasc Med 2005;2:536–43.

34. Unger RH. Minireview: weapons of lean body mass destruction: the role of ectopic lipids in the metabolic syndrome. Endocrinology 2003;144:5159–65.

35. Lee Y, Hirose H, Ohneda M, et al. Beta-cell lipotoxicity in the pathogenesis of non-insulin-dependent diabetes mellitus of obese rats: impairment in adipocyte–beta-cell relationships. Proc Natl Acad Sci U S A 1994;91:10878–82.

36. McGavrock JM, Victor RG, Unger RH, et al. Adiposity of the heart, revisited. Ann Intern Med 2006;144:517–24.

37. Ezekowitz MD. Atrial fibrillation: the epidemic of the new millennium. Ann Intern Med 1999;131:537–8.

38. Go AS, Hylek EM, Phillips KA, et al. Prevalence of diagnosed atrial fibrillation in adults: national implication of rhythm management and stroke prevention: the Anticoagulation and Risk Factors in Atrial Fibrillation (ATRIA) study. JAMA 2001;285:2370–5.

39. Wang TJ, Parise H, Levy D, et al. Obesity and the risk of new-onset atrial fibrillation. JAMA 2004;292:2471–7.

40. Pritchett AM, Jacobsen SJ, Mahoney DW, et al. Left atrial volume as an index of left atrial size: a population-based study. J Am Coll Cardiol 2003;41:1036–43.

41. Frost L, Juul Hune L, Vestergaard P. Overweight and obesity as risk factors for atrial fibrillation or flutter: the Danish Diet, Cancer, and Health study. Am J Med 2005;118:489–95.

42. Gami AS, Caples SM, Somers VK. Obesity and obstructive sleep apnea. Endocrinol Metab Clin North Am 2003;32:869–94.

43. Bozkurt B, Deswal A. Obesity as a prognostic factor in chronic symptomatic heart failure. Am Heart J 2005;150:1233–9.

44. Curtis JP, Selter JG, Wang Y, et al. The obesity paradox. Arch Intern Med 2005;165:55–61.

45. Lopez-Jimenez F, Jacobson SJ, Reeder GS, et al. Prevalence and secular trends of excess body weight and impact on outcomes after myocardial infarction in the community. Chest 2004;125(4):1205–12.

46. Uretsky S, Messerli FH, Bangalore S, et al. Obesity paradox in patients with hypertension and coronary artery disease. Am J Med 2007;120:863–70.

47. Gruberg L, Mercado N, Milo S, et al. Impact of body mass index on the outcome of patients with multivessel disease randomized to either coronary artery bypass

grafting or stenting in the ARTS trial: the obesity paradox II? Am J Cardiol 2005; 95:439–44.

48. Nikolsky E, Stone GW, Grines CL, et al. Impact of body mass index on outcomes after primary angioplasty in acute myocardial infarction. Am Heart J 2006;151: 168–75.

49. Curtis JP, Selter JG, Wang Y, et al. The obesity paradox: body mass index and outcomes in patients with heart failure. Arch Intern Med 2005;165(1):55–61.

50. Romero-Corral A, Montori VM, Somers VK, et al. Association of bodyweight with total mortality and with cardiovascular events in coronary artery disease: a systematic review of cohort studies. Lancet 2006;368:666–78.

51. Kaplan RC, Heckbert SR, Furburg CD, et al. Predictors of subsequent coronary events, stroke, and death among survivors of first hospitalized myocardial infarction. J Clin Epidemiol 2002;55:654–64.

52. Grum HS, Whitlow PL, Kip KE. The impact of body mass index on short-term and long-term outcomes inpatients undergoing coronary revascularization. (BARI). J Am Coll Cardiol 2002;39:834–40.

53. Lissin LW, Gauri AJ, Froelicher VF, et al. The prognostic value of body mass index and standard exercise testing in male veterans with congestive heart failure. J Card Fail 2002;8:206–15.

54. King H, Aubert RE, Herman WH. Global burden of diabetes, 1995–2025: prevalence, numerical estimates, and projections. Diabetes Care 1998;21:1414–31.

55. Mokdad AH, Ford ES, Bowman BA, et al. Prevalence of obesity, diabetes, and obesity-related health risk factors, 2001. JAMA 2003;289:76–9.

56. Roper NA, Bilous RW, Kelly WF, et al. Excess mortality in a population with diabetes and the impact of material deprivation: longitudinal, population based study. BMJ 2001;332:1389–93.

57. Gu K, Cowie CC, Harris MI. Diabetes and decline in heart disease mortality in US adults. JAMA 1999;281:1291–7.

58. Huxley R, Barzi F, Woodward M. Excess risk of fatal coronary heart disease associated with diabetes in men and women: meta-analysis of 37 prospective cohort studies. BMJ 2006;332:73–8.

59. National Cholesterol Education Program, Adult Treatment Panel III. Executive summary of the third report of the National Cholesterol Education Program (NCEP) Expert Panel on Detection, Evaluation and Treatment of High Blood Cholesterol in Adults. JAMA 2001;285(19):2486–98.

60. Natham DM, Cleary PA, Backlund JY, et al. for the Diabetes Control and Complications Trial/Epidemiology of Diabetes Interventions and Complications (DCCT/EDIC) study research group. Intensive diabetes treatment and cardiovascular disease in patients with type 1 diabetes. N Engl J Med 2005;353:2643–53.

61. Gaede P, Vedel P, Larsen N, et al. Multifactorial intervention and cardiovascular disease in patients with type 2 diabetes. N Eng J Med 2003;348:383–93.

62. Pan XR, Li GW, Hu YH, et al. Effects of diet and exercise in preventing NIDDM in people with impaired glucose tolerance. The Da Qing IGT and Diabetes Study. Diabetes Care 1997;20:537–44.

63. Tuomilehto J, Lindstrom J, Eriksson JG, et al. Finnish Diabetes Prevention Study Group. Prevention of type 2 diabetes mellitus by changes in lifestyle among subjects with impaired glucose tolerence. N Engl J Med 2002;346:393–403.

64. Knowler WC, Barnett-Connor E, Fowler SE, et al. Reduction in the incidence of type 2 diabetes with lifestyle intervention. N Eng J Med 2002;346:393–403.

65. Garrison RJ, Kannel WB, Stokes ME, et al. Incidence and precursors of hypertension in young adults: the Framingham offspring study. Prev Med 1987;16:235–51.

66. El-Atat F, Aneja A, Mcfarlane S, et al. Obesity and hypertension. Endocinol Metab Clin North Am 2003;32:832–54.
67. Engeli S, Sharma AM. Emerging concepts in the pathophysiology and treatment of obesity-associated hypertension. Curr Opin Cardiol 2002;17:355–9.
68. Toto RD. Treatment of hypertension in chronic kidney disease. Semin Nephrol 2005;25:435–9.
69. Lewington S, Clarke R, Qizilbash N, et al. Prospective Studies Collaboration. Age-specific relevance of usual blood pressure to vascular mortality: a meta-analysis of individual data for one million adults in 61 prospective studies. Lancet 2002;360:1903–13.
70. Stamler J, Stamler R, Neaton JD. Blood pressure systolic and diastolic and cardiovascular risks. US population data. Arch Intern Med 1993;153:598–615.
71. Frohlich ED, Epstein C, Chobanian AV, et al. The heart in hypertension. N Engl J Med 1992;327:998–1008.
72. Hall JE, Hildebrandt DA, Kuo J. Obesity hypertension: role of leptin and sympathetic nervous system. Am J Hypertens 2001;14:103S–15S.
73. He J, Whelton PK. Elevated systolic blood pressure and risk of cardiovascular and renal disease: overview of evidence from observational epidemiologic studies and randomized controlled trials. Am Heart J 1999;138:211–9.
74. Chobanian AV, Bakris GL, Black HR, et al. The National High Blood Pressure Education Program Coordinating Committee. Seventh report of the Joint National Committee on Prevention, Detection, Evaluation, and Treatment of High Blood Pressure. Hypertension 2003;42:1206–52.
75. Heart Outcomes Prevention Evaluation Study Investigators. Effects of ramipril on cardiovascular and microvascular outcomes in people with diabetes mellitus: results of the HOPE study and MICRO-HOPE substudy. Lancet 2000;355:253–9.
76. Yusuf S, Sleight P, Pogue J, et al. Effects of an angiotensin-converting-enzyme inhibitor, ramipril, on cardiovascular events in high-risk patients. The Heart Outcomes Prevention Evaluation Study Investigators. N Eng J Med 2000; 342(3):145–53.
77. Pedersen TR. Six-year follow-up of the Norwegian Multicenter Study on timolol after acute myocardial infarction. N Eng J Med 1985;313:1055–8.
78. Tuck ML. Obesity, the sympathetic nervous system, and essential hypertension. Hypertension 1992;19:167–77.
79. Genest JJ, Martin-Munley SS, McNamara JR, et al. Familial lipoprotein disorders in patients with premature coronary artery disease. Circulation 1992;85(6):2025–33.
80. Austin MA, Hokanson JE, Edwards KL. Hypertriglyceridemia as a cardiovascular risk factor. Am J Cardiol 1998;81(Suppl):7B–12B.
81. Garber AM, Alvins AL. Triglyceride concentration and coronary heart disease. Not yet proved of value as a screening test. BMJ 1994;309(6946):2–3.
82. Austin MA, King MC, Vranizan KM, et al. Atherogenic lipoprotein phenotype. A proposed genetic marker for coronary heart disease risk. Circulation 1990; 82(2):495–506.
83. Anderson TJ, Meredith IT, Charbonneau F, et al. Endothelium-dependent coronary vasomotion relates to the susceptibility of LDL to oxidation in humans. Circulation 1996;93(9):1647–50.
84. Griffin JH, Fernandez JA, Deguchi H. Plasma lipoproteins, hemostasis and thrombosis. Thromb Haemost 2001;86(1):386–94.
85. Grundy SM, Cleeman JI, Mez CN, et al. Implications of recent clinical trials for the National Cholesterol Education Program Adult Treatment Panel III guidelines. Circulation 2004;110:227–39.

86. Nesto RW. Beyond low-density lipoprotein: addressing the atherogenic lipid triad in type 2 diabetes mellitus and metabolic syndrome. Am J Cardiovasc Drugs 2005;5:379–87.

87. Robins SJ, Rubins HB, Faas FH, et al, for the VA-HIT Study Group. Insulin resistance and cardiovascular events with low HDL cholesterol. The Veterans Affairs HDL Intervention trial (VA-HIT). Diabetes Care 2003;26:1513–7.

88. Keech A, Simes RJ, Barter P, et al. for the FIELD study investigators. Effects of long-term fenofibrate therapy on cardiovascular events in 9795 people with type 2 diabetes mellitus (the FIELD study) randomized controlled trial. Lancet 2005; 366:1849–61.

89. Goff DC, Gerstein HC, Ginsberg HN, et al. Prevention in cardiovascular disease in persons with type 2 diabetes mellitus: current knowledge and rationale for the Action to Control Cardiovascular Risk in Diabetes (ACCORD) trial. Am J Cardiol 2007;99(Suppl):4i–20i.

90. Ford ES, Giles WH, Dietz WH. Prevalence of the metabolic syndrome among US adults: findings from the Third National Health and Nutritional Examination Survey. JAMA 2002;287(3):356–9.

91. Sattar N, Gaw A, Scherbakova O, et al. Metabolic syndrome with and without C-reactive protein as a predictor of coronary heart disease and diabetes in the West of Scotland Coronary Prevention Study. Circulation 2003;108:414–9.

92. Isomaa B, Almgren P, Tuomi T, et al. Cardiovascular morbidity and mortality associated with the metabolic syndrome. Diabetes Care 2001;24:683–9.

93. Hunt KJ, Resendez RG, Williams K, et al. National cholesterol education program versus World Health Organization metabolic syndrome in relation to all-cause and cardiovascular mortality in the San Antonio Heart Study. Circulation 2004;110:1251–7.

94. Forseca VA. Rationale for the use of insulin sensitizers to prevent cardiovascular events in type 2 diabetes. Am J Med 2007;120:S18–25.

95. Després J-P, Lamrche B, Mauriége P, et al. Hyperinsulinemia as an independent risk factor for ischemic heart disease. N Engl J Med 1996;334:952–7.

96. Olefsky JM, Farqunar JW, Reaven GM. Reappraisal of the role of insulin in hypertriglyceridemia. Am J Med 1974;57:551–60.

97. Miller WM, Nori Janosz KE, Yanez J, et al. Effects of weight loss and pharmacotherapy on inflammatory markers of cardiovascular disease. Expert Rev Cardiovasc Ther 2005;3(4):743–59.

98. Juonala M, Viikari JS, Laitinen T, et al. Interrelations between brachial endothelial function and carotid intima-media thickness in young adults: the Cardiovascular Risk in Young Finns study. Circulation 2004;110:2918–23.

99. Eschwege E, Richard JL, Thibult N, et al. Coronary heart disease mortality in relation with diabetes, blood glucose and plasma insulin levels: the Paris Prospective Study, ten years later. Horm Metab Res Suppl 1985;15:41s–6s.

100. Foneseca V, Desouza C, Asnani S, et al. Nontraditional risk factors for cardiovascular disease in diabetes. Endocr Rev 2004;25:153–75.

101. Mazzone T, Meyer PM, Feinstein SB, et al. Effect of pioglitazone compared with glimipiride on carotid-media thickness in type 2 diabetes. JAMA 2006;296:2572–81.

102. Tenenbaum A, Motro M Fisman EZ. Dual and panperoxisome proliferators-activated receptors (PPAR) co-agonism: the benzafibrate lessons. Cardiovasc Diabetol 2005;4:14–9.

103. Keane WF, Eknoyan G. Proteinuria, Albuminuria, Risk Assessment, Detection, Elimination (PARADE): a position paper of the National Kidney Foundation. Am J Kidney Dis 1999;33:1004–10.

104. Yudkin JS. Hyperinsulinemia, insulin resistance, microalbuminuria and the risk of coronary heart disease. Ann Med 1996;28:433–8.
105. Mykkanen L, Zaccaro DJ, Wagenknecht LE, et al. Microalbuminuria is associated with insulin resistance in nondiabetic subjects: the Insulin Resistance Atherosclerosis Study. Diabetes 1998;47:793–800.
106. deZeeuw D, Remuzzi G, Parving HH, et al. Albuminuria, a therapeutic target for cardiovascular protection in type 2 diabetic patients with nephropathy. Circulation 2004;110:921–7.
107. Grassi G, Seravalle G, Dell'Oro R, et al. Comparative effects of candesartan and hydrochlorothiazide on blood pressure, insulin sensitivity and sympathetic drive in obese hypertensive individuals: results of the CROSS study. J Hypertens 2003;21:1761–9.
108. Lefebre AM, Laville M, Vega N, et al. Depot-specific differences in adipose tissue gene expression in lean and obese subjects. Diabetes 1998;47:98–103.
109. Rosito GA, D'Agostino RB, Massaro J, et al. Association between obesity and a prothrombotic state: the Framingham offspring study. Thromb Haemost 2004;91:683–9.
110. Kohler HP, Grant PJ. Plasminogen-activating inhibitor type 1 and CAD. N Engl J Med 2000;342:1792–801.
111. Ridker PM, Cushman M, Stamfer MJ, et al. Inflammation, aspirin and the risk of cardiovascular disease in apparently healthy men. N Eng J Med 1997;336:973–9.
112. Pearson TA, Mensah GA, Alexander RW, et al. American heart association guide for improving cardiovascular health at the community level: a statement for public health practitioners, healthcare providers and health policy makers from the American heart association expert panel on population and prevention science. Circulation 2003;107:645–51.
113. Ridker PM, for the JUPITTER Study group. Rosuvastatin in the primary prevention of cardiovascular disease among patients with low levels of low-density lipoprotein cholesterol and elevated high-sensitivity C-reactive protein: rationale and design of the JUPITER trial. Circulation 2003;108:2292–7.
114. McConnell JP, Hoefner DM. Lipoprotein-associated phospholipase A2. Clin Lab Med 2006;26(3):679–97.
115. Grunstein K, Wilcox I, Yang T-S, et al. Snoring and sleep apnea in men: association with central obesity and hypertension. Int J Obes 1993;17:533–40.
116. Malhotra A, White DP. Obstructive sleep apnea. Lancet 2002;360(9328):237–45.
117. Young T, Palta M, Dempsey J, et al. The occurrence of sleep-disordered breathing among middle-aged adults. N Eng J Med 1993;328(17):1230–5.
118. Blankfield RP, Hudgel DW, Tapolyai AA, et al. Bilateral leg edema, obesity pulmonary hypertension and obstructive sleep apnea. Arch Intern Med 2000;160:2357–62.
119. Young T, Peppard P, Palta M, et al. Population-based study of sleep-disordered breathing as a risk factor for hypertension. Arch Intern Med 1997;157:1746–52.
120. Gami AS, Pressman G, Caples SM, et al. Association of atrial fibrillation and obstructive sleep apnea. Circulation 2004;110:364–7.
121. Shahar E, Whitney CW, Redline S, et al. Sleep-disordered breathing and cardiovascular disease: cross-sectional results of the Sleep Heart Health study. Am J Respir Crit Care Med 2001;163:19–25.
122. Peker Y, Kraiczi H, Hedner J, et al. An independent association between obstructive sleep apnea and coronary artery disease. Eur Respir J 1999;14(1):179–84.
123. Dyken ME, Somers VK, Yamanda T, et al. Investigating the relationship between stroke and obstructive sleep apnea. Stroke 1996;27:401–7.

The Dietary Treatment of Obesity

Gal Dubnov-Raz, MD, MSc[a],*, Elliot M. Berry, MD, FRCP[b]

KEYWORDS

• Diet • Weight • Obesity • Glycemic index • Fat • Calcium

Talking of a man who was grown very fat, so as to be incommoded by corpulency, Dr. Johnson said, "He eats too much, Sir."
BOSWELL: "I don't know, Sir, you will see one man fat who eats moderately, and another lean who eats a great deal."
JOHNSON: "Nay, Sir, whatever may be the quantity that a man eats, it is plain that if he is too fat, he has eaten more than he should have done."
[Boswell's Life of Samuel Johnson. Part IX, 1782–1783]

The obesity epidemic is a "huge" reality. For centuries, mankind has known that eating too much and/or exercising too little is hazardous to one's health. This fact was even known in times when infectious diseases and malnutrition took their toll and reduced human lifespan to nearly a half what it is today. For example, 800 years ago, Maimonides asserted that one should never eat unless hungry, the stomach should only be filled to three-quarters full, and when one exercises and works, he will not become sick and his strength will increase. As early as the 6th century, the Roman Catholic Church included gluttony and sloth among the seven deadly sins.

During the past decades, a dramatic increase in the rate of obesity occurred throughout the Western world.[1–5] This rapid increase cannot be explained through changes in metabolism or genetics, *pace* the "thrifty" genotype,[6] and must necessarily be caused by an obesogenic or toxic environment promoting a positive energy balance.

The burden of obesity-associated diseases paralleled this increase,[7] and occurred despite numerous studies, national statements, and position stands of professional organizations stating that obesity must be addressed seriously, prevented, and treated.[8] More than ever, multilevel, multidisciplinary strategies seem to be needed, with combined forces of the major stakeholders, including governments, communities, health care services, medical societies, industry, and media, and of course obese individuals.[9,10]

A version of this article appeared in the 37:4 issue of the *Endocrinology and Metabolism Clinics of North America*.
^a Pediatric Obesity, Exercise and Sport Medicine, Department of Pediatrics, Mount Scopus, Hadassah-Hebrew University Medical Center, Jerusalem, Israel 91120
^b Department of Human Nutrition and Metabolism, The Braun School of Public Health and Community Medicine, Hadassah-Hebrew University Medical Center, Jerusalem, Israel 91120
* Corresponding author.
E-mail address: gal-d@bezeqint.net

Treatment of obesity obviously must lead to a negative energy balance, preferably through both reducing food intake and increasing energy expenditure. Even though this strategy sounds simple in theory (according to the first law of thermodynamics), decades of advocating weight loss have failed to stop the obesity epidemic. This article discusses contemporary issues in the dietary treatment of obesity and future research directions.

Because of the numerous medical complications of obesity (eg, diabetes, hypertension, hypercholesterolemia, cardiovascular disease, cancer) and the profound effect that many nutrients have on all of them, this discussion must be narrowed to weight loss per se in adults.

INCREASING PHYSICAL ACTIVITY OR DECREASING FOOD INTAKE?

A negative energy balance can be attained through either eating less, exercising more, or both. A deficiency of 500 kcal/d is recommended to achieve a weight loss rate of approximately 1 lb ($\sim$ 0.5 kg) per week.[8,11,12] However, the major question arises whether it matters if this energy deficit comes from decreasing food intake or increasing physical activity. Several studies have addressed this question. The same energy deficit obtained through either increased exercise or a dietary restriction seems to yield similar changes in body weight, but the composition of lost tissue differs. On average, the composition of weight loss is approximately 70% fat and 30% lean body mass, whereas loss of the latter causes a decrease in the resting metabolic rate. Exercise aids in minimizing the loss of lean body mass, thereby reducing the decrease in metabolic rate (for increased efficiency) that accompanies any loss in body weight.[13,14]

Several investigators examined the differences between two methods of energy deficit: diet restriction or increased exercise. In the first study, 52 obese men were randomly assigned to one of four study groups (diet-induced weight loss, exercise-induced weight loss, exercise without weight loss, and control).[15] After 3 months, weight decreased by 8% in the diet-induced and exercise-induced weight loss groups, and changes in abdominal obesity, visceral fat, and insulin resistance were also comparable (because of a higher unplanned energy deficit in the exercise group, these values were corrected for energy deficit). A second, similar study was conducted among 54 premenopausal women using a similar protocol.[16] This study showed that the exercise-induced weight loss group had a greater reduction in total and abdominal fat compared with the diet-induced group.

A recent, randomized controlled trial tested the effect of 6 months of a 25% energy deficit through diet alone or diet plus exercise (12.5% reduction of intake, 12.5% increase in energy expenditure) on body composition and fat distribution in 35 overweight individuals.[17] The calculated energy deficit across the intervention was not different between the groups, as opposed to many of the previous studies. Study participants lost approximately 10% of body weight, 24% of fat mass, and 27% of abdominal visceral fat in both groups.

Finally, a 1-year randomized trial comparing the effects of increased energy expenditure of approximately 300 kcal/d (equivalent to walking 60 minutes) with an isocaloric deficit of energy intake found a similar fat mass loss of 25% and comparable reductions in heart disease risk factors, namely plasma low-density lipoprotein (LDL) C concentration, total cholesterol/high-density lipoprotein (HDL) C ratio, C-reactive protein (CRP) concentrations, and insulin resistance.[18] The concept that exercise in obese patients is beneficial even without weight loss has also been shown in type 2 diabetics.[19]

Collectively, these randomized, well-controlled studies suggest that, when comparing the effects of an energy deficit through increased physical activity or decreased dietary intake on body fat, "a calorie is a calorie," whether burned by increased physical activity or never consumed at all.

However, physical activity exerts additional health benefits other than pure physical weight loss. Physical activity seems to be able to improve the metabolic complications of obesity even without weight loss,[15,16] while also preventing numerous chronic diseases, such as heart disease,[20] cancer,[21] obesity,[22] and diabetes,[23] and improving mood through many mechanisms.[24] Many metabolic effects are independent of body composition,[25,26] and therefore it may be said that "fat and fit may be better than being lean and lazy."

Furthermore, adding physical activity to weight loss programs is crucial to maintain the reduced weight, and therefore the authors firmly believe it must be an integral part of any weight-loss diet (see article elsewhere in this issue). However, to obtain the desired energy deficit for weight loss under normal circumstances, caloric intake must be reduced; it is much easier to reduce caloric intake by 500 kcal/d, for example, than to increase expenditure of that magnitude. Examples of activities that use approximately 500 kcal of energy, for a person weighing approximately 80 kg, are an hour of jogging at 5 km/h, or 35 minutes of jump-rope. Given that dietary intervention is a crucial part of weight loss, the question now arises whether some diets are more effective in weight loss than others.

ARE ALL DIETS CREATED EQUAL?

For many years, researchers and clinicians debated what the optimal diet for weight loss is, and if such a diet actually exists. The fundamental question is again, "is a calorie a calorie?"; that is, do different compositions of isocaloric diets have different effects on weight loss. The major controversy seems to be between low-fat (LF) and low-carbohydrate (LC) diets. Two additional contemporary issues concern the benefits of using a diet with a low glycemic index or a diet rich in dairy products and calcium.

Low-Fat Versus Low-Carbohydrate Diets

LF diets are those that restrict fat intake to less than 25% to 35% of daily energy intake.[12,27,28] LC diets are those that advocate minimizing carbohydrate intake (~20–100 g/d, depending on the type of diet and its stage), with the additional calories needed originating from protein and fat. An in-depth review of the constituents of common diets is available.[29]

The first man to undergo an LC diet and report its success, nearly 150 years ago, seemed to be William Banting,[30] a relative of Sir Frederick Banting, the codiscoverer of insulin. In 1972, Robert Atkins published his book "Dr. Atkins' Diet Revolution,"[31] which widely publicized the concept of LC diets for weight loss, but was also immediately criticized.[32] Studies showing either superiority or inferiority over LF diets sparked decade-long disputes between promoters of both nutrition regimens.[33]

Numerous studies comparing the two approaches for weight loss have been conducted, accompanied by many editorial comments, reviews, and meta-analyses.[34–48] This article focuses on the larger longer-term, randomized trials. Recent systematic reviews and meta-analyses[42–44] summarized the conclusions from the many papers comparing the two diet types. Apparently in the long-term (at least 1 year), LC diets do not induce more weight loss than LF diets, and no difference occurs in blood pressure, lipid profile, or glucose/insulin changes; attrition rates are also similar. Only the meta-analysis of the more recent randomized controlled trials[44] concluded that total cholesterol and LDL levels decreased more after LF diets, but HDL and triglyceride values changed more after LC diets.

Four studies comparing various diet regimens for weight loss are of particular interest. Dansinger and colleagues[45] randomized 160 overweight participants to one of four diets for 1 year: Atkins (carbohydrate restriction), Zone (macronutrient balance), Weight Watchers (calorie restriction), or Ornish (fat restriction). All diets resulted in modest weight loss at 1 year, with no statistically significant differences among diets, and no meaningful differences in heart disease risk factors and insulin resistance. No adverse effects or deterioration of heart disease risk factors were noted. Of the subjects, 60% completed the study year, but compliance decreased significantly and similarly between the diet groups.

In a similar study, Truby and colleagues[46] randomized 293 overweight participants to one of five diet groups for a 6-month trial: Atkins, Slim-Fast plan, Weight Watchers, a precooked meal program (Rosemary Conley's), and a control group. All diets resulted in significant but similar loss of body fat and weight at the end, despite lack of control of total energy intake by the researchers. Fasting glucose levels and cholesterol improved only in the Weight Watchers group. Adherence to the diet for another 6 months (total of 1 year) resulted in a similar approximately 10% weight loss in all diets.

Gardner and colleagues[47] randomized 311 overweight women to follow the Atkins, Zone, LEARN (LF diet, based on national guidelines), or Ornish diets. At 12 months, weight loss was greater in the Atkins diet group compared with the other diet groups (–4.7 kg, –1.6 kg, –2.6 kg, and –2.2 kg, respectively), but significantly different only from the Zone diet. The lipid profile and blood pressure changes were better in the Atkins group. Attrition rate was relatively low at 20%.

Finally, a recent workplace-based study conducted in Israel among 322 overweight and obese employees compared the effect of an LC, an LF, or a Mediterranean-style diet on weight loss and cardiovascular risk factors.[48] After 2 years, among the 272 participants who adhered with the program (85%), the LC and Mediterranean diets were associated with greater weight loss than the LF (−0.5 body mass index [BMI] units in LC and Mediterranean diets versus LF). In addition, beneficial changes were seen in some metabolic markers: lipid profile improved best in the LC group; the inflammatory marker CRP decreased by more than 20% only in the LC and Mediterranean diet groups; and among the subgroup of diabetics, only the Mediterranean diet decreased plasma glucose levels. This study suggests that LC and Mediterranean diets can be beneficial over an LF diet in some circumstances, and emphasizes the ability of the workplace in promoting lifestyle changes.

These four studies stand out because they used several diet compositions, as opposed to those comparing LC and LF alone. The discrepancies in results between the study by Gardner and colleagues[47] and that by Shai and colleagues,[48] which found the Atkins diet to be superior to three other nutritional regimens, can be explained by either the population studied or the higher support provided by the study staff or spouse, as reflected in the high adherence rate. Nevertheless, these studies continue to maintain the ongoing debate over whether LC diets are superior to the nationally recommended LF diets.

Several mechanisms have been suggested for the possible added value of LC diets in promoting weight loss, including (1) higher amounts of protein, which promotes satiety more than carbohydrates, (2) ongoing gluconeogenesis to compensate for the body's carbohydrate needs, which is an energy-consuming process, (3) increased diuresis, (4) loss of glycogen stores and their associated water, (5) high levels of circulating ketones, which suppress appetite, (6) limited food choices, or (7) underreporting of food intake by the LF group.[49–53]

A final issue is safety. A systematic review of more than 100 studies identified no adverse effects or unwarranted metabolic changes, especially renal function.[43] Recently, a life-threatening complication of an Atkins diet, in the form of severe ketoacidosis, was described.[54] Because most studies were conducted among healthy volunteers, and only a few among diabetics, insufficient data exists on LC diets in populations with underlying diseases.

In summary, despite several beneficial properties of LC over LF diets, even the high-quality studies continue to generate conflicting results. Future studies will surely help identify the best proportions between macronutrients for weight loss and metabolic improvements. A recent summary that attempted to define the optimum dietary composition for a weight-loss diet suggested moderate carbohydrate (35%–50%) and fat intake (25%–35%), with protein contributing the remainder at 25% to 30% (which is relatively high).[52] One wonders whether this is a variation of the adage "Moderation in all things, including moderation." However, the overriding factor determining the success of any diet is long-term compliance, which is an individual choice that cannot be manipulated easily by investigators.

Low Glycemic Index Diets

The glycemic index is a measure of glucose availability in food,[55] and is calculated as the percentage of the area under the plasma glucose response curve measured during the 2 hours after ingestion of the food in question, relative to the same amount of carbohydrate taken as glucose/white bread. Foods with a high glycemic index (HGI) (>70), such as white bread, potatoes, or corn flakes, whose glucose is readily digested and absorbed, cause a rapid increase in plasma glucose levels. Foods with a low glycemic index (LGI) (<50), such as pasta, fruits, and beans, cause a much slower increment in plasma glucose levels.

Experts have postulated that fat reduction has failed to combat the current obesity epidemic because of the carbohydrate content: substitution of fat with HGI foods merely causes increased hunger, anabolism of adipose tissue, and weight gain.[56] The rapid absorption of sugar from an HGI causes a large surge in insulin secretion, which then exerts its anabolic effects. In addition, the high insulin levels decrease blood glucose levels, causing more hunger in the few hours after an HGI meal.

In an insulin-resistant person, this high demand from the β cell might potentially result in β-cell secretion defects and apoptosis, leading to type 2 diabetes. In an LGI diet, the ambient insulin secretion is lower, without large swings, and these unwanted effects are moderated. Therefore, it is better to eat little and often than to fast and feast – nibbling is preferable to gorging, despite a similar total daily energy intake.

A prospective cohort study of 6-year follow-up was conducted among 185 men and 191 women, examining the role of glycemic index in future weight and fat-mass changes.[57] Using questionnaires for food frequency and various confounders, the authors concluded that, in women only, an HGI diet was associated with increases in BMI and fat mass. Another observational study among 572 healthy adults also showed that changes in BMI were positively associated with dietary intake of carbohydrates and the glycemic index.[58]

However, as in most fields of medicine, this concept is controversial. Advocates of using an LGI diet for weight loss[59] and their opponents[60] both raise convincing explanations supporting their views. In light of the existing, although not unanimous, observational evidence that HGI diets can increase weight gain, several interventional studies have examined whether lowering the glycemic index can affect weight loss. This article focuses on data from the longer-term randomized trials.

A recent review of the highest-quality randomized studies examining the effect of LGI diets on weight loss concluded that they produce larger decreases in BMI, fat mass, and total and LDL cholesterol.[61] Because studies were generally short-term, further research with longer-term follow-up was recommended.

Results of a large 18-month study comparing weight loss effects of LGI versus HGI diets was published concurrently.[62] This study, conducted in Brazil where beans are a common food (very low GI), randomized 203 healthy women who had a BMI ranging from 23 to 30 kg/m^2 to an LGI or HGI diet, differing by 40 glycemic index points. Intake was high in carbohydrates (60% of energy) and low in fat (26%–28% of energy), and individuals were given a small energy restriction (−100–300 kcal/d). Outcome measures were weight change during 18 months, hunger, and fasting serum insulin and lipids. Although the LGI group showed a slightly greater weight loss in the first 2 months of follow-up, both groups began to regain weight after 12 months, and at 18 months, the small weight change maintained (−260 and −400 g for LGI and HGI) was not significantly different between groups. A greater reduction was observed in the LGI diet group for triacylglycerol and very low-density lipoprotein (VLDL) cholesterol, with no differences in measures of hunger. Hence, this study did not support the benefit of an LGI diet for weight loss.

In another recent study, researchers randomized 34 healthy overweight adults to diets with 30% caloric deficiency and either an HGI or an LGI.[63] All food was provided for 6 months, and subjects self-administered the diet plans for another 6 months. The LGI diet had 40% daily energy as carbohydrates (compared with 60% in the HGI) and a glycemic index lower by 33 units. Primary and secondary outcomes included energy intake, body weight and fatness, hunger, satiety, and resting metabolic rate, none of which differed between the groups at end of study. An additional study, conducted among 39 obese subjects randomized to hypocaloric diets (−760 kcal/d) with LGI, HGI, or high fat, concluded that the glycemic index had no effect on weight loss.[64]

In summary, high-quality randomized trials continue to raise conflicting results regarding the role of the glycemic index in weight loss and maintenance. The authors suggest that more studies be conducted in free-living conditions, where the presumed higher satiety of an LGI diet can be translated into a lower reduction of energy intake; in a controlled trial, holding the energy intake constant in both LGI and HGI groups might blunt one of the possible benefits of an LGI diet. In addition, they suggest that the effect of LGI and HGI meals on hunger and satiety be examined in the clinic on an individual basis, to see if lowering the glycemic index may assist in the reduced calorie diet.

Calcium and Dairy Products

In 1984, McCarron[65] reported an inverse relationship between dietary calcium intake and body weight. Since then, several observational studies and interventions have assessed the reproducibility, magnitude, and mechanisms of this phenomenon. Studies conducted in this field show conflicting results regarding diets with a higher calcium or dairy intake, showing either reduced weight or increased weight loss,[66–75] no effect,[75–80] or even increased weight or weight gain.[80–82]

A systematic review of 13 randomized trials involving supplementation of either calcium or dairy products again found controversial results, and summarized that these product had no mean effect on weight loss.[83] Several differences in methodology can explain these discrepancies. One pitfall in eating dairy products for increased weight loss might be the increased caloric intake, should the eager weight-loser try to maximize this mechanism. The added energy in consuming three dairy products per day averaged approximately 200 kcal/d in one study,[84] a meaningful increase in the long-term. Data from the Health Professionals Follow-Up Study showed that men who had the largest increase in high-fat dairy products gained significantly more weight than those who decreased their intake. Therefore, total energy consumption must be considered to prevent its counteracting of possible beneficial effects of dairy products on weight.[80] Similar findings were observed in children and older adults.[79,81]

Several mechanisms for the effect of calcium and dairy foods on cell metabolism and adiposity have been identified.[85,86] The major mechanism seems to be a suppression of intracellular calcium, which then enhances lipolysis, with an interesting greater effect of dairy products than calcium supplements. Possible explanations are the presence of additional bioactive compounds, such as angiotensin converting enzyme inhibitors or branched chain amino acids, which act synergistically with calcium to attenuate adiposity.

Increased fecal fat loss is another mechanism through which calcium may aid in weight loss. However, in this case, further increasing calcium intake should enhance weight loss, but a large observational study did not find any benefit in increasing the daily intake more than 800 mg/d,[87] which is even below the minimal recommended intake for adults. In addition, different dairy products were recently found to affect body weight differently, thereby suggesting that pooling all "dairy products" in questionnaires or diet recommendations may be erroneous.[88] In this large study, researchers examined the association between changes in dairy product consumption and weight change over 9 years among 19,352 women, while addressing differential intakes of whole milk (3% fat), medium-fat milk (1.5% fat), low-fat milk ($\leq$0.5% fat), whole sour milk (3% fat), low-fat sour milk (0.5% fat), cheese, and butter (80% fat). Findings were that increasing intakes of dairy products and calcium did not universally affect weight gain, despite whether these increases involved low-fat milk or cheese and butter. Subjects who complied with their consumption of more than one dairy portion of milk with 3% fat had a statistically significant relative risk of 0.85 for weight gain, whereas those who maintained high cheese intake had a risk of 0.70. These results were not affected by correction for calcium or energy intake. Therefore, not all milk products are created equal, and future studies are needed to identify the more beneficial dairy products in assisting weight loss.

WEIGHT MAINTENANCE AND THE REDUCED OBESE

Why is treating obesity so difficult, and why do so many different treatments exist?

A clue may be found when studying a "rare" clinical subject: a reduced obese person who has succeeded in losing weight and maintaining the new body weight for more than a year. The National Weight Control Registry documented the metabolic and behavioral cost of maintaining a reduced obese state for more than 5 years. The average weight loss was 30 kg and minimum maintenance 13.6 kg. The results are instructive.[89] Both men and women consumed a low-fat diet (24%) and exercised to use 470 and 360 kcal/d, respectively. The net energy balance was 918 kcal/d for women and 1225 kcal/d for men. These reduced obese subjects ate an average of five meals a day and conducted a very regimented existence.

Anyone with clinical experience in weight management knows that adopting such a lifestyle is extremely hard. which perhaps explains why combating obesity is such a difficult task. Other studies usually show a much milder amount of weight loss. A recent meta-analysis summarizing 80 clinical trials of long-term weight loss through combinations of diet, exercise, or medications showed that in the long-term (3–4 years), weight loss averaged 3 kg with diet alone, or nearly 4 kg with diet and exercise.[90]

The importance of the reduced obese is that if one only uses an experimental paradigm comparing normal-weight and obese subjects, then whether any abnormal finding such as (for example) hyperglycemia or hyperinsulinemia is either primary (causative) or secondary to the obese state cannot be known; this may only be determined after the person loses weight. If after weight reduction the abnormalities are reversed (such as in the examples above), then they must be secondary; however, parameters that are normal in the obese state but abnormal after weight reduction may be relevant to the induction of obesity or its perpetuation.

One such finding is that reduced obese subjects have diminished energy requirements for maintaining body weight compared with similar-weight never-obese subjects.[13] This discovery suggests that weight reduction leads to an increase in metabolic efficiency, perhaps mediated through altered catecholamine and thyroid sensitivity.[14] In the former study,[13] 26 obese subjects, with an average weight of 152.5 kg, were hospitalized in a metabolic ward and fed a formula so that their weight did not change beyond $\pm$ 0.5 kg over a week. Caloric requirements were then calculated to determine how many calories per meter squared per day they required.

The same experiment was repeated in a similar number of controls to determine how many calories were needed to keep in balance a person who was never obese. The obese subjects had their weight brought down to an average of 100 kg and the same calculation was performed. On average, the obese subjects required 1432 kcal/m^2/d. The never-obese subjects weighing 62 kg required 1341 kcal/m^2/d.

No significant difference was seen between nonobese and obese people, although in absolute terms the obese ate more because of their larger surface areas. However, the reduced obese at 100 kg, still obese, had a dramatic reduction in the amount of energy for maintaining caloric requirements at 1050 kcal/m^2/d. This decreased energy expenditure continued for 1 to 2 years after weight loss. Hence, in metabolic terms, the reduced obese were much more efficient in using less energy for weight maintenance.

The body systems responding to energy metabolism are the adrenosympathetic system and the thyroid. This system was then investigated through testing the hemodynamic and metabolic responses to exogenous and endogenous epinephrine after insulin-induced hypoglycemia.[14] Three groups were examined: obese, reduced obese, and never-obese. In all three groups, hemodynamic and glucose responses were similar. However, when glycerol release was recorded, the obese and never-obese were found to react similarly, but the reduced obese responded excessively despite secreting fewer catecholamines. The obese acted like the normal subjects, whereas the reduced obese (who are now believed to be "normal"), were in fact abnormal.

After endogenous epinephrine infusion, the same response profiles were recorded. Again, the obese responded like the controls, and the reduced obese had a very attenuated response but seemed to be very sensitive to the effects of catecholamines, as shown from exaggerated glycerol release. The enhanced sensitivity to the metabolic effects of epinephrine suggests that in the reduced obese, adrenal medullary activity may be reduced, with secondary up-regulation of peripheral β receptors (or down-regulation of α). The reduced obese also seem to have low T$_3$ concentrations, perhaps in an attempt to conserve energy. This physiologic understanding may help in the development of new treatment modalities for weight maintenance.

FACILITATING WEIGHT LOSS AND DIETING

The roles of society, the media (targeting both adults and children), the food industry (pricing, quality, labeling, and portion sizes), and safe community infrastructure for exercise in providing an enabling environment for weight loss are essential parts of national programs in combating obesity, but are beyond the scope of this article. These areas are extensively discussed elsewhere.[9,10] All programs must include increased motivation to exercise in the home, community, and workplace. Furthermore, obesity is greater in lower socioeconomic sectors of the population, and therefore programs must be suitably tailored to the needs and economic constraints of these groups.

SUMMARY

In no sector of therapeutics is the theory so simple as in weight control. The major gap lies in translating this theory into practice. In the final analysis, the answer lies in personal choice, because many diets seem to work, but not universally in all studies. A reduced calorie diet is obviously essential, although the composition remains to be individually tailored. For this, health care professionals must become "personal trainers" and realize the importance of lifestyle prescriptions with regard to diet and exercise in all consultations, fitting them to the needs of patient. It may be argued that medical practitioners do not have the necessary time or behavioral skills for these long-term interventions, which might be better handled by a team of other health professionals.

Prevention is, of course, better than treatment, and therefore a major effort must be made to target children, from breast feeding to education throughout schooling. No more surveys are needed; "we know the enemy and it is us."

In the words of the *Lancet* editorial concerning obesity:[91] "Our public health leaders must replace prevarication with imagination."

REFERENCES

1. Li C, Ford ES, McGuire LC, et al. Increasing trends in waist circumference and abdominal obesity among US adults. Obesity 2007;15:216–24.
2. Wardle J, Boniface D. Changes in the distributions of body mass index and waist circumference in English adults, 1993/1994 to 2002/2003. Int J Obes (Lond) 2007;32:527–32.
3. Berg C, Rosengren A, Aires N, et al. Trends in overweight and obesity from 1985 to 2002 in Goteborg, West Sweden. Int J Obes (Lond) 2005;29:916–24.
4. Bendixen H, Holst C, Sorensen TI, et al. A. Major increase in prevalence of overweight and obesity between 1987 and 2001 among Danish adults. Obes Res 2004;12:1464–72.
5. Koziel S, Szklarska A, Bielicki T, et al. Changes in the BMI of Polish conscripts between 1965 and 2001: secular and socio-occupational variation. Int J Obes (Lond) 2006;30:1382–8.
6. Neel JV. Diabetes mellitus: a "thrifty" genotype rendered detrimental by "progress"? Am J Hum Genet 1962;14:353–62.
7. Ford ES, Giles WH, Mokdad AH. Increasing prevalence of the metabolic syndrome among US adults. Diabetes Care 2004;27:2444–9.
8. National Institutes of Health. Clinical guidelines on the identification, evaluation, and treatment of overweight and obesity in adults - The evidence report. Obes Res 1998;6:S51–210.

9. Global strategy on diet, physical activity and health. A framework to monitor and evaluate implementation. Geneva (Switzerland): World Health Organization; 2006.

10. Branca F, Nikogosian H, Lobstein T, editors. The challenge of obesity in the WHO European region and the strategies for response. Copenhagen (Denmark): World Health Organization; 2007.

11. Avenell A, Sattar N, Lean M. ABC of obesity. Management: Part I - Behaviour change, diet, and activity. BMJ 2006;333:740–3.

12. Klein S, Sheard NF, Pi-Sunyer X, et al. Weight management through lifestyle modification for the prevention and management of type 2 diabetes: rationale and strategies. A statement of the American Diabetes Association, the North American Association for the Study of Obesity, and the American Society for Clinical Nutrition. Am J Clin Nutr 2004;80:257–63.

13. Leibel RL, Hirsch J. Diminished energy requirements in reduced-obese patients. Metabolism 1984;33:164–70.

14. Leibel RL, Berry EM, Hirsch J. Metabolic and hemodynamic responses to endogenous and exogenous catecholamines in formerly obese subjects. Am J Physiol 1991;260:R785–91.

15. Ross R, Dagnone D, Jones PJ, et al. Reduction in obesity and related comorbid conditions after diet-induced weight loss or exercise-induced weight loss in men. A randomized, controlled trial. Ann Intern Med 2000;133:92–103.

16. Ross R, Janssen I, Dawson J, et al. Exercise-induced reduction in obesity and insulin resistance in women: a randomized controlled trial. Obes Res 2004;12: 789–98.

17. Redman LM, Heilbronn LK, Martin CK, et al. Effect of calorie restriction with or without exercise on body composition and fat distribution. J Clin Endocrinol Metab 2007;92:865–72.

18. Fontana L, Villareal DT, Weiss EP, et al. Calorie restriction or exercise: effects on coronary heart disease risk factors. A randomized, controlled trial. Am J Physiol Endocrinol Metab 2007;293(1):E197–202.

19. Lee S, Kuk JL, Davidson LE, et al. Exercise without weight loss is an effective strategy for obesity reduction in obese individuals with and without type 2 diabetes. J Appl Physiol 2005;99(3):1220–5.

20. Haskell WL, Lee IM, Pate RR, et al. Physical activity and public health: updated recommendation for adults from the American College of Sports Medicine and the American Heart Association. Circulation 2007;116:1081–93.

21. Kushi LH, Byers T, Doyle C, et al. American Cancer Society Guidelines on Nutrition and Physical Activity for cancer prevention: reducing the risk of cancer with healthy food choices and physical activity. CA Cancer J Clin 2006;56:254–81.

22. Saris WH, Blair SN, van Baak MA, et al. How much physical activity is enough to prevent unhealthy weight gain? Outcome of the IASO 1st stock conference and consensus statement. Obes Rev 2003;4:101–14.

23. Sigal RJ, Kenny GP, Wasserman DH, et al. Physical activity/exercise and type 2 diabetes: a consensus statement from the American Diabetes Association. Diabetes Care 2006;29:1433–8.

24. Dubnov G, Berry EM. Physical activity and mood: the endocrine connection. In: Warren MP, Constantini N, editors. Sports endocrinology. Totowa (NJ): Humana Press; 2000. p. 421–32.

25. Lee CD, Blair SN, Jackson AS. Cardiorespiratory fitness, body composition, and all-cause and cardiovascular disease mortality in men. Am J Clin Nutr 1999;69: 373–80.

26. Wei M, Kampert JB, Barlow CE, et al. Relationship between low cardiorespiratory fitness and mortality in normal-weight, overweight, and obese men. JAMA 1999; 282:1547–53.
27. Third Report of the National Cholesterol Education Program (NCEP) Expert Panel on Detection, Evaluation, and Treatment of High Blood Cholesterol in Adults (Adult Treatment Panel III) final report. Circulation 2002;106:3143–421.
28. American Heart Association Nutrition Committee. Diet and lifestyle recommendations revision 2006: a scientific statement from the American Heart Association Nutrition Committee. Circulation 2006;114:82–96.
29. Freedman MR, King J, Kennedy E. Popular diets: a scientific review. Obes Res 2001;9(Suppl 1):1S–40S.
30. Banting W. Letter on corpulence, addressed to the public. 3rd edition. London: Harrison; 1869.
31. Atkins RC. Dr Atkins Diet Revolution. New York: David McKay Co. NY; 1972.
32. A critique of low-carbohydrate ketogenic weight reduction regimens. A review of Dr. Atkins' diet revolution. JAMA 1973;224:1415–9.
33. Well-Known Diet Gurus Square off at ACC 2001. American College of Cardiology 50th Annual Scientific Session. Scientific Session News 2001;19:5.
34. Brehm BJ, Seeley RJ, Daniels SR, et al. A randomized trial comparing a very low carbohydrate diet and a calorie-restricted low fat diet on body weight and cardiovascular risk factors in healthy women. J Clin Endocrinol Metab 2003;88(4):1617–23.
35. McAuley KA, Hopkins CM, Smith KJ, et al. Comparison of high-fat and high-protein diets with a high-carbohydrate diet in insulin-resistant obese women. Diabetologia 2005;48(1):8–16.
36. Stern L, Iqbal N, Seshadri P, et al. The effects of low-carbohydrate versus conventional weight loss diets in severely obese adults: one-year follow-up of a randomized trial. Ann Intern Med 2004;140(10):778–85.
37. Yancy WS Jr, Olsen MK, Guyton JR, et al. A low-carbohydrate, ketogenic diet versus a low-fat diet to treat obesity and hyperlipidemia: a randomized, controlled trial. Ann Intern Med 2004;140(10):769–77.
38. Foster GD, Wyatt HR, Hill JO, et al. A randomized trial of a low-carbohydrate diet for obesity. N Engl J Med 2003;348(21):2082–90.
39. Samaha FF, Iqbal N, Seshadri P, et al. A low-carbohydrate as compared with a low-fat diet in severe obesity. N Engl J Med 2003;348(21):2074–81.
40. Segal-Isaacson CJ, Johnson S, Tomuta V, et al. A randomized trial comparing low-fat and low-carbohydrate diets matched for energy and protein. Obes Res 2004;12(Suppl 2):130S–40S.
41. Volek JS, Sharman MJ, Gomez AL, et al. Comparison of a very low-carbohydrate and low-fat diet on fasting lipids, LDL subclasses, insulin resistance, and postprandial lipemic responses in overweight women. J Am Coll Nutr 2004;23(2):177–84.
42. Pirozzo S, Summerbell C, Cameron C, et al. Advice on low-fat diets for obesity. Cochrane Database Syst Rev 2002;2:CD003640.
43. Bravata DM, Sanders L, Huang J, et al. Efficacy and safety of low-carbohydrate diets: a systematic review. JAMA 2003;289(14):1837–50.
44. Nordmann AJ, Nordmann A, Briel M, et al. Effects of low-carbohydrate vs low-fat diets on weight loss and cardiovascular risk factors: a meta-analysis of randomized controlled trials. Arch Intern Med 2006;166(3):285–93.
45. Dansinger ML, Gleason JA, Griffith JL, et al. Comparison of the Atkins, Ornish, Weight Watchers, and Zone diets for weight loss and heart disease risk reduction: a randomized trial. JAMA 2005;293(1):43–53.

46. Truby H, Baic S, deLooy A, et al. Randomised controlled trial of four commercial weight loss programmes in the UK: initial findings from the BBC "diet trials". BMJ 2006;332:1309–14.

47. Gardner CD, Kiazand A, Alhassan S, et al. Comparison of the Atkins, Zone, Ornish, and LEARN diets for change in weight and related risk factors among overweight premenopausal women: the A TO Z Weight Loss Study: a randomized trial. JAMA 2007;297(9):969–77.

48. Shai I, Schwarzfuchs D, Henkin Y, et al. Weight loss with a low-carbohydrate, Mediterranean, or low-fat diet. N Engl J Med 2008;359:229–41.

49. Astrup A, Meinert Larsen T, et al. Atkins and other low-carbohydrate diets: hoax or an effective tool for weight loss? Lancet 2004;364(9437):897–9.

50. Feinman RD, Fine EJ. "A calorie is a calorie" violates the second law of thermodynamics. Nutr J 2004;28(3):9.

51. Buchholz AC, Schoeller DA. Is a calorie a calorie? Am J Clin Nutr 2004;79: S899–906.

52. Schoeller DA, Buchholz AC. Energetics of obesity and weight control: does diet composition matter? J Am Diet Assoc 2005;105:S24–8.

53. Brehm BJ, Spang SE, Lattin BL, et al. The role of energy expenditure in the differential weight loss in obese women on low-fat and low-carbohydrate diets. J Clin Endocrinol Metab 2005;90(3):1475–82.

54. Chen TY, Smith W, Rosenstock JL, et al. A life-threatening complication of Atkins diet. Lancet 2006;367:958.

55. Jenkins DJ, Wolever TM, Taylor RH, et al. Glycemic index of foods: a physiological basis for carbohydrate exchange. Am J Clin Nutr 1981;34:362–6.

56. Brand-Miller JC, Holt SH, Pawlak DB, et al. Glycemic index and obesity. Am J Clin Nutr 2002;76(1):281S–5S.

57. Hare-Bruun H, Flint A, Heitmann BL. Glycemic index and glycemic load in relation to changes in body weight, body fat distribution, and body composition in adult Danes. Am J Clin Nutr 2006;84(4):871–9.

58. Ma Y, Olendzki B, Chiriboga D, et al. Association between dietary carbohydrates and body weight. Am J Epidemiol 2005;161(4):359–67.

59. Pawlak DB, Ebbeling CB, Ludwig DS. Should obese patients be counselled to follow a low-glycaemic index diet? Yes. Obes Rev 2002;3(4):235–43.

60. Raben A. Should obese patients be counselled to follow a low-glycaemic index diet? No. Obes Rev 2002;3(4):245–56.

61. Thomas DE, Elliott EJ, Baur L. Low glycaemic index or low glycaemic load diets for overweight and obesity. Cochrane Database Syst Rev 2007;18(3):CD005105.

62. Sichieri R, Moura AS, Genelhu V, et al. An 18-mo randomized trial of a low-glycemic-index diet and weight change in Brazilian women. Am J Clin Nutr 2007;86(3):707–13.

63. Das SK, Gilhooly CH, Golden JK, et al. Long-term effects of 2 energy-restricted diets differing in glycemic load on dietary adherence, body composition, and metabolism in CALERIE: a 1-y randomized controlled trial. Am J Clin Nutr 2007;85(4):1023–30.

64. Raatz SK, Torkelson CJ, Redmon JB, et al. Reduced glycemic index and glycemic load diets do not increase the effects of energy restriction on weight loss and insulin sensitivity in obese men and women. J Nutr 2005;135(10):2387–91.

65. McCarron DA. Dietary calcium as an antihypertensive agent. Nutr Rev 1984;42: 223–5.

66. Davies KM, Heaney RP, Recker RR, et al. Calcium intake and body weight. J Clin Endocrinol Metab 2000;85:4635–8.

67. Lin YC, Lyle RM, McCabe LD, et al. Dairy calcium is related to changes in body composition during a two year exercise intervention in young women. J Am Coll Nutr 2000;19:754–60.

68. Zemel MB, Shi H, Greer B, et al. Regulation of adiposity by dietary calcium. FASEB J 2000;14:1132–8.

69. Pereira MA, Jacobs DR, Van Horn L, et al. Dairy consumption, obesity, and the insulin resistance syndrome in young adults. The CARDIA study. JAMA 2002; 287:2081–9.

70. Mirmiran P, Ezmaillzadeh A, Azizi F. Dairy consumption and body mass index: an inverse relationship. Int J Obes Relat Metab Disord 2005;29:115–21.

71. Jacqmain M, Doucet E, Despres JP, et al. Calcium intake, body composition, and lipoprotein-lipid concentrations in adults. Am J Clin Nutr 2003;77:1448–52.

72. Shahar DR, Abel R, Elhayany A, et al. Does dairy calcium intake enhance weight loss among overweight diabetic patients? Diabetes Care 2007;30:485–9.

73. Lovejoy JC, Champagne CM, Smith SR, et al. Ethnic differences in dietary intakes, physical activity, and energy expenditure in middle-aged, premenopausal women: the Healthy Transitions Study. Am J Clin Nutr 2001;74:90–5.

74. Loos RJ, Rankinen T, Leon AS, et al. Calcium intake is associated with adiposity in black and white men and white women of the HERITAGE Family Study. J Nutr 2004;134:1772–8.

75. Lorenzen JK, Mølgaard C, Michaelsen KF, et al. Calcium supplementation for 1 y does not reduce body weight or fat mass in young girls. Am J Clin Nutr 2006;83: 18–23.

76. Phillips SM, Bandini LG, Cyr H, et al. Dairy food consumption and body weight and fatness studied longitudinally over the adolescent period. Int J Obes Relat Metab Disord 2003;27:1106–13.

77. Venti CA, Tataranni PA, Salbe AD. Lack of relationship between calcium intake and body size in an obesity-prone population. J Am Diet Assoc 2005;105: 1401–7.

78. Gunther CW, Legowski PA, Lyle RM, et al. Dairy products do not lead to alterations in body weight or fat mass in young women in a 1-y intervention. Am J Clin Nutr 2005;81:751–6.

79. Snijder MB, van der Heijden AA, van Dam RM, et al. Is higher dairy consumption associated with lower body weight and fewer metabolic disturbances? The Hoorn Study. Am J Clin Nutr 2007;85:989–95.

80. Kamycheva E, Joakimsen RM, Jorde R. Intakes of calcium and vitamin D predict body mass index in the population of Northern Norway. J Nutr 2003; 133:102–6.

81. Rajpathak SN, Rimm EB, Rosner B, et al. Calcium and dairy intakes in relation to long-term weight gain in US men. Am J Clin Nutr 2006;83:559–66.

82. Berkey CS, Rockett HR, Willett WC, et al. Milk, dairy fat, dietary calcium, and weight gain: a longitudinal study of adolescents. Arch Pediatr Adolesc Med 2005;159:543–50.

83. Trowman R, Dumville JC, Hahn S, et al. A systematic review of the effects of calcium supplementation on body weight. Br J Nutr 2006;95(6):1033–8.

84. Hollis JH, Mattes RD. Effect of increased dairy consumption on appetitive ratings and food intake. Obesity (Silver Spring) 2007;15(6):1520–6.

85. Zemel MB. The role of dairy foods in weight management. J Am Coll Nutr 2005; 24(Suppl 6):537S–46S.

86. Teegarden D. The influence of dairy product consumption on body composition. J Nutr 2005;135(12):2749–52.

87. Boon N, Koppes LL, Saris WH, et al. The relation between calcium intake and body composition in a Dutch population: The Amsterdam Growth and Health Longitudinal Study. Am J Epidemiol 2005;162(1):27–32.

88. Rosell M, Håkansson NN, Wolk A. Association between dairy food consumption and weight change over 9 y in 19,352 perimenopausal women. Am J Clin Nutr 2006;84:1481–8.

89. Klem ML, Wing RR, McGuire MT, et al. A descriptive study of individuals successful at long-term maintenance of substantial weight loss. Am J Clin Nutr 1997;66: 239–46.

90. Franz MJ, VanWormer JJ, Crain AL, et al. Weight-loss outcomes: a systematic review and meta-analysis of weight-loss clinical trials with a minimum 1-year follow-up. J Am Diet Assoc 2007;107:1755–67.

91. The catastrophic failures of public health. Lancet 2004;363:745.

Exercise and the Treatment of Diabetes and Obesity

Donal J. O'Gorman, PhD[a], Anna Krook, PhD[b],*

KEYWORDS

- Exercise • Skeletal muscle • Insulin resistance
- Substrate metabolism • Gene expression • AMPK

Lifestyle intervention programs encompassing exercise and healthy diets are an option for the treatment and management of obesity and Type 2 diabetes and have long been known to exert beneficial effects on whole-body metabolism, in particular leading to enhanced insulin-sensitivity. As evident from other articles in this issue, obesity is associated with increased risk of several illnesses and premature mortality. However, physical inactivity is itself associated with a number of similar risks, independently of body-mass index,[1] and is an independent risk factor for more than 25 chronic diseases, including Type 2 diabetes and cardiovascular disease.[2] Because obesity, with or without overt Type 2 diabetes, and physical inactivity very often coexist in the same individual when being discussed,[3] there has been debate recently regarding the relative effects of physical exercise itself and the effect of exercise-induced weight loss.

EXERCISE INTERVENTION PROGRAMS

In obese individuals, a low level of physical fitness is a better predictor of all-cause mortality than cholesterol levels, smoking status, or blood pressure and is similar to having had a previous cardiovascular event.[4] Exercise training has many cardiovascular and metabolic benefits, including decreased blood pressure,[5] plasma lipoprotein and triglyceride levels,[6] and improvements in glycemic control,[7] insulin sensitivity,[8] vascular structure, and endothelial function.[9] The goal of exercise and lifestyle modification programs is to combine education, dietary awareness, supervised physical activity, and social support to assist participants in making permanent lifestyle

A version of this article appeared in the 37:4 issue of the *Endocrinology and Metabolism Clinics of North America*.

This work was supported by Grants from the Swedish Research Council, Novo Nordisk Foundation, and the Hedlunds Foundation.

[a] School of Health and Human Performance, Dublin City University, Dublin, Ireland
[b] Integrative Physiology, Department of Physiology and Pharmacology, von Eulers väg 4a, Karolinska Institutet, 171 77 Stockholm, Sweden
* Corresponding author.
E-mail address: anna.krook@ki.se

Med Clin N Am 95 (2011) 953–969
doi:10.1016/j.mcna.2011.06.007
0025-7125/11/$ – see front matter © 2011 Elsevier Inc. All rights reserved.

changes.[10] Exercise training increases insulin sensitivity[8] and results in lower fasting insulin concentrations. Studies using the hyperinsulinemic-euglycemic clamp demonstrate that for the same circulating insulin concentration, glucose disposal rates are higher and endogenous glucose production rates are lower in exercise-trained subjects.[11,12] This benefit can be maintained in those who exercise throughout their lifespan, as master athletes have a similar glucose and insulin response to an oral glucose tolerance test as young athletes, and a significantly better insulin response than young sedentary subjects. Therefore, exercise training has a positive impact on insulin sensitivity, glucose disposal, and insulin secretion in normal glucose-tolerant subjects.

Exercise training also increases whole-body insulin-mediated glucose disposal in obese Type 2 diabetic patients.[13] The clinical profiles of subjects with impaired glucose tolerance,[14–17] or with relatively newly diagnosed diabetes[18] have been successfully improved using exercise intervention programs. In larger studies however, patient compliance is a major challenge, especially as the obesity itself—as well as other common associated ailments—make regular exercise programs both difficult and unsafe.[19] One hurdle for exercise programs is that successful implementation of exercise and lifestyle-modification programs in patients with long-standing disease or complications has been more challenging.[20,21] However, lifestyle modifications can be successful in subjects with more long-standing disease. The authors have shown that a 31-week residential lifestyle-modification program significantly improved several clinical parameters in overweight Type 2 diabetic subjects, with significant improvements in glycemic control, oxygen uptake, blood pressure, and cholesterol.[22] At the same time, average weight loss was modest (2 kg–3 kg reduction from an average starting weight of approximately 100 kg). Importantly, subjects also reported increased well being and reduced stress.[22] Participants were referred to the program by their physicians and were not volunteers who would perhaps be more likely to comply with dietary and exercise advice. Instead, most of these patients had not responded to previous lifestyle advice and pharmacologic interventions. Thus, lifestyle-modification programs are a powerful treatment option to reduce risk factors associated with obesity and diabetes, even in patients who have not responded to conventional therapy.

EXERCISE-MEDIATED EFFECTS IN SKELETAL MUSCLE

Exercise and muscle contraction per se leads to alteration in skeletal muscle metabolism and alters the metabolic capacity of the muscle. Contraction may also lead to the release of circulatory factors from the muscle, which could exert influence on other organs. In response to exercise training (that is, several repeated exercise bouts) muscle growth is increased.[23] There are also accompanying changes in the metabolic profile of the muscle, such that there is an increased reliance on lipid oxidation, even under higher work-loads. Another well-characterized response to exercise and contraction is enhanced skeletal muscle insulin sensitivity. These changes are reversible, and thus the opposite effects are noted in response to inactivity. A section later in the this article discusses some of the molecular changes in skeletal muscle following exercise and contraction, and which may be important in mediating the beneficial exercise effects.

Metabolic Response to Exercise

Exercise is a metabolic stress that acutely increases the demand for energy production. While lipid and carbohydrate oxidation are both increased during exercise, the limitation of oxygen availability favors carbohydrate as the preferential substrate. Skeletal muscle glucose uptake is increased during exercise and blood-glucose concentrations are maintained by hepatic glycogenolysis and gluconeogenesis and indirectly by an increased rate of muscle glycogen utilization. Prolonged or high-intensity exercise has been shown to deplete both liver[24] and muscle glycogen,[25] resulting in reduced carbohydrate oxidation and blood-glucose concentration. The after-exercise period is characterized by an increased rate of glucose uptake to replenish muscle glycogen concentrations.[26]

Lipid oxidation is especially important during prolonged low-intensity exercise where oxygen availability is sufficient for β-oxidation, when carbohydrate stores are depleted, and in the after-exercise recovery. Exercise training also results in an increase in the relative contribution of lipid to total oxidation during submaximal exercise.[27] The regulation of lipolysis and the relative contribution of plasma nonesterified fatty acids (NEFA), plasma triglycerides, and intramuscular triglycerides (IMTG) to skeletal muscle fat oxidation are also influenced by the exercise conditions. Exercise training improves the insulin sensitivity of lipolysis[28] and increases the rate of glycerol and NEFA appearance at rest.[29] However, during low-intensity exercise, the rate of lipolysis does not change following exercise training,[11,30] and as the rate of NEFA appearance exceeds that of fat oxidation,[31,32] it is likely that the increased lipid oxidation following training is caused by IMTG oxidation.[30,33,34] Endurance exercise training increases the accumulation and turnover of IMTG.[33,34]

Immediate Effects of a Single Bout of Exercise

An acute bout of exercise leads to an immediate increase in glucose transport in skeletal muscle, mediated via an insulin-independent translocation of glucose transporter (GLUT)-4 to the cell surface.[35–38] The work performed by the muscle leads to a reduction of ATP relative to AMP levels, leading to the activation of the AMP-sensitive protein kinase (AMPK).[39] Activation of AMPK stimulates glucose uptake and lipid oxidation to produce energy, while turning off energy-consuming processes, including glucose and lipid production, to restore intracellular energy balance. AMPK activation is also central in mediating some of the long-term effects of exercise, as discussed below.

Exercise and Substrate Oxidation in Obesity and Type 2 Diabetes

Impairments have been noted in skeletal muscle glucose and fatty acid metabolism in obesity and Type 2 diabetes in the resting state.[40–43] This is evident by impaired post-receptor insulin signaling, reduced glucose uptake, and rates of glycogen synthesis.[44,45] Abnormal fatty acid metabolism leads to increased accumulation of IMTGs[46] and decreased lipid oxidation during fasting and insulin-stimulated conditions.[47] Thus, exercise-mediated enhancement of substrate oxidation is especially important in the treatment of obesity and Type 2 diabetes, as these conditions are associated with impaired skeletal muscle lipid utilization. An acute bout of exercise increases lipid oxidation in overweight and obese subjects, but it is not clear if total lipid oxidation is less than[48] or greater than lean controls.[49] Glucose disposal and plasma NEFA oxidation during 60 minutes of exercise at 50% VO_2peak has been found to be similar in lean and obese subjects, although the contribution of muscle glycogen was reduced in obese subjects, with the balance presumably coming from an increase in nonsystemic lipid oxidation.[49] It has been challenging to clearly understand the response of obese subjects to exercise because of the inherent heterogeneity of this group. Phenotypic differences may partly explain the variable response, as plasma lipid availability is reported to be greater in men with visceral adiposity compared with those with subcutaneous adiposity,[50] and exercise training has a greater impact on fat oxidation in subjects with upper body but not lower body obesity.[51] It is also important to note that, while weight gain is associated with insulin resistance, the degree of insulin resistance varies greatly and can subsequently influence substrate selection. For example, total carbohydrate oxidation and muscle glycogen utilization has been found to be lower in overweight insulin-resistant women as compared with insulin-sensitive women, consistent with a greater contribution of lipid oxidation to energy production during exercise.[52]

The effect of exercise training on substrate oxidation is not as clear in obese and Type 2 diabetic populations, as in lean populations. While resting fat oxidation may not change in obese subjects after training at either low or high intensity (40% or 70% VO_{2max}), fat oxidation during exercise increases at lower intensity.[53] In this study, the absolute rate of fat oxidation was similar in both high- and low-intensity training groups after training, the respiratory exchange ratio for the high-intensity group was greater before training, giving a high basal fat oxidation rate and a lower training adaptation.[53] In studies that have combined energy restriction with exercise training, the exercise is associated with increased resting fat oxidation,[27] insulin sensitivity[27,54] and mitochondrial adaptations.[55,56]

The accumulation of IMTG in obesity is most likely caused by a reduction in lipid oxidation with similar or increased NEFA uptake. Energy restriction and exercise training do not decrease IMTG in obese subjects,[57] though an increase in IMTG turnover could contribute to enhanced insulin sensitivity. The inconclusive results for training-related changes in lipid oxidation for obese individuals may be related to subject heterogeneity, as explained previously, or study design. In many exercise intervention protocols the exercise intensity is relatively low, and training frequency is usually 3 to 4 days per week. This leads to a total increase in energy expenditure of approximately 1,000 kcal per week. This is significantly less than a typical energy restriction protocol of 500 to 1,000 kcal per day. Recent evidence, which will be discussed later, indicates that weekly energy expenditure in excess of 2,000 kcal may be required to prevent weight gain and even more may be necessary for weight loss. It is also possible that the lipid oxidation rates may not increase following training because there may be an upper limit of skeletal muscle fat oxidation.[53] In line with this, maximal oxygen uptake increased in young obese—but not young obese Type 2 diabetics—following a 12-week exercise training program.[58] Thus, intrinsic factors in the muscle that regulate oxidation may not be responsive to exercise training in some populations; whether this is a disease-related factor or reflects underlying genetic differences in exercise response is discussed below.

Carbohydrate oxidation rates appear to be similar in lean, obese, and Type 2 diabetic groups during exercise.[59,60] However, if excess lipid availability alters substrate utilization in obese subjects, the combination of elevated glucose and lipid levels in Type 2 diabetes leads to further metabolic difficulties. In response to one-legged aerobic exercise training in subjects with Type 2 diabetes or nondiabetic controls, glucose oxidation tended to decrease in both groups during exercise, while increased fat oxidation was only noted in the nondiabetic group.[61] Sixteen hours after the last training bout, the rate of carbohydrate oxidation had increased in both groups, but significantly more in the nondiabetic group, thus indicating an impaired exercise response in subjects with Type 2 diabetes.[61] Furthermore, in normo-glycemic insulin-resistant offspring of Type 2 diabetics, carbohydrate oxidation rates were proportionally decreased, and there was no increase in response to an acute bout or 6-weeks of exercise training.[62] Based on the current literature it is difficult to draw conclusions regarding substrate utilization in obese and Type 2 diabetes subjects; however, it is likely that the elevated fasting glucose and lipids result in different metabolic responses than in lean controls. These changes may result in altered exercise response, differential regulation of the insulin-signaling cascade, and regulation of gene expression and protein synthesis.

MOLECULAR MECHANISMS UNDERLYING EXERCISE EFFECTS IN SKELETAL MUSCLE

Insulin Resistance and Metabolic Dysfunction in Skeletal Muscle

Evidence suggests that decreased insulin-mediated glucose transport is a primary defect in skeletal muscle.[63,64] Insulin resistance is characterized by decreased insulin receptor and insulin receptor substrate-1 (IRS-1) tyrosine phosphorylation, and decreased phosphatidylinositol 3-kinase (PI3-kinase) activity following insulin stimulation.[65] A potential mechanism for the down-regulation of the insulin-signaling cascade involves the regulation of lipid metabolism. The accumulation of IMTG is correlated with insulin resistance and is thought to be related to a decrease in mito-chondrial oxidative activity[66] resulting from a reduction in the activity of oxidative enzymes[67] and the electron transport chain.[68] Accumulation of IMTG may be the result of a decrease in mitochondrial fatty acid oxidation, resulting in an increase in cytosolic long-chain fatty acyl CoA (reviewed in Lowell and Shulman[69]). Diacylglycerol (DAG) accumulation also occurs and is associated with an increase in the activity of protein kinase C ϵ and θ isoforms, which are known to increase the serine phosphor-ylation of the insulin receptor and IRS-1. Reduced expression of DAG kinase delta has been noted in skeletal muscle from Type 2 diabetic subjects,[70] which could contribute to an increased DAG accumulation. Interestingly, exercise leads to enhanced skeletal muscle expression of DAG kinase delta.[71,72]

Although it is probable that many different factors underlie and contribute to the disturbances in metabolism, altered mitochondrial function would affect both lipid and glucose metabolism. Skeletal muscle is highly dependent on oxidative phos-phorylation for energy production. Reduced expression of enzymes important for mitochondrial oxidative phosphorylation have been found in skeletal muscle from obese subjects.[73] Alternatively, the decrease in mitochondrial oxidative phosphory-lation in insulin resistance could be because of changes in mitochondrial structure. The size and number of mitochondria are decreased and there is evidence of degen-erated mitochondria in insulin-resistant conditions, such as obesity and Type 2 diabetes.[68] Thus, recent evidence points to a strong association between insulin resistance and mitochondrial dysfunction in skeletal muscle. The identification of mechanisms that increase mitochondrial biogenesis, oxidative enzyme activity, and glucose transport have important implications for increasing substrate utilization and insulin sensitivity.

Skeletal Muscle Contraction and the Regulation of Gene Expression

Muscle contraction is known to produce a multitude of physiologic adaptations, including an increase in insulin-mediated glucose disposal,[38] and therefore provides a novel model for identifying cellular and molecular mechanisms of insulin resistance. In addition to the many physiologic adaptations, exercise training increases skeletal muscle mitochondria size and number[74] in an intensity-dependent manner.[75] This is coupled with an increase in Krebs cycle, β-oxidation, and electron transport-chain activity, facilitating a shift in cellular substrate utilization toward greater free fatty acid oxidation.[74] Interestingly, a lifestyle modification involving both weight loss and increased physical activity in previously sedentary obese subjects led to an increase in both mitochondrial size and number.[76] The changes noted in mitochondria were also associated with improvements in insulin resistance.[76] This indicates that reduced mitochondrial number associated with obesity is reversible.

Thus skeletal muscle contraction not only increases energy expenditure but is also a key regulator of gene and protein expression. The impact on protein synthesis extends beyond the mitochondria to include a broad range of proteins involved in carbohydrate metabolism (GLUT-4, hexokinase, glycogen synthase), lipid metabolism (lipoprotein lipase, CD36, carnitine palmitoyltransferase I) insulin-signaling intermediates (PI3-kinase activity), and angiogenic regulators.[61,77–82] As a corollary, the absence of regular physical activity will lead to decreased rates of protein synthesis and over time contribute to impaired metabolic function.

Recent work on the mechanisms responsible for enhanced NEFA oxidation suggest that exercise-mediated up-regulation of gene expression associated with peroxisome proliferator-activated receptor alpha and gamma (PPARα/γ) and PPARγ coactivator-1α (PGC-1α) may be responsible.[83,84] Short term exercise training increases lipid oxidation and this is associated with an increased expression of FAT/CD36, regulating NEFA uptake across the plasma membrane, and CPT-1, regulating mitochondrial NEFA uptake.[84]

Although there is compelling evidence for exercise-mediated regulation of mitochondrial function, it is also important to point out that the role of mitochondrial impairments in mediating the metabolic phenotypes associated with Type 2 diabetes and obesity has been challenged. In human subjects harboring mitochondrial mutations, diabetes often develops as a result of impairments in beta cell function, while peripheral insulin sensitivity is maintained and obesity rarely develops.[85] Mice with a targeted reduction in mitochondrial function are protected against diabetes and obesity, suggesting that the reduction in oxidative phosphorylation noted in the muscle of insulin resistant subjects could be a compensatory mechanism.[86]

Which Exercise-Regulated Pathways Mediate Changes in Muscle Metabolism?

The contractile process is an important mechanical stimulus for the regulation of cellular signals controlling gene expression and mitochondrial biogenesis. Mitochondrial biogenesis is a complex process requiring the coordinated expression of nuclear- and mitochondrion-encoded proteins and the import and assembly of these proteins into a functional organelle. There is strong evidence to suggest that intracellular calcium flux ($[Ca^{2+}]_i$) and ATP turnover (which leads to AMPK activation) are the major contraction-mediated signaling cascades contributing to changes in gene expression and mitochondrial biogenesis.[87,88]

The activation of these signaling cascades culminates in the expression and activation of transcription factors, including CREB and MEF2, and promotes PGC-1α gene expression.[89] Calcium binds to calmodulin (CaM) before activating Ca^{2+}/CaM-dependent kinases (CaMK). CaMKIV increases mitochondrial biogenesis via PGC-1α in mouse skeletal muscle[90] but is not expressed in human skeletal muscle.[91] Calcium signaling in human muscle may be mediated via CaMKII, which is activated in a dose-dependent manner by contraction.[91]

AMPK is required for mitochondrial biogenesis in skeletal muscle in response to chronic energy deprivation.[92] AMPK increases mitochondrial biogenesis by activation of NRF-1,[87,93] and by directly increasing gene expression by colocalizing to the nucleus.[93] However, the mechanism of AMPK-regulated gene expression is not fully understood as it increases the expression of some, but not all, mitochondrial enzymes.[94] AMPK also directly binds to, and phosphorylates, PGC-1α[95] and may have a more important role as a regulator of protein activation and function.

It has become clear that nuclear receptor-mediated transactivation requires interaction with coactivators. PGC-1α is a well-characterized coactivator of a wide array of transcription factors and, when over-expressed in myotubes, there is an increase in oxygen consumption, the expression of genes in oxidative phosphorylation, and mito-chondrial biogenesis,[96] all of which are characteristic adaptations associated with endurance exercise training. PGC-1α is believed to be a master regulator of metabolic gene expression as it regulates transcription factors involved in the expression of nuclear encoded mitochondrial proteins, mitochondrial DNA transcription, GLUT-4 biogenesis, and fatty acid oxidation (reviewed in Lin and colleagues[97]). PGC-1α expression is attenuated in obesity and diabetes, contributing to metabolic dysfunc-tion, with decreased mitochondrial content, energy expenditure, and increased IMTGs and insulin resistance.[98–100] Obese Zucker rats have a greater rate of palmitate incor-poration into IMTG and decreased expression of PGC-1α in comparison to lean controls.[101] The regulation of PGC-1α expression and the subsequent execution of cell-specific transcriptional programs are important for metabolic homeostasis.

Because many aspects of exercise-trained muscle are similar to properties associ-ated with type 1/oxidative muscle fibers, including enhanced insulin sensitivity and increased number of mitochondria, the study of fiber-type determination using trans-genic mice has been illustrative in identification of genes that are also important in response to exercise. For example, in transgenic mice, over-expression PGC-1α leads to an increased proportion of type IIA and type I skeletal muscle fibers.[102] Similarly in mice, transgenic expression of an activated form of PPARδ also increased the propor-tion of type I fibers.[103] The expression of a highly homologous receptor, PPARα, has been shown to be controlled by exercise and metabolic status in skeletal muscle.[104–106] Because PGC1 is a cofactor for both PPARδ and PPARα, there is collective evidence for the importance of these signaling events in regulation of muscle metabolic phenotype.

Expression of PGC-1α is increased 2 to 3 hours following an acute bout of exercise[107–111] and after exercise training.[107,112–114] There is a positive relationship between the expression of PGC-1α and maximal oxygen consumption, as well as oxidative phosphorylation activity in human skeletal muscle.[115] While there is strong evidence to support a contraction-mediated increase in PGC-1α expression following exercise, the regulation of PGC-1α target genes is less clear. NRF-1 expression is unchanged following an acute bout of exercise[108,116] and exercise training[112] despite an increase in PGC-1α. Therefore, it is important to consider the importance of PGC-1α activation, the role of other transcription coregulators, and muscle fiber character-istics in the regulation exercise-mediated mitochondrial biogenesis.

In addition to signals mediated via PPARα, PPARδ, and PGC-1α, expression and activity of the Ca^{2+} sensitive enzyme calcineurin has also been implicated as playing an important role in fiber-type transformation, using muscle-targeted expression of Calcinuerin Aα.[117–120] Compared to transgenic mice over-expressing PPARδ or PGC-1, the calcineurin transgenic mice have a more modest increase in type 1 fiber content, suggesting that calcineurin activity alone is not sufficient to drive the slow-fiber phenotype.[118] Thus, data from transgenic mice and functional genomics impli-cate PPARα, PPARδ, PGC-1α, and Calcineurin as the basis of a signaling network controlling skeletal muscle fiber-type transformation and metabolism in rodents.

Given the substantial differences between rodent and human skeletal muscle,[74] in particular as regards skeletal muscle adaptation and fiber-type transformation, trans-lational studies in human beings are important. Elite athletes have an increased 24-hour skeletal muscle metabolism, enhanced whole-body insulin sensitivity, and an increased proportion of type I fibers.[121] In contrast, following spinal cord injury, alterations in neuronal input are associated with changes in skeletal muscle pheno-type, with decreased fiber size, increased percentage of mATPase type IIB fibers, and dramatic loss of type I fibers to near undetectable levels.[122,123] When comparing these two groups to a group of age-matched healthy sedentary subjects, the authors could show that expression of PPARα, PPARδ, PGC-1α, but not Calcineurin Aα correlated with the exercise status and type I fiber content in skeletal muscle *vastus lateralis* biopsies, providing evidence for the relevance of these genes implicated in controlling skeletal muscle fiber-type transformation and metabolism in human beings as well.[124]

Genetic Variation May Determine Exercise Response

Although exercise exerts many positive effects in the majority of subjects, there is also a wide range of individual response to exercise. There is increasing evidence that an individual's genetic make-up will influence the subsequent response to exercise, and that some individuals may be inherently less able to respond to training. Differences in mRNA profiles in skeletal muscle have been mapped between groups of subjects who show marked difference in the improvement in glucose tolerance as a response to the same amount of 20-week exercise training, demonstrating the existence of "exercise resistance."[72]

A proline for alanine substitution at position 12 (Pro12Ala polymorphism) in the gene encoding PPARγ *(PPARG)* has been related with obesity directly, as well as physical activity level,[125] while variations at Gly482Ser predict exceptional endurance capacity.[126] Carriers homozygous for the Ser482 variants have been shown to be more capable of improving cardio-respiratory fitness when physically active, suggesting that Gly482Ser could explain some of the between-person variance in adaptation after exercise training.[127]

Exercise training leads to increased skeletal muscle expression of PPARδ in both animals[104] and human beings.[71] Up-regulation of skeletal muscle PPARδ protein expression has been linked to improvements in clinical parameters in diabetic subjects following an exercise intervention, such that subjects where there was no change in PPARδ did not experience the metabolic improvements observed in subjects where PPARδ increased.[71] A further indication that the ability to up-regulate PPARδ may be necessary for exercise to mediate positive effects on metabolism come from studies linking genetic variations at the *PPARD* locus with change in aerobic physical fitness and insulin sensitivity during lifestyle intervention. Genetic variation at the *PPARD*, *PPARGC1A*,[128,129] and *PPARG*[130] have also been linked to exercise response loci. Variations at *PPARD*, and *PPARGC1A* have both additive[129] and independent effects.[128,129] The association of genetic variation at the loci of the above genes with the ability to benefit from physical exercise further highlight PPAR-PGC1 regulated genes and pathways as key in mediating exercise adaptation.

EXERCISE RECOMMENDATIONS IN THE MANAGEMENT OF OBESITY AND TYPE 2 DIABETES

Physical inactivity is undoubtedly a major contributing factor to weight gain and the development of Type 2 diabetes. It has been argued that exercise is necessary to maintain normal metabolic function because of the important regulatory control on gene expression, mitochondrial biogenesis, oxygen consumption, and energy expenditure.[2] One of the challenges faced by clinicians and exercise specialists is to reintroduce physical activity into daily living, in place of sedentary behaviors adopted by advances in technology. In an attempt to encourage physical activity, the recommendations developed over a decade ago focused on the minimal amounts of physical activity required to maintain or improve cardiovascular health.[131] While this approach had many merits, the recommendations quickly became adopted as general guidelines for population health and the treatment of clinical conditions. It has recently been proposed that these guidelines may not be adequate to prevent weight gain or optimize the use of exercise to treat clinical conditions. This has caused a certain amount of conflict between those who promote practical and achievable guidelines in a modern society and those who wish to optimize the therapeutic benefits of exercise.

There have been relatively few randomized, controlled trials to evaluate the impact of exercise on weight reduction.[132] Many of the published articles adopted an exercise protocol of approximately 150 minutes per week, based on an exercise recommendation of 30 minutes of physical activity on all or most days of the week.[131] This is equivalent to 150-kcal to 200-kcal energy expenditure per day or approximately 700 kcal to 1,000 kcal per week. Therefore, the magnitude of weight loss for exercise alone, or the additional benefit of exercise to an energy-restricted diet has been modest.[133] This is not surprising if one considers that energy-restricting protocols often result in a 500 kcal per day energy deficit, equivalent to 3,500 kcal per week. There have only been two studies that have matched the energy expenditure of exercise with that of an energy-restricting protocol. When 500 kcal[134] or 700 kcal[135] per day was expended by exercise, the magnitude of weight loss was similar to that of an isocaloric energy-restricting diet for 12 weeks. Therefore, exercise is an effective weight-loss strategy but the accumulated energy expenditure required for weight reduction may be greater than the general recommendations.

Recently, the United States Institute of Medicine (IoM) and the International Association for the Study of Obesity (IASO) have recommended that 45 to 60 minutes per day of physical activity may be required to prevent weight gain.[136,137] The IoM developed this recommendation from the evidence in their Doubly Labeled Water database, which indicated that those who maintained a normal body-mass index across the lifespan had a total daily energy expenditure that was 1.7 times their basal metabolic rate,[136] and the data indicated that 60 minutes of daily physical activity would be required for an individual to move from a sedentary to an active lifestyle. The IASO estimated that for a sedentary individual to become active they would require an additional 490 kcal of daily energy expenditure,[137] which is considerably more than the 150 kcal to 200 kcal per day accumulated with the general exercise guidelines. It is likely that this increased recommendation will pose difficulties for public health guidelines and for professionals who promote exercise adherence, but it is necessary to distinguish between general health and therapeutic benefits of exercise and to establish more specific strategies.

A more targeted approach has recently been taken for the role of exercise in the treatment of Type 2 diabetes. In a review of the evidence base for exercise modality, intensity and frequency, Praet and van Loon[138] have proposed exercise guidelines based on the clinical characteristics of the patient. In particular, they differentiate the exercise prescription on the basis of the duration of diabetes, the initial fitness of the individual, their body mass index, and the length of time they have been exercise training. They have also provided guidelines for endurance, resistance, and interval training, all of which have been shown to improve insulin sensitivity and glycemic control.[138] To advance the therapeutic use of exercise in the treatment of obesity and Type 2 diabetes, it will be necessary to conduct more randomized, controlled trials and to clearly differentiate between the general health and clinical benefits of exercise.

SUMMARY

An active lifestyle increases general health and is protects from a number of different conditions, including exercise and obesity. There is emerging evidence that exercise by itself exerts clinically beneficial effects in both lean and obese subjects, even in the absence of effects on weight.[1] Recent results have brought an increasing understanding of the molecular mechanisms underlying the beneficial effects of exercise at the level of metabolism and changes in gene expression. There is a significant dose-response to the effect of exercise, and the current guidelines regarding exercise amount may need to be revised upwards. Furthermore, this treatment option should not be overlooked.

REFERENCES

1. Pedersen BK. Body mass index-independent effect of fitness and physical activity for all-cause mortality. Scand J Med Sci Sports 2007;17:196–204.
2. Booth FW, Chakravarthy MV, Gordon SE, et al. Waging war on physical inactivity: using modern molecular ammunition against an ancient enemy. J Appl Physiol 2002;93:3–30.
3. Adams SA, Der Ananian CA, DuBose KD, et al. Physical activity levels among overweight and obese adults in South Carolina. South Med J 2003;96:539–43.
4. Wei M, Kampert JB, Barlow CE, et al. Relationship between low cardiorespiratory fitness and mortality in normal-weight, overweight, and obese men. JAMA 1999;282:1547–53.
5. Iyawe VI, Ighoroje AD, Iyawe HO. Changes in blood pressure and serum cholesterol following exercise training in Nigerian hypertensive subjects. J Hum Hypertens 1996;10:483–7.
6. Despres JP, Lamarche B. Low-intensity endurance exercise training, plasma lipoproteins and the risk of coronary heart disease. J Intern Med 1994;236:7–22.
7. Boule NG, Haddad E, Kenny GP, et al. Effects of exercise on glycemic control and body mass in type 2 diabetes mellitus: a meta-analysis of controlled clinical trials. JAMA 2001;86:1218–27.
8. Kirwan JP, del Aguila LF, Hernandez JM, et al. Regular exercise enhances insulin activation of IRS-1-associated PI3-kinase in human skeletal muscle. J Appl Physiol 2000;88:797–803.
9. Steiner S, Niessner A, Ziegler S, et al. Endurance training increases the number of endothelial progenitor cells in patients with cardiovascular risk and coronary artery disease. Atherosclerosis 2005;181:305–10.
10. Bergström K, Barany P, Holm I. An educational programme for persistent lifestyle changes in patients with chronic renal disease. EDTNA ERCA J 1999;25: 42–4.
11. Dela F, Mikines KJ, von Linstow M, et al. Effect of training on insulin-mediated glucose uptake in human muscle. Am J Physiol 1992;263:E1134–43.
12. King DS, Dalsky GP, Staten MA, et al. Insulin action and secretion in endurance-trained and untrained humans. J Appl Physiol 1987;63:2247–52.
13. O'Gorman DJ, Karlsson HKR, McQuaid S, et al. Exercise training increases insulin-stimulated glucose disposal and GLUT4 (SLC2A4) protein content in patients with type 2 diabetes. Diabetologia 2006;49:2983–92.
14. Eriksson J, Lindström J, Valle T, et al. Prevention of Type II diabetes in subjects with impaired glucose tolerance: the Diabetes Prevention Study (DPS) in Finland. Study design and 1-year interim report on the feasibility of the lifestyle intervention programme. Diabetoloiga 1999;42:793–801.
15. Eriksson K, Lindgarde F. Prevention of type 2 (non-insulin-dependent) diabetes mellitus by diet and physical exercise: the 6-year Malmö feasibility study. Diabetologia 1991;34:891–8.

16. X Pan, Li G, Hu Y, et al. Effects of diet and exercise in preventing NIDDM in people with impaired glucose tolerance: the Da Qing IGT and Diabetes Study. Diabetes Care 1997;20:537–44.
17. Tuomilehto J, Lindstrom J, Eriksson JG, et al. Prevention of Type 2 diabetes mellitus by changes in lifestyle among subjects with impaired glucose tolerance. N Engl J Med 2001;344:1343–50.
18. Uusitupa MI. Early lifestyle intervention in patients with non-insulin-dependent diabetes mellitus and impaired glucose tolerance. Annu Mediaev 1996;28: 445–9.
19. Hamdy O, Goodyear LJ, Horton ES. Diet and exercise in type 2 diabetes mellitus. Endocrinol Metab Clin North Am 2001;30:883–907.
20. Ligtenberg PC, Hoekstra JBL, Bol E, et al. Effects of physical training on metabolic control in elderly type 2 diabetes mellitus patients. Clin Sci (Colch) 1997; 93:127–35.
21. Skarfors ET, Wegener TA, Lithell H, et al. Physical training as treatment for type 2 (non-insulin-dependent) diabetes in elderly men. A feasibility study over 2 years. Diabetologia 1987;30:930–3.
22. Krook A, Holm I, Pettersson S, et al. Reduction of risk factors following lifestyle modification programme in subjects with type 2 (non-insulin dependent) diabetes mellitus. Clin Physiol Funct Imaging 2003;23:21–30.
23. Holloszy JO, Booth FW. Biochemical adaptations to endurance exercise in muscle. Annu Rev Physiol 1976;38:273–91.
24. Bruce CR, Lee JS, Hawley JA. Postexercise muscle glycogen resynthesis in obese insulin-resistant Zucker rats. J Appl Physiol 2001;91:1512–9.
25. Price TB, Rothman DL, Taylor R, et al. Human muscle glycogen resynthesis after exercise: insulin-dependent and -independent phases. J Appl Physiol 1994;76: 104–11.
26. Greiwe JS, Hickner RC, Hansen PA, et al. Effects of endurance exercise training on muscle glycogen accumulation in humans. J Appl Physiol 1999;87:222–6.
27. Goodpaster BH, Katsiaras A, Kelley DE. Enhanced fat oxidation through physical activity is associated with improvements in insulin sensitivity in obesity. Diabetes 2003;52:2191–7.
28. DiPietro L, Dziura J, Yeckel CW, et al. Exercise and improved insulin sensitivity in older women: evidence of the enduring benefits of higher intensity training. J Appl Physiol 2006;100:142–9.
29. Romijn JA, Klein S, Coyle EF, et al. Strenuous endurance training increases lipolysis and triglyceride-fatty acid cycling at rest. J Appl Physiol 1993;75:108–13.
30. Klein S, Coyle EF, Wolfe RR. Fat metabolism during low-intensity exercise in endurance-trained and untrained men. Am J Physiol 1994;267:E934–40.
31. Horowitz JF, Klein S. Lipid metabolism during endurance exercise. Am J Clin Nutr 2000;72:558S–63S.
32. Smekal G, von Duvillard SP, Pokan R, et al. Effect of endurance training on muscle fat metabolism during prolonged exercise: agreements and disagreements. Nutrition 2003;19:891–900.
33. Hurley BF, Nemeth PM, Martin WH 3rd, et al. Muscle triglyceride utilization during exercise: effect of training. J Appl Physiol 1986;60:562–7.
34. Larson-Meyer DE, Newcomer BR, Hunter GR. Influence of endurance running and recovery diet on intramyocellular lipid content in women: a 1H NMR study. Am J Physiol Endocrinol Metab 2002;282:E95–106.
35. Douen AG, Ramlal T, Rastogi SA, et al. Exercise induces recruitment of the "insulin responsive" glucose transporter. Evidence for distinct intracellular

insulin- and exercise-recruitable transporter pools in skeletal muscle. J Biol Chem 1990;265:13427–30.

36. Kristiansen S, Hargreaves M, Richter EA. Exercise-induced increase in glucose transport, GLUT-4, and VAMP-2 in plasma membrane from human muscle. Am J Physiol Endocrinol Metab 1996;270:E197–81.

37. Lund S, Holman GD, Schmitz O, et al. Contraction stimulates translocation of glucose transporter GLUT4 in skeletal muscle through a mechanism distinct from that of insulin. Proc Natl Acad Sci U S A 1995;92:5817–21.

38. Zierath JR. Exercise effects of muscle insulin signaling and action: invited review: exercise training-induced changes in insulin signaling in skeletal muscle. J Appl Physiol 2002;93:773–81.

39. Long YC, Zierath JR. AMP-activated protein kinase signaling in metabolic regulation. J Clin Invest 2006;116:1776–83.

40. Kelley DE, Mintun MA, Watkins SC, et al. The Effect of non-insulin-dependent diabetes mellitus and obesity on glucose transport and phosphorylation in skeletal muscle. J Clin Invest 1996;97:2705–13.

41. Kelley DE, Simoneau J-A. Impaired free fatty acid utilization by skeletal muscle in non-insulin-dependent diabetes mellitus. J Clin Invest 1994;94:2349–56.

42. Zierath JR. In vitro studies of human skeletal muscle. hormonal and metabolic regulation of glucose transport. Acta Physiol Scand 1995;155:1–96.

43. Zierath JR, He L, Guma A, et al. Insulin action on glucose transport and plasma membrane GLUT4 content in skeletal muscle from patients with NIDDM. Diabetologia 1996;39:1180–9.

44. Krook A, Björnholm M, Jiang X-J, et al. Characterization of signal transduction and glucose transport in skeletal muscle from Type 2 (non-insulin-dependent) diabetic patients. Diabetes 2000;49:284–92.

45. Shulman GI, Rothman DL, Jue T, et al. Quantitation of muscle glycogen synthesis in normal subjects and subjects with non-insulin-dependent diabetes by 13C nuclear magnetic resonance spectroscopy. N Engl J Med 1990;322:223–8.

46. Goodpaster BH, Theriault R, Watkins SC, et al. Intramuscular lipid content is increased in obesity and decreased by weight loss. Metabolism 2000;49: 467–72.

47. Blaak EE, Wagenmakers AJL, Glatz JFC, et al. Plasma FFA utilization and fatty acid-binding protein content are diminished in type 2 diabetic muscle. Am J Physiol Endocrinol Metab 2000;279:E146–54.

48. Mittendorfer B, Fields DA, Klein S. Excess body fat in men decreases plasma fatty acid availability and oxidation during endurance exercise. Am J Physiol Endocrinol Metab 2004;286:E354–62.

49. Goodpaster BH, Wolfe RR, Kelley DE. Effects of obesity on substrate utilization during exercise. Obes Res 2002;10:575–84.

50. Numao S, Hayashi Y, Katayama Y, et al. Effects of obesity phenotype on fat metabolism in obese men during endurance exercise. Int J Obes 2006;8: 1189–96.

51. van Aggel-Leijssen DP, Saris WH, Wagenmakers AJ, et al. The effect of low-intensity exercise training on fat metabolism of obese women. Obes Res 2001;9:86–96.

52. Braun B, Sharoff C, Chipkin SR, et al. Effects of insulin resistance on substrate utilization during exercise in overweight women. J Appl Physiol 2004;97:991–7.

53. van Aggel-Leijssen DP, Saris WH, Wagenmakers AJ, et al. Effect of exercise training at different intensities on fat metabolism of obese men. J Appl Physiol 2002;92:1300–9.

54. Menshikova EV, Ritov VB, Toledo FG, et al. Effects of weight loss and physical activity on skeletal muscle mitochondrial function in obesity. Am J Physiol Endocrinol Metab 2005;288:E818–25.

55. Menshikova EV, Ritov VB, Ferrell RE, et al. Characteristics of skeletal muscle mitochondrial biogenesis induced by moderate-intensity exercise and weight loss in obesity. J Appl Physiol 2007;103:21–7.

56. Ritov VB, Menshikova EV, He J, et al. Deficiency of subsarcolemmal mitochondria in obesity and type 2 diabetes. Diabetes 2005;54:8–14.

57. Malenfant P, Tremblay A, Doucet E, et al. Elevated intramyocellular lipid concentration in obese subjects is not reduced after diet and exercise training. Am J Physiol Endocrinol Metab 2001;280:E632–9.

58. Burns N, Finucane FM, Hatunic M, et al. Early-onset type 2 diabetes in obese white subjects is characterised by a marked defect in beta cell insulin secretion, severe insulin resistance and a lack of response to aerobic exercise training. Diabetologia 2007;50:1500–8.

59. Giacca A, Groenewoud Y, Tsui E, et al. Glucose production, utilization, and cycling in response to moderate exercise in obese subjects with type 2 diabetes and mild hyperglycemia. Diabetes 1998;47:1763–70.

60. Kang J, Kelley DE, Robertson RJ, et al. Substrate utilization and glucose turnover during exercise of varying intensities in individuals with NIDDM. Med Sci Sports Exerc 1999;31:82–9.

61. Dela F, Larsen JJ, Mikines KJ, et al. Insulin-stimulated muscle glucose clearance in patients with NIDDM. Effects of one-legged physical training. Diabetes 1999; 44:1010–20.

62. Perseghin G, Price TB, Petersen KF, et al. Increased glucose transport-phosphorylation and muscle glycogen synthesis after exercise training in insulin-resistant subjects. N Engl J Med 1996;335:1357–62.

63. Cline GW, Petersen KF, Krssak M, et al. Impaired glucose transport as a cause of decreased insulin-stimulated muscle glycogen synthesis in type 2 diabetes. N Engl J Med 1999;341:240–6.

64. Krook A, Wallberg-Henriksson H, Zierath JR. Sending the signal: molecular mechanisms regulating glucose uptake. Med Sci Sports Exerc 2004;36:1212–7.

65. Krook A, Bjornholm M, Galuska D, et al. Characterization of signal transduction and glucose transport in skeletal muscle from type 2 diabetic patients. Diabetes 2000;49:284–92.

66. Petersen KF, Dufour S, Befroy D, et al. Impaired mitochondrial activity in the insulin-resistant offspring of patients with type 2 diabetes. N Engl J Med 2004;350:664–71.

67. Simoneau JA, Kelley DE. Altered glycolytic and oxidative capacities of skeletal muscle contribute to insulin resistance in NIDDM. J Appl Physiol 1997;83: 166–71.

68. Kelley DE, He J, Menshikova EV, et al. Dysfunction of mitochondria in human skeletal muscle in Type 2 diabetes. Diabetes 2002;51:2944–50.

69. Lowell BB, Shulman GI. Mitochondrial dysfunction and type 2 diabetes. Science 2005;307:384–7.

70. Chibalin AV, Leng Y, Vieira E, et al. Down-Regulation of diacylglycerol kinase delta contributes to hyperglycemia-induced insulin resistance. Cell 2008;132: 375–86.

71. Fritz T, Krämer DK, Karlsson HKR, et al. Low-intensity exercise increases skeletal muscle protein expression of PPAR delta and UCP3 in type 2 diabetic patients. Diabetes Metab Res Rev 2006;22:492–8.

72. Teran-Garcia M, Rankinen T, Koza RA, et al. Endurance training-induced changes in insulin sensitivity and gene expression. Am J Physiol Endocrinol Metab 2005;288:E1168–78.

73. Simoneau J-A, Kelley DE. Altered glycolytic and oxidative capacities of skeletal muscle contribute to insulin resistance in NIDDM. J Appl Physiol 1997;83: 166–71.

74. Holloszy JO, Coyle EF. Adaptations of skeletal muscle to endurance exercise and their metabolic consequences. J Appl Physiol 1984;56:831–8.

75. Dudley GA, Abraham WM, Terjung RL. Influence of exercise intensity and duration on biochemical adaptations in skeletal muscle. J Appl Physiol 1982;53: 844–50.

76. Toledo FG, Watkins S, Kelley DE. Changes induced by physical activity and weight loss in the morphology of intermyofibrillar mitochondria in obese men and women. J Clin Endocrinol Metab 2006;91:3224–7.

77. Chibalin AV, Yu M, Ryder JW, et al. Exercise-induced changes in expression and activity of proteins involved in insulin-signal-transduction in skeletal muscle: differential effects on IRS-1 and IRS-2. Proc Natl Acad Sci U S A 2000;97:38.

78. Houmard JA, Egan PC, Neufer PD, et al. Elevated skeletal muscle glucose transporter levels in exercise-trained middle-aged men. Am J Physiol 1991; 261:E437–43.

79. Hughes VA, Fiatarone MA, Fielding RA, et al. Exercise increases muscle GLUT4-levels and insulin action in subjects with impaired glucose tolerance. Am J Physiol 1993;264:E855–62.

80. Ploug T, Stallknecht BM, Pedersen O, et al. Effect of endurance training on glucose transport capacity and glucose transporter expression in rat skeletal muscle. Am J Physiol 1990;259:E778–86.

81. Ren J-M, Semenkovich CF, Gulve EA, et al. Exercise induces rapid increases in GLUT4 expression, glucose transport capacity, and insulin-stimulated glycogen storage in muscle. J Biol Chem 1994;269:14396–401.

82. Yu M, Blomstrand E, Chibalin AV, et al. Exercise-associated differences in an array of proteins involved in signal transduction and glucose transport. J Appl Physiol 2001;90:29–34.

83. Horowitz JF, Leone TC, Feng W, et al. Effect of endurance training on lipid metabolism in women: a potential role for PPARalpha in the metabolic response to training. Am J Physiol Endocrinol Metab 2000;279:E348–55.

84. Tunstall RJ, Mehan KA, Wadley GD, et al. Exercise training increases lipid metabolism gene expression in human skeletal muscle. Am J Physiol Endocrinol Metab 2002;283:E66–72.

85. Maassen JA, t Hart LM, Janssen GM, et al. Mitochondrial diabetes and its lessons for common Type 2 diabetes. Biochem Soc Trans 2006;34:819–23.

86. Freyer C, Larsson N. Is Energy Deficiency Good in Moderation? Cell 2007;131: 448–50.

87. Bergeron R, Ren JM, Cadman KS, et al. Chronic activation of AMP kinase results in NRF-1 activation and mitochondrial biogenesis. Am J Physiol Endocrinol Metab 2001;281:E1340–6.

88. Ojuka EO, Jones TE, Han DH, et al. Raising Ca2+ in L6 myotubes mimics effects of exercise on mitochondrial biogenesis in muscle. FASEB J 2003;17: 675–81.

89. Handschin C, Rhee J, Lin J, et al. An autoregulatory loop controls peroxisome proliferator-activated receptor gamma coactivator 1alpha expression in muscle. PMID 2003;100:7111–6.

90. Wu H, Kanatous SB, Thurmond FA, et al. Regulation of mitochondrial biogenesis in skeletal muscle by CaMK. Science 2002;296:349–52.
91. Rose AJ, Hargreaves M. Exercise increases Ca2+-calmodulin-dependent protein kinase II activity in human skeletal muscle. J Physiol 2003;553:303–9.
92. Zong H, Ren JM, Young LH, et al. AMP kinase is required for mitochondrial biogenesis in skeletal muscle in response to chronic energy deprivation. PMID 2002;99:15983–7.
93. McGee SL, Howlett KF, Starkie RL, et al. Exercise increases nuclear AMPK alpha2 in human skeletal muscle. Diabetes 2003;52:926–8.
94. Winder WW, Holmes BF, Rubink DS, et al. Activation of AMP-activated protein kinase increases mitochondrial enzymes in skeletal muscle. J Appl Physiol 2000;88:2219–26.
95. Jager S, Handschin C, St-Pierre J, et al. AMP-activated protein kinase (AMPK) action in skeletal muscle via direct phosphorylation of PGC-1alpha. PMID 2007;104:12017–22.
96. Wu Z, Puigserver P, Andersson U, et al. Mechnisms controlling mitochondrial biogenesis and respiration through the thermogenic coactivator PGC-1. Cell 1999;98:115–24.
97. Lin J, Handschin C, Spiegelman BM. Metabolic control through the PGC-1 family of transcription coactivators. Cell Metab 2005;1:361–70.
98. Crunkhorn S, Dearie F, Mantzoros C, et al. Peroxisome proliferator activator receptor gamma coactivator-1 expression is reduced in obesity: potential pathogenic role of saturated fatty acids and p38 mitogen-activated protein kinase activation. J Biol Chem 2007;282:15439–50.
99. Mootha VK, Lindgren CM, Eriksson KF, et al. PGC-1alpha-responsive genes involved in oxidative phosphorylation are coordinately downregulated in human diabetes. Nat Genet 2003;34:267–73.
100. Patti ME, Butte AJ, Crunkhorn S, et al. Coordinated reduction of genes of oxidative metabolism in humans with insulin resistance and diabetes: potential role of PGC1 and NRF1. PNAS 2003;100:8466–71.
101. Benton CR, Han XX, Febbraio M, et al. Inverse relationship between PGC-1alpha protein expression and triacylglycerol accumulation in rodent skeletal muscle. J Appl Physiol 2006;100:377–83.
102. Lin J, Wu H, Tarr PT, et al. Transcriptional co-activator PGC-1 alpha drives the formation of slow-twitch muscle fibres. Nature 2002;418:797–801.
103. Wang YX, Zhang CL, Yu RT, et al. Regulation of muscle fiber type and running endurance by PPARdelta. PLoS Biol 2004;2:e294.
104. Kannisto K, Chibalin A, Glinghammar B, et al. Differential expression of peroxisomal proliferator activated receptors alpha and delta in skeletal muscle in response to changes in diet and exercise. Int J Mol Med 2006;17:45–52.
105. Russell AP, Hesselink MK, Lo SK, et al. Regulation of metabolic transcriptional co-activators and transcription factors with acute exercise. FASEB J 2005;19:986–8.
106. Watt MJ, Southgate RJ, Holmes AG, et al. Suppression of plasma free fatty acids upregulates peroxisome proliferator-activated receptor (PPAR) alpha and delta and PPAR coactivator 1alpha in human skeletal muscle, but not lipid regulatory genes. J Mol Endocrinol 2004;33:533–44.
107. Baar K, Wende AR, Jones TE, et al. Adaptations of skeletal muscle to exercise: rapid increase in the transcriptional coactivator PGC-1. FASEB J 2002;16:1879–86.
108. Cartoni R, Leger B, Hock MB, et al. Mitofusins 1/2 and ERRalpha expression are increased in human skeletal muscle after physical exercise. J Physiol 2005;567:349–58.

109. Mahoney DJ, Parise G, Melov S, et al. Analysis of global mRNA expression in human skeletal muscle during recovery from endurance exercise. FASEB J 2005;19:1498–500.

110. Pilegaard H, Osada T, Andersen LT, et al. Substrate availability and transcriptional regulation of metabolic genes in human skeletal muscle during recovery from exercise. Metab Clin Exp 2005;54:1048–55.

111. Vissing K, Andersen JL, Schjerling P. Are exercise-induced genes induced by exercise? FASEB J 2005;19:94–6.

112. Pilegaard H, Saltin B, Neufer PD. Exercise induces transient transcriptional activation of the PGC-1alpha gene in human skeletal muscle. J Physiol 2003;546:851–8.

113. Russell AP, Feilchenfeldt J, Schreiber S, et al. Endurance training in humans leads to fiber type-specific increases in levels of peroxisome proliferator-activated receptor-gamma coactivator-1 and peroxisome proliferator-activated receptor-alpha in skeletal muscle. Diabetes 2003;52:2874–81.

114. Short KR, Vittone JL, Bigelow ML, et al. Impact of aerobic exercise training on age-related changes in insulin sensitivity and muscle oxidative capacity. Diabetes 2003;52:1886.

115. Garnier A, Fortin D, Zoll J, et al. Coordinated changes in mitochondrial function and biogenesis in healthy and diseased human skeletal muscle. FASEB J 2005;19:43–52.

116. Norrbom J, Sundberg CJ, Ameln H, et al. PGC-1alpha mRNA expression is influenced by metabolic perturbation in exercising human skeletal muscle. J Appl Physiol 2004;96:189–94.

117. Naya FJ, Mercer B, Shelton J, et al. Stimulation of slow skeletal muscle fiber gene expression by calcineurin in vivo. J Biol Chem 2000;275:4545–8.

118. Oh M, Rybkin II, Copeland V, et al. Calcineurin Is necessary for the maintenance but not embryonic development of slow muscle fibers. Mol Cell Biol 2005;25:6629–38.

119. Ryder JW, Bassel-Duby R, Olson EN, et al. Skeletal muscle reprogramming by activation of calcineurin improves insulin action on metabolic pathways. J Biol Chem 2003;278:44298–304.

120. Schiaffino S, Serrano A. Calcineurin signaling and neural control of skeletal muscle fiber type and size. Trends Pharmacol Sci 2002;23:569–75.

121. Saltin B, Henriksson J, Nygaard E, et al. Fiber types and metabolic potentials of skeletal muscles in sedentary man and endurance runners. Ann NY Acad Sci 1977;301:3–29.

122. Aksnes AK, Hjeltnes N, Wahlstrom EO, et al. Intact glucose transport in morphologically altered denervated skeletal muscle from quadriplegic patients. Am J Physiol 1996;271:E593–600.

123. Grimby G, Broberg C, Krotkiewska I, et al. Muscle fiber composition in patients with traumatic cord lesion. Scand J Rehabil Med 1976;8:37–42.

124. Kramer DK, Ahlsen M, Norrbom J, et al. Human skeletal muscle fibre type variations correlate with PPARα, PPARδ and PGC-1α mRNA. Acta Physiologica 2006;188:207–16.

125. Franks PW, Luan J, Browne PO, et al. Does peroxisome proliferator-activated receptor gamma genotype (Pro12ala) modify the association of physical activity and dietary fat with fasting insulin level? Metabolism 2004;53:11–6.

126. Lucia A, Gómez-Gallego F, Barroso I, et al. PPARGC1A genotype (Gly482Ser) predicts exceptional endurance capacity in European men. J Appl Physiol 2005;99:344–8.

127. Franks PW, Barroso I, Luan J, et al. PGC-1alpha genotype modifies the association of volitional energy expenditure with [OV0312]O2max. Med Sci Sports Exerc 2003;35:1998–2004.

128. Andrulionyte L, Peltola P, Chiasson JL, et al. Single nucleotide polymorphisms of PPARD in combination with the Gly482Ser substitution of PGC-1A and the Pro12Ala substitution of PPARG2 predict the conversion from impaired glucose tolerance to Type 2 diabetes: the stop-NIDDM trial. Diabetes 2006;55:2148–52.

129. Stefan N, Thamer C, Staiger H, et al. Genetic variations in PPARD and PPARG-C1A determine mitochondrial function and change in aerobic physical fitness and insulin sensitivity during lifestyle intervention. J Clin Endocrinol Metab 2007;92:1827–33.

130. Adamo KB, Sigal RJ, Williams K, et al. Influence of Pro12Ala peroxisome proliferator-activated receptor gamma2 polymorphism on glucose response to exercise training in type 2 diabetes. Diabetologia 2005;48:1503–9.

131. Pate RR, Pratt M, Blair SN, et al. Physical activity and public health. A recommendation from the Centers for Disease Control and Prevention and the American College of Sports Medicine. JAMA 1995;273:402–7.

132. Ross R, Janssen I. Physical activity, total and regional obesity: dose-response considerations. Med Sci Sports Exerc 2001;33:S521–9.

133. Catenacci VA, Wyatt HR. The role of physical activity in producing and maintaining weight loss. Nature clinical practice. Endocrinology 2007;3:518–29.

134. Sopko G, Leon AS, Jacobs DR Jr, et al. The effects of exercise and weight loss on plasma lipids in young obese men. Metab Clin Exp 1985;34:227–36.

135. Ross R, Dagnone D, Jones PJ, et al. Reduction in obesity and related comorbid conditions after diet-induced weight loss or exercise-induced weight loss in men. A randomized, controlled trial. Ann Intern Med 2000;133:92–103.

136. Brooks GA, Butte NF, Rand WM, et al. Chronicle of the Institute of Medicine physical activity recommendation: how a physical activity recommendation came to be among dietary recommendations. Am J Clin Nutr 2004;79:921S–30S.

137. Saris WH, Blair SN, van Baak MA, et al. How much physical activity is enough to prevent unhealthy weight gain? Outcome of the IASO 1st Stock Conference and consensus statement. Obes Rev 2003;4:101–14.

138. Praet SF, van Loon LJ. Optimizing the therapeutic benefits of exercise in Type 2 diabetes. J Appl Physiol 2007;103:1113–20.

Cognitive and Behavioral Approaches in the Treatment of Obesity

Brent Van Dorsten, PhD[a],*, Emily M. Lindley, PhD[b]

KEYWORDS

- Cognitive • Behavioral • Obesity • Weight loss • Energy gap
- Treatment

The worldwide increase in the prevalence of overweight and obesity constitutes a global health epidemic.[1–3] Despite increased public and professional awareness of the issues associated with increased body weight, the prevalence of obesity doubled from 1980 to 2002 in United States adults, while overweight prevalence tripled in children and adolescents in this same period.[4,5] In tracking this rapid proliferation, Mokdad and colleagues[6] reported a 5.6% 1-year increase (2000–2001) in the adult prevalence of obesity, and Flegal and colleagues[4] reported that 64.5% and 30.5% of the adult United States population had, respectively, reached the threshold of overweight (body mass index or BMI $\geq$25 kg/m^2) and obese (BMI $\geq$30.0 kg/m^2). Subsequently, Ogden and colleagues[7] reported the prevalence of obesity for adult United States males significantly increased from 27.5% (1999–2000) to 31.1% (2003–2004), but no significant change was recorded for female adults in this time period. Embedded within these data are documented increases in the prevalence of obesity across gender, age groups, socioeconomic status, and ethnicity.

Obesity is associated with several major adverse health conditions, including diabetes, hypertension, hypercholesterolemia, certain cancers, sleep apnea, congestive heart failure, and stroke.[8–13] In the medical literature, the close affiliation between obesity and type 2 diabetes is apparent,[14,15] and it is currently estimated that 19.3 million United States adults have diabetes (9.3% of the population total), with one-third of this number remaining undiagnosed.[16,17] Previous 5-year observational data reported that overweight, no-treatment control adults gain 1 kg to 1.5 kg per

A version of this article appeared in the 37:4 issue of the *Endocrinology and Metabolism Clinics of North America*.

[a] Department of Physical Medicine and Rehabilitation, Campus Box 6511, Mail Stop F-493, University of Colorado Denver, 1635 North Ursula Street, Aurora, CO 80045-0511, USA
[b] Department of Orthopedics, Campus Box 6511, Mail Stop F-493, University of Colorado Denver, 1635 North Ursula Street, Aurora, CO 80045-0511, USA
* Corresponding author.
E-mail address: brent.vandorsten@uchsc.edu

Med Clin N Am 95 (2011) 971–988
doi:10.1016/j.mcna.2011.06.008
0025-7125/11/$ – see front matter © 2011 Elsevier Inc. All rights reserved.

medical.theclinics.com

year,[18] and even a 1-kg increase has been associated with a 9% relative increase in the prevalence of diabetes.[19] Upon examining trends in the number of deaths attributable to the six leading causes of death in United States adults, Jemel and colleagues[20] reported a 45% increase in deaths related to diabetes from 1987 to 2002. Again related to the increased prevalence in obesity during this same time, Fontaine and colleagues[9] reported obesity to be strongly associated with a reduction of life expectancy in young adults, and several investigators have reported an increased burden of functional disability in obese persons.[8,21,22]

COGNITIVE BEHAVIORAL MODIFICATION AND WEIGHT LOSS

A variety of published recommendations encourage overweight persons (eg, BMI of 25.0 kg/m^2–29.9 kg/m^2) who have two or more health risk factors to consume a low-calorie diet and increase physical activity to achieve the United States Surgeon General's recommendation for 30 minutes or more per day most days of the week.[23,24] Behaviorally based weight-loss interventions have been shown to produce a 0.5 kg to 1.0 kg average weekly weight loss, or an approximate 8.5 kg to 9.0 kg decrease (8%–10% of total body weight) from before to after treatment, with drop-out rates less than 20%.[25,26] Consistent with the emerging conceptualization of overweight and obesity as a chronic condition requiring long-term care, Wadden and colleagues[27] reported that average weight losses have more than doubled over the past 30 years as treatment lengths have more than tripled. Despite improved weight losses, weight regain continues to plague long-term treatment results, as most individuals regain one-third of lost weight within 1 year, with nearly half having returned to their original weight within 5 years.[25,27,28] To successfully maintain weight loss, a considerable amount of literature supports the necessity for greater durations of exercise (eg, $\geq$200–300 minutes per week) than those recommended to reduce health risk.[29–32]

Behavioral modification has comprised the fundamental component of weight-loss treatment for decades, and has traditionally involved weekly instructional sessions focusing on dietary change, activity increase, and instruction in behavior change techniques. Treatment programs have increased to over 40 weeks in length over the past two decades,[26,33] with the active instructional phases typically lasting 16 to 26 weeks and follow-ups extended to 1 or more years. Dietary recommendations encourage the development a nutritional diet of 1,200 kcal to 1,800 kcal per day, with no more than 20% to 30% of calories from fat.[34,35] Behavior change curricula are delivered in groups of 10 to 20 participants and address dietary intake, increasing physical activity, and modifying intrapersonal or environmental factors that support undesirable health practices. Physical activity goals include progressively achieving 30 to 40 minutes of moderate intensity activity on most days per week (eg, $\geq$150 minutes of moderate intensity walking per week), with increased amounts of exercise necessary to facilitate long-term weight-loss maintenance.[34,36]

Despite the emergence of multiple published recommendations for diet and exercise in the promotion of weight loss, little evidence exists to support that these recommendations are used by persons trying to lose weight outside of formal programs. Bish and colleagues[37] reported from Behavioral Risk Factor Surveillance System (2000) data that 46% of United States women and 33% of men acknowledged currently trying to lose weight, yet only 19% of women and 22% of men reported using both caloric restriction and increased exercise as their primary weight-loss strategy. Only one-fifth of respondents were noted to be achieving the minimal requirements for each as stated above.

Most published weight-loss programs are conducted in university-based settings and provide instruction in behavioral modification strategies, while the cognitive component—concentrating on the assessment and modification of thoughts, beliefs, emotions, self-attributions, self-esteem, and self-efficacy relative to weight loss—has received comparatively little attention. In fact, two recent large scale behaviorally-based investigations of lifestyle change intended to produce long-term weight loss used empiric interventions in which less than 30% of the lifestyle curriculum was specifically devoted to cognitive or affective issues.[38,39]

This article is intended to provide an overview of the unique cognitive and behavioral components of lifestyle interventions for weight loss, and to investigate potential psychosocial and metabolic factors contributing to the published difficulties in achieving long-term weight-loss maintenance.

BEHAVIORAL MODIFICATION FOR WEIGHT LOSS

Behavior modification consists of a set of behavior change strategies derived from the experimental analysis of human behavior and designed to incrementally develop and sustain desirable behaviors or to decrease the frequency of undesirable behaviors.[40,41] The basic tenet in behavioral modification for weight loss is that learned behaviors contributing to excessive food intake, poor dietary choices or habits, or sedentary activity habits are predominate, but can be modified and restructured to produce weight reduction.[42] Brownell and colleagues[43] proposed three distinct phases of behavior change, including identifying motivation for change, implementing change strategies, and developing relapse-prevention strategies to ensure long-term durability of change.

There are multiple publications describing the commonly employed behavioral modification strategies for dietary change, increasing physical activity, and preventing relapse.[44–48] Establishing objective treatment goals, self-monitoring of diet and exercise behaviors, making changes to the environment to support positive changes, using stimulus control techniques to cue the occurrence of desired behaviors, and relapse-prevention planning are among the techniques used in modifying behaviors associated with weight loss. A brief synopsis of the goal and purpose of these various behavioral strategies follows.

Goal Setting

The development of realistic and attainable weight loss goals before beginning treatment is critical to facilitating personal acceptance and maintenance of losses achieved. Behavior goals in obesity treatment may include selecting a specific weight-loss target and metabolic or psychosocial improvements. Establishing moderate weight-loss goals may be associated with greater levels of achievement and maintenance.[49] Overall weight-loss goals should be subdivided into weekly 1 to 1.5 pound losses via specifying the specific behaviors to be performed to achieve this goal, and predetermined rewards to be administered for successful accomplishment of incremental goals.

Self-Monitoring

Self-monitoring entails the systematic recording of an operationally defined target behavior. This strategy has been purported as the single most important tool used by persons attempting weight loss,[50] and a host of literature exists to support its efficacy in improving both initial weight loss and weight maintenance.[51–53] Self-monitoring can be used to record a variety of factors in weight loss, including calories or fat grams consumed, walking minutes or number of pedometer steps, and any of a host of subjective factors affecting weight (eg, motivation, obstacles, or emotional factors). Self-recording can assist in establishing accurate baseline values of a behavior, increase awareness of maladaptive behavior patterns, and provide feedback and reinforcement for initial changes in the phenomenon being recorded. Increasing accuracy of subjective estimates of target behaviors (eg, number of calories eaten per day) is critical as the published error in estimates of caloric intake and energy expenditure has been as high as 50%.[54–57] Wadden and colleagues[58] reported that frequent and thorough monitoring of food intake was associated with twice as much weight loss as infrequent monitoring. If behavioral fatigue occurs and the frequency or intensity of monitoring falters, self-recording may be used incrementally (eg, 1–2 weeks per month) to maintain accuracy of estimates, and may be targeted to those specific behaviors the person is performing well to act as reinforcement to continue efforts.

Stimulus Control

Behavioral interventions for dietary change are based upon the premise that food intake is prompted by internal and external cues (eg, antecedents) that become associated with the target behavior of eating.[59] Stimulus control is a behavior-change technique designed to identify and modify cues associated with food or activity patterns. Environmental cues that prompt overeating or sedentary behaviors may be modified to those that more adaptively prompt and support improved eating habits or physical activity.[60] Simple cues can be placed in a person's home or work environments to prompt medication adherence or increased episodes of walking, certain foods can be eliminated from the environment to remove cues for unhealthy eating, or an individual may remove themselves from a high-risk environment loaded with cues to overeat (eg, buffets, happy hours). While a 167-to-1 ratio may be considered mathematically weak, this ratio may represent the "best case scenario" in weight-loss treatment.[46] Specifically, if a person attempting weight loss meets for 1 hour per week with a behavioral counselor, there are an additional 167 hours in this same week for them to navigate the array of cues, prompting unhealthy eating and sedentary behavior, to successfully achieve an incremental goal. Manipulating environmental "prompts" to cue the performance of adaptive new behaviors can increase long-term success.

Changing the Environment

Assuming that home and work environments can contribute to inactivity and unhealthy eating by providing multiple unhealthy prompts (eg, snack foods, late-night television advertising) and a dearth of healthy prompts (eg, inaccessible exercise equipment, unavailable walking shoes), considerable environmental change is likely necessary to facilitate lifestyle change efforts when one begins weight loss. Altering shopping habits to increase the availability of fruits and vegetables, providing for healthy snacks, decreasing the availability of undesirable foods, making access to exercise equipment convenient, and re-arranging home or work schedules to allow for activity time can all contribute to success in weight loss. Changing an environment that tolerates an unhealthy lifestyle also includes changing one's social environment to increase exposure to others who are supportive and encouraging of weight-loss efforts to improve health.

Problem Solving

A valuable component of behavioral modification for weight loss and weight-loss maintenance is instructing individuals in a multistep problem-solving strategy to sustain efforts to lose weight. Problem solving techniques consist of five fundamental steps: (1) identifying and operationally defining a specific challenge; (2) rostering an array of potential alternative behaviors; (3) evaluating the benefits and disadvantages of each option; (4) selecting and implementing an option with a high probability for success; and (5) evaluating the relative success of this new option. This problem-solving process can be used to address environmental (eg, work schedule conflicts, transportation issues, adverse weather, minor physical injuries, eating in restaurants), and intrapersonal challenges (eg, amotivation, mood issues, or negative self-talk). As it is implausible to assume that any person might accurately anticipate the vast array of challenges they might face in performing a desired behavior over an extended period of time, flexible problem-solving skills can be critical in sustaining long-term performance.[61]

Relapse Prevention

The contemporary weight-loss literature accurately emphasizes the persistent problems with long-term maintenance following weight reduction.[60,62,63] However, several factors have been identified as contributing to successful weight maintenance. Long-term contact with treatment providers has widely been identified as an important factor facilitating weight maintenance.[64–66] Long-term follow-up contacts can be equally accomplished face-to-face or via telephone, Internet, or e-mail.[32,67–73] While the optimal frequency of maintenance contacts is largely unknown, frequency of weighing is another factor identified by successful weight-loss maintainers.[52,73,74] Provision of personal trainers and monetary incentives for weight loss[75,76] and group-contingent work site competitions[77,78] have also been shown to successfully stimulate long-term participation with weight-loss programs.

COGNITIVE THERAPY FOR WEIGHT LOSS

Cognitive therapy, most commonly referred to as cognitive-behavioral therapy (CBT), was derived in the 1960s from the work of Aaron Beck and postulated that erroneous and negatively biased interpretations of internal and external events lie at the core of negative perceptions of one's self, one's future, and the world in general.[79] These interpretational errors or cognitive distortions may produce enduring dysfunctional beliefs that increase one's vulnerability to mood or behavioral disorders. Among the various cognitive distortions potentially impacting health and illness, are magnifying negative aspects of ourselves or a circumstance, failing to recognize or minimizing positives, personalizing negative events, and dichotomous thinking, which polarizes experiences as excessively positive or negative.[80,81] Cognitive therapy is founded upon the premise that the manner in which a person thinks about themselves or a given event impacts how they will emotionally and behaviorally respond to the event.[82] When an expectation of failure exists, many individuals will not engage in goal-directed behaviors and in turn interpret this "inevitable" lack of success as "evidence" of personal incompetence. Considering patients with many prior failed efforts to lose weight and maintain weight losses, a bevy of cognitive distortions may exist and adversely flavor attempts to lose weight.

The term "cognitive-behavioral therapy" is often used interchangeably with "behavior modification" or "behavior therapy," but actually offers some subtle distinction in practice. Cognitive approaches to weight loss focus on identifying behavioral and thought patterns that affect eating and have the potential to be useful in weight-loss treatment by identifying and modifying thoughts or self-perceptions associated with maladaptive diet and exercise patterns, prior relapses, or prior treatment failures.[83,84] A number of publications have highlighted the impact of cognitive thoughts and beliefs on body weight and weight loss, and have recommended increasing the focus on cognitive change to enhance weight loss and weight-loss maintenance.[83,85–87]

Cognitive Strategies in Weight Treatment

A variety of strategies may be used to increase awareness of negative thought processes influencing body weight, including self-monitoring of negative cognitions, problem-solving alternatives to negative self-talk, and cognitive restructuring to challenge the validity of negative self-attributions. Additionally, preintervention strategies can include motivational interviewing and establishing reasonable and objective expectations for treatment outcome.

Motivational readiness

Cognitive and behavioral modification strategies can be applied in weight management well before a person begins their first overt efforts to lose weight.[46] When attempting to evaluate readiness for change, health care professionals are increasingly using motivational interviewing (MI) techniques[88] to assess personal motivations to commit to losing weight, to validate ambivalence patients may feel about making this commitment, to explore obstacles to be encountered in this effort, and to elucidate personal resources to navigate these obstacles. Establishing readiness for change has shown to predict sustained change efforts.[89,90] In a review of the use of MI in weight loss, Van Dorsten[91] reported that current literature supports the efficacy of several adaptations of MI for producing weight loss and weight-loss maintenance, increasing physical activity, and improving regimen adherence. A variety of additional published studies have found motivational interviewing strategies, when used in combination with other behavioral interventions, to be associated with increased reported physical exercise, dietary change, eating disorder treatment, and improved treatment adherence.[92–96]

Patient expectations for treatment

While a 5% to 10% reduction in body weight is considered sufficient to improve many health-risk factors,[34] previous research has suggested that many patients pursuing weight-loss treatment find this amount of weight loss to be inconsequential and disappointing. Foster and colleagues[97] assessed the before-treatment weight-loss goals for 45 obese women randomized to a behaviorally based weight-loss treatment. While prior behavioral treatment research suggests a positive outcome would be an 8% to 10% reduction in before-treatment body weight, this subject group identified a 32% reduction as their average weight-loss goal. During a 48-week treatment, participants lost an average 16 kg (16% total body weight), but collectively considered this loss to be "disappointing." Subsequent studies have demonstrated equally unreasonable weight-loss goals for patients seeking weight loss via behavioral treatment, bariatric surgery, and pharmacologic treatments.[98,99] In attempting to curb unrealistic before-treatment weight-loss expectations, Wadden and colleagues[100] provided participants with both verbal and written empiric information regarding expected weight loss with 1 year of weight-loss medication use, yet this information had minimal influence on repeated unreasonable expectations throughout weight-loss treatment. This literature emphasizes the dramatic need to clarify patient expectations for treatment and the rationale behind these expectations, and to re-evaluate changes in these expectations over the course of treatment.

Cognitive restructuring

Emotional factors can have considerable impact on a person's dedication to weight change and may be a strong antecedent to overeating or abandoning activity.[46] Most people seeking weight loss have endured many prior unsuccessful attempts, often with loss and regain, and this history may be an important factor in predicting future weight-loss efforts via the production of negative self-perceptions (eg, "can't do it, will never succeed"). As such, using strategies to self-monitor negative thoughts and their impact on food intake or physical activity, problem-solving to create alternative responses to negative thoughts, and self-reinforcement strategies to reward oneself for making changes can all contribute to restructuring of behavioral habits that are prompted by cognitive events.

In their cognitive behavioral recommendations for weight loss, Cooper and Fairburn[85] suggested that weight treatment focus on teaching individuals to appreciate the significance of even minor weight changes and to develop an action plan to enact when weight increases. These investigators stated that weight-loss patients need to gradually acquire the belief that they are capable of implementing strategies to appropriately control their weight (eg, self-efficacy).

Evidence of Efficacy of Cognitive-Behavioral Treatment

It is difficult to succinctly evaluate the efficacy of "cognitive behavioral management" of obesity, as this term is used to encompasses all facets of treatment except for medication-only or surgery. Considering the multiple variations of diet, physical activity, and CBT packages published in the literature—and adding adherence techniques, meal replacements, motivational interviewing adaptations, and medication to this matrix—an exponential number of combinations exist against which to assess the success of treatment. However, systematic reviews of the efficacy of cognitive behavioral lifestyle-change interventions provide considerable support for the contributions of these interventions in weight-loss treatment.[101,102] Shaw and colleagues[101] reported collective results for two studies[103,104] testing psychologic interventions for weight treatment and concluded that CBT, when added to diet and exercise interventions, produced superior weight losses (7.3 kg) than diet and exercise treatment alone (2.4 kg). Similarly, Painot and colleagues[105] investigated the efficacy of CBT plus diet and exercise interventions versus CBT alone in 70 overweight adults. Results indicated weight losses of 1.9 kg (standard deviation or SD = 0.6 kg) for the combined treatment group versus weight gain of 0.5 kg (SD = 0.6 kg) for the CBT-alone group at 3-month follow-up. Sbrocco and colleagues[106] reported a study comparing CBT versus BT weight loss interventions for 24 overweight subjects. Significant between-group results ($P<.01$) indicated weight losses of 7 kg (SD = 2.0) and 10 kg (SD = 3.4) for CBT participants at 6 and 12 months, compared with 4.5 kg (SD = 2.6) and 4.3 kg (SD = 2.5) for the BT group. Norris and colleagues[102] reported conclusions from a systematic review of 22 studies of overweight or obese adults with type 2 diabetes evidencing small-to-moderate results for diet, exercise, and CBT interventions in producing weight loss of sufficient magnitude to be associated with improved health outcomes. These investigators concluded that the small-to-moderate changes detected for treatment were somewhat minimized by moderate weight losses of up to 10 kg in comparison populations.

A host of additional articles and meta-analyses support the superiority of diet-plus-exercise interventions versus diet alone in producing weight loss and long-term weight-loss maintenance.[28,36,107,108] Several large-scale national studies provide additional support that behavioral lifestyle interventions can produce moderate sustained weight loss that have been shown to associate with decreased health risks in overweight or obese adults with type 2 diabetes, and to prevent or delay onset of type 2 diabetes in those at risk.[109–111]

It is equally difficult to succinctly pare apart cognitive and behavioral components of treatment packages for the purpose of determining a unique contribution by either in lifestyle-based weight-loss interventions, given varying compilations of both in published weight-loss curricula. However, several recent publications have demonstrated an important impact of emotions and thoughts on the weight-loss process. Starhe and Hallstrom[112] investigated the efficacy of a cognitive group treatment program on 105 obese female subjects. Sixty-five subjects were randomized to treatment, with 43 randomized to wait-list control. Treatment subjects attended 10 weekly 3-hour group sessions consisting of cognitive therapy, psychoeducation, and information on dietary intake and nutrition. The purpose of the treatment program groups was to discuss factors influencing personal eating patterns, as well as information that could be useful in changing eating behaviors. Treatment participants were provided a 1, 200-kcal to 1,300-kcal diet recommendation tailored to individual preferences and without food restrictions. The cognitive treatment program addressed causes of underlying disordered eating, self-control, low self-esteem, and reaction to stress. Sessions investigated personal reactions to stressful events, emotions related to dysfunctional eating patterns, and ways in which alternative thoughts might positively influence eating behaviors. Homework assignments included personally implementing new insights with emphasis on the impact of specific thoughts and beliefs on personal eating patterns. No booster sessions were offered following the 10-week intervention. Control subjects remained on the waiting list for nonsurgical treatment of obesity at a university-based obesity-treatment program. All participants had weight measured at baseline, end of treatment, and 6-, 12- and 18-month follow-up.

Results were reported for only the 34 (60%) of randomized treatment subjects and 31 (72%) control subjects who completed 18-month follow-up. At the end of treatment, the CBT-intervention group produced an 8.5-kg (SD = 16.1) weight loss, which actually increased to 10.7 kg at 12 months. No comparative raw data were reported for control subjects but graphic weight comparisons review minimal weight change for control subjects, producing significant ($P<.01$) differences between groups at all follow-ups. At 18-month follow-up, treatment subjects showed a mean weight reduction of 10.4 kg, while the control group showed a 2.4-kg weight increase ($P<.001$). The investigators concluded that this short-term cognitive treatment may have contributed to significant weight loss and weight-loss maintenance in treatment subjects, and that long-term treatment may not be necessary to produce sustained weight loss.

Stahre and colleagues[84] followed this initial effort with a randomized, controlled trial comparing a similar cognitively based weight-loss intervention against a more traditional behaviorally based weight-loss intervention (eg, "control" condition) in 54 obese females. This subject population identified themselves as "perpetual dieters" and each had previously been involved with numerous individual or group weight-loss programs. Those assigned to the cognitive group treatment program (CT) received instruction in 10 weekly 2-hour sessions intended to inform subjects about possible causes of dysfunctional eating patterns and provide information that could be used to change eating behaviors. Specific attention was devoted to the issues of self-esteem, self-control, and stress management. Additionally, this group received nutrition instructions with a 1,200 kcal to 1,300 kcal per day goal. Participants assigned to the behavioral "control" condition (BT) received similar length instruction designed to achieve behavioral change in diet, stress management, and physical activity. This control program consisted of lectures, group discussions, and practical demonstrations. Data are presented for the 15 subjects completing the CT program and 13 completing an 18-month follow-up, and for 20 completing the BT program and 16 completing the 18-month follow-up. Significant differences in group weight losses were observed at completion of the 10-week programs, with 8.6 kg (SD = 2.9) reported for the CT group and 0.7 kg (SD = 1.2) for the BT group (P<.01). As might be expected, subjects in the CT group scored higher on topics related to cognitive influences on body weight and lower on behavioral issues of nutrition and physical activity on an end-of-treatment knowledge examination. Additional significant weight differences were observed at 18-month follow-up, with the CT group recording 5.9-kg (SD = 5.4) maintained losses versus a 0.03-kg (SD = 4.3) weight gain in the BT group. These investigators acknowledged that the weight losses in the CT group in this study were sizably less than in their original investigation, but reported a modified intervention from 30 to 20 hours of contact and fewer participants with BMI greater than 35 as potential explanations.

Rapoport and colleagues[113] reported the results of a study using a modified CBT intervention (MCBT) versus standard CBT (SCBT) for producing weight loss in 63 overweight women. Both treatment groups involved 10 weekly 2-hour group meetings led by a dietician and health psychologist with training in CBT. The primary goal of the MCBT arm was weight maintenance (ie, no weight gain), and emphasized instruction in healthy eating and exercise as a means of reducing the psychosocial and medical risks of obesity. Motivational interviewing and encouragement to monitor food intake and distance walked via use of pedometers was included. Weight loss was specifically not identified as a treatment goal and participants were discouraged from restrictive dieting. In contrast, the main goal of the SCBT arm was gradual weight loss (eg, 1–2 pounds per week) achieved via a moderate calorie-restriction diet, increased energy expenditure, and instruction in behavioral change techniques. As such, while the fundamental goals of each arm differed, a vast similarity in methods is observed. Results at end of treatment demonstrated a 3.9-kg weight loss for the 38 subjects in the SCBT group versus 1.3-kg weight loss for the 37 MCBT subjects. At 1-year follow-up, mean weight loss in the SCBT group was 3.6 kg, while weight loss had increased to 2.0 kg in the MCBT group. As such, while weight loss from baseline was significant in the SCBT group but not MCBT group at end of treatment, both groups showed small but significant changes from baseline to week 52, with no differences between groups. Additional 1-year follow-up findings included significant changes for both groups on metabolic measures (eg, cholesterol, blood pressure, waist circumference), physical activity, psychologic factors (eg, self-esteem, depression, eating patterns), and diet composition. The investigators concluded the MCBT intervention to be successful from a general physical and psychologic health improvement standpoint, and in producing modest sustained weight loss. However, in terms of psychosocial variables, the predicted advantage of MCBT was not achieved. In all, several investigators have emphasized the need to equally address cognitive and motivational factors when pursuing weight loss with patients who likely have several failed prior attempts. While cognitive issues have received less attention than strict behavioral measures, initial data suggests that systematically addressing cognitive factors may enhance long-term weight-loss results.

THE COMPLEXITIES OF WEIGHT-LOSS MAINTENANCE

When an individual's body achieves a state of energy balance, such that energy intake and expenditure are relatively equal, a stable body weight can be maintained. Weight gain occurs when a positive energy balance occurs (ie, energy intake is greater than energy expenditure), and weight loss can result when energy balance becomes negative, with energy expenditure exceeding intake. Weight loss can be reasonably accomplished via any combination of reduced intake and increased expenditure. While numerous studies have shown that obese individuals are able to lose weight by producing a negative energy balance via food restriction, there is little data to support successful long-term weight-loss maintenance in this population. Some reports have suggested that as few as 2% of individuals participating in weight-loss programs maintain a substantial weight loss over several years.[114,115] However, when successful weight loss maintenance is defined as a loss of at least 10% of body weight for at least 1 year, then the number of successful maintainers may exceed 20%.[116] Despite the documented success of weight-loss programs and the lack of such documentation for long-term weight maintenance, the primary focus of obesity research remains on weight loss rather than strategies to promote and achieve long-term maintenance. Weight-loss maintenance is often viewed as a permanent extension of the negative energy balance that led to initial weight loss. Sustaining a negative-energy balance indefinitely is a lofty challenge, particularly in the face of compensatory metabolic changes associated with weight loss.

The Energy Gap

Hill and colleagues[117] coined the term "energy gap" to describe the changes in energy requirements that occur as a result of weight loss. As described above, to maintain a stable body weight, energy input and expenditure must be equally opposing. However, when individuals lose body mass their total energy requirements also decrease. This results in lower energy expenditure, which creates an energy gap that biases the body toward regaining lost weight. Thus, a greater understanding of how metabolic changes influence weight-loss maintenance is necessary to define appropriate strategies for achieving energy balance and a stable body weight after significant weight loss.

Examples of the Energy Gap in Research

An essential component of energy balance is resting metabolic rate (RMR), as it is representative of the energy expenditure of metabolically active tissue. A number of studies have suggested that weight loss in human beings is associated with a reduction in RMR, which contributes to the energy gap described above.[118–121] There remains some dispute as to whether the change in RMR is appropriate for the new leaner body mass or whether the RMR becomes disproportionately low. While human bariatric studies are informative, they possess innate limitations, such as the inability to measure metabolic rates before and after obesity onset. In human studies, the RMR of after-weight loss subjects is most often compared with control subjects that have never been obese. It is possible that this comparison is not reflective of the true metabolic changes that take place in obese individuals over the course of obesity onset and subsequent weight loss. Furthermore, there are issues of inconsistent methodology across the studies used to assess RMR and other metabolic indices. To overcome these limitations, rat models of obesity have been developed to allow investigators to monitor changes in metabolic rate at each stage of weight gain and loss.[122–124] In these studies, obesity-prone rats were first allowed free access to a high-fat diet for 16 weeks to establish obesity, and were then placed on a low-calorie diet for 2 weeks to produce a 10% to 15% reduction in body weight. For the next 8 to 16 weeks, the rats either remain on the low-calorie diet or are again allowed ad libitum feeding, resulting in weight regain. In these studies, weight loss significantly suppresses metabolic rate in obese rats to a greater extent than would be expected for the change in body mass and reduction in energy intake. Furthermore, when rats are maintained at a reduced body weight, the elevated metabolic efficiency does not return over time to the before-weight loss metabolic rate, but have been shown to return to baseline after 8 weeks of weight regain.[123,124] When rats are allowed to regain lost weight, several peripheral metabolic responses occur, including preferential lipid accumulation in adipose tissue via hyperplasia and the presence of two humoral adiposity factors that underestimate peripheral adiposity.[122] This underestimation of peripheral adiposity likely signals the central nervous system to positively skew the energy balance. These findings support the existence of a compensatory metabolic response to weight loss that opposes weight-loss maintenance and instead encourages the body to regain lost weight. Moreover, this homeostatic feedback system does not appear to readjust over time as a function of weight-loss maintenance.

Consequences of the Energy Gap

These studies indicate that the issues surrounding weight loss maintenance may be much broader than that of individual motivation and self-control. Because RMR decreases after significant weight loss, the resulting energy gap shifts the balance between energy intake and expenditure requirements. With lower energy expenditure, it becomes more difficult for individuals to achieve the energy balance necessary for weight-loss maintenance. According to Hill, a weight loss of 40 pounds would result in an energy gap of 300 kcal to 350 kcal.[125] Thus, to maintain weight loss, an individual would have to either permanently reduce their energy intake by an additional 300 kcal to 350 kcal per day or increase their energy expenditure by 300 kcal to 350 kcal per day. This would roughly equate to taking an additional 6,000 steps or 3 miles per day. Although possible, both of these options pose difficult life-long challenges to weight maintenance. This highlights the challenge caused by the energy gap in weight maintenance and the importance of viewing weight loss and weight maintenance as two separate issues with separate underlying processes.

NATIONAL WEIGHT CONTROL REGISTRY INSIGHTS ON WEIGHT MAINTENANCE

In 1994, the National Weight Control Registry (NWCR) was established to study weight loss and the weight-maintenance strategies of successful weight-loss maintainers. Participants in this registry must have maintained at least a 30-pound weight loss for a minimum of 1 year. Although registry participants have reported using a variety of approaches to lose weight, several common strategies appear for promoting weight-loss maintenance.[51,52,126,127] First, a large proportion of NWCR participants eat a moderately low-fat, high-carbohydrate diet with approximately 24% of total energy from fat. Second, almost 80% of NWCR participants report that they eat breakfast daily, which is consistent with growing evidence that eating breakfast is associated with healthy body weight.[128] NWCR participants also consistently self-monitor and record their body weight, food intake, and physical activity. Lastly, participants in the NWCR engage in high levels of physical activity, equivalent to roughly 1 hour of moderate intensity physical activity per day. These results suggest that NWCR participants maintain their weight loss by achieving energy balance through a combination of reduced energy intake and increased energy expenditure, thus overcoming the energy gap.

SUMMARY

The research reviewed within this article provides support for both the cognitive and behavioral components of cognitive behavioral weight-loss interventions. Lifestyle-based treatments have produced markedly improved results in the past 20 years, in part attributable to changes in treatment structure. Use of pretreatment participant preparation strategies, extended treatment periods with clearly defined weight-loss goals, combining multiple dietary and physical activity strategies, and increasing emphasis on long-term provider contact and relapse prevention have modestly improved long-term weight maintenance. Several investigators have emphasized the need to incorporate additional cognitive components into the cognitive-behavioral treatment of obesity to improve both short- and long-term outcomes.[85–87] Furthermore, continued insights into metabolic changes producing an energy gap after weight loss should no doubt continue to refine insights into the behavioral requirements of long-term weight loss.

Despite increased awareness and behavioral treatment advances, the worldwide prevalence of obesity and weight-related chronic illnesses continues to expound. Behavioral treatment is inherently challenging and time-consuming, and readily available to only a fraction of the population who may benefit from inclusion. Several investigators have cautioned that individual or small group-based interventions are insufficient to serve the population masses requiring treatment, and that continued development of community or Web-based programs, and community-development tactics to increase healthy lifestyles, are needed.[67,129]

The call has been sounded to conceptualize obesity as a chronic health condition requiring lifelong treatment.[130] As such, the conceptualization of cognitive-behavioral therapies as a one-time treatment is passé. As the current number of obesity specialists and behaviorally trained professionals is insufficient to combat this problem[46,131]; an increased emphasis upon training nontraditional weight specialists and nonbehavioral community providers is obviated.

REFERENCES

1. Popkin BM, Doak CM. The obesity epidemic is a worldwide phenomenon. Nutr Rev 1998;56:106–14.
2. Van Dorsten B. Behavioral modification in the treatment of obesity. In: Barnett AH, Kumar S, editors. Obesity and diabetes. London: John Wiley & Sons; 2004. p. 111–30.
3. Wadden TA, Brownell KD, Foster GD. Obesity: responding to the global epidemic. J Consult Clin Psychol 2002;70:510–25.
4. Flegal KM, Carroll MD, Ogden CL, et al. Prevalence and trends in obesity among US adults, 1999–2000. JAMA 2002;288:1723–7.
5. Hedley AA, Ogden LC, Johnson CL, et al. Prevalence of overweight and obesity among US children, adolescents, and adults 1999–2002. JAMA 2004;291: 2847–50.
6. Mokdad AH, Ford ES, Bowman BA, et al. Prevalence of obesity, diabetes, and obesity-related health risk factors: 2001. JAMA 2003;289:76–9.
7. Ogden DCL, Carroll MD, Curtin LR, et al. Prevalence of overweight and obesity in the United States, 1999–2004. JAMA 2006;295:1549–55.
8. Alley DE, Chang VW. The changing relationship of obesity and disability, 1988–2004. JAMA 2007;298:2020–6.
9. Fontaine KR, Redden DT, Wang C, et al. Years of life lost due to obesity. JAMA 2003;289:187–93.
10. Hainer V, Toplak H, Mitrakou A. Treatment modalities of obesity: what fits whom? Diabetes Care 2008;31:S269–77.
11. Klein S, Burke LE, Bray G, et al. Clinical implications of obesity with special focus on cardiovascular disease. Circulation 2004;110:2952–67.

12. Labib M. The investigation and management of obesity. J Clin Pathol 2003;56: 17–25.
13. Must A, Spadano J, Coakley EH, et al. The disease burden associated with overweight and obesity. JAMA 1999;282:1523–9.
14. Gregg EW, Guralnik JM. Is disability obesity's price of longevity? JAMA 2007; 298:2066–7.
15. Gregg EW, Cheng YJ, Cadwell BL, et al. Secular trends in cardiovascular disease risk factors according to body mass index in US adults. JAMA 2005;293:1868–74.
16. Cowie CC, Rust KF, Byrd-Holt DD, et al. Prevalence of diabetes and impaired fasting glucose in adults in the U.S. population: National Health And Nutrition Survey 1999–2002. Diabetes Care 2006;29:1263–8.
17. Norris SL, Kansagara D, Bougatsos C, et al. Screening adults for Type 2 diabetes: a review of the evidence for the U.S. Preventive Services Task Force. Ann Intern Med 2008;148:855–68.
18. Rothacker DQ. Five-year self-management of weight using meal replacements: comparison with matched controls in rural Wisconsin. Nutrition 2000;16:344–8.
19. Mokdad A, Ford E, Bowman B, et al. Diabetes trends in the US: 1990–1998. Diabetes Care 2000;23:1278–83.
20. Jemel A, Ward E, Hao Y, et al. Trends in leading causes of death in the United States, 1970–2002. JAMA 2005;294:1255–9.
21. Al Snih S, Ottenbacher KJ, Markides KS, et al. The effect of obesity on disability vs mortality in older Americans. Arch Intern Med 2007;167:774–80.
22. Weil E, Wachterman M, McCarthy EP, et al. Obesity among adults with disabling conditions. JAMA 2002;288:1265–8.
23. National Heart, Lung, and Blood Institute (NHLBI) & North American Association for the Study of Obesity (NAASO). Practical Guide to the Identification, Evaluation, and Treatment of Overweight and Obesity in Adults. Bethesda (MD): National Institutes of Health; 2000.
24. United States Department of Health and Human Services. Physical activity and health: a report of the Surgeon General. Atlanta (GA): Centers for Disease Control; 1996.
25. Perri MG, Corsica JA. Improving the maintenance of weight lost in behavioral treatment of obesity. In: Wadden TA, Stunkard AJ, editors. Handbook of obesity treatment. New York: Guilford Press; 2002. p. 357–79.
26. Wing RR. Behavioral weight control. In: Wadden TA, Stunkard AJ, editors. Handbook of obesity treatment. New York: Guilford Press; 2002. p. 301–16.
27. Wadden TA, Butryn ML, Wilson C. Lifestyle modification for the management of obesity. Gastroenterology 2007;132:2226–38.
28. Curioni CC, Lourenco PM. Long-term weight loss after diet and exercise: a systematic review. Int J Obes 2005;29:1168–74.
29. American College of Sports Medicine. Appropriate intervention strategies for weight loss and prevention of weight regain for adults. Med Sci Sports Exerc 2001;33:2145–56.
30. Jakicic J. The role of physical activity in prevention and treatment of body weight gain in adults. J Nutr 2002;132:S3826–9.
31. Jakicic JM, Otto AD. Physical activity considerations for the treatment and prevention of obesity. Am J Clin Nutr 2005;82:S226–9.
32. Jakicik JM, Marcus BH, Lang W, et al. Effect of exercise on 24-month weight loss maintenance in overweight women. Arch Intern Med 2008;168:1550–9.
33. Perri MG, Nezu AM, Patti ET, et al. Effect of length of treatment on weight loss. J Consult Clin Psychol 1989;57:450–2.

34. Jakicic JM, Clark K, Coleman E, et al. Appropriate intervention strategies for weight loss and prevention of weight gain for adults. Med Sci Sports Exerc 2001;33:2145–56.

35. Lichtenstein AH, Appel LJ, Brands M, et al. Diet and lifestyle recommendations: revision 2006. Circulation 2006;114:82–96.

36. Volek JS, VanHeest JL, Forsythe CE. Diet and exercise for weight loss: a review of current issues. Sports Med 2005;35:1–9.

37. Bish CL, Michels-Blanck H, Serdula MK, et al. Diet and physical activity behaviors among Americans trying to lose weight: 2000 behavioral risk factor surveillance system. Obes Res 2005;13:596–607.

38. Diabetes Prevention Program Research Group. The Diabetes Prevention Program (DPP). Description of the lifestyle intervention. Diabetes Care 2002; 25:2165–71.

39. LookAHEAD Research Group. The Look AHEAD Study: a description of the lifestyle intervention and the evidence supporting it. Obesity 2006;14:737–52.

40. Miltenberger RG. Behavior modification: principles and procedures. Pacific Grove (CA): Brooks/Cole Publishing Company; 1997.

41. Kazdin AE. Behavioral modification in applied settings. Pacific Grove (CA): Brooks/Cole Publishing Company; 1994.

42. Jeffery RW, Epstein L, Wilson GT, et al. Long-term maintenance of weight loss: current status. Health Psychol 2000;19:5S–16S.

43. Brownell KD, Marlatt GA, Lichtenstein E, et al. Understanding and preventing relapse. Am Psychol 1986;41:765–82.

44. Brownell KD. The LEARN program for weight management. Dallas (TX): American Health; 2000.

45. Poston WSC, Foreyt JP. Successful management of the obese patient. Am Fam Physician 2000;61:3615–22.

46. Van Dorsten B. Behavior change components of obesity treatment. In: Barnett AH, Kumar S, editors. Diabetes and obesity. New York: Blackwell Publishing, in press.

47. Van Dorsten B. Behavior change strategies for increasing exercise in diabetes. In: Regensteiner J, Stewart K, Veves A, et al, editors. Diabetes and exercise. Totowa, NJ: Humana Press, in press.

48. Wing RR. Behavioral approaches to the treatment of obesity. In: Bray G, Bouchard C, James WPT, editors. Handbook of obesity. New York: Marcel Dekker; 1998. p. 855–73.

49. Jeffrey RW, Wing RR, Mayer RR. Are smaller weight losses or more achievable weight loss goals better in the long term for obese patients? J Consult Clin Psychol 1998;66:641–5.

50. Cobain MR, Foreyt JP. Designing "lifestyle interventions" with the brain in mind. Neurobiol Aging 2005;26S:S85–7.

51. Butryn ML, Phelan S, Hill JO, et al. Consistent self-monitoring of weight: a key component of successful weight loss maintenance. Obesity 2007;15:3091–6.

52. Klem ML, Wing RR, McGuire MT, et al. A descriptive study of individuals successful at long-term maintenance of substantial weight loss. Am J Clin Nutr 1997;66:239–46.

53. Boutelle KN, Kirschenbaum DS. Further support for consistent self-monitoring as a vital component of successful weight control. Obes Res 1998;6:219–24.

54. Bandini LG, Schoeller DA, Cyr HN, et al. Validity of reported energy intake in obese and non-obese adolescents. Am J Clin Nutr 1990;52:421–5.

55. Irwin ML, Ainsworth BE, Conway JM. Estimation of energy expenditure from physical activity measures: determinants of accuracy. Obes Res 2001;9:517–25.

56. Lichtman SW, Pisarska K, Berman ER, et al. Discrepancy between self-reported and actual caloric intake and exercise in obese subjects. N Engl J Med 1992; 327:1893–8.
57. Jakicic JM, Polley BA, Wing RR. Accuracy of self-reported exercise and the relationship with weight loss in overweight women. Med Sci Sports Exerc 1998;30: 634–8.
58. Wadden TA, Berkowitz RI, Womble LG, et al. Randomized trial of lifestyle modification and pharmacotherapy for obesity. N Engl J Med 2005;353:2111–20.
59. Foster GD. Clinical implications for the treatment of obesity. Obesity 2006;14: 182S–5S.
60. Foreyt JP, Goodrick GK. Factors common to successful therapy for the obese patient. Med Sci Sports Exerc 1991;23:292–7.
61. Perri MG, Nezu AM, McKelvey WF, et al. Relapse prevention training and problem-solving therapy in the long-term management of obesity. J Consult Clin Psychol 2001;69:722–6.
62. DePue JD, Clark MM, Ruggiero L, et al. Maintenance of weight loss: a needs assessment. Obes Res 1998;3:241–7.
63. Perri MG. The maintenance of treatment effects in the long-term management of obesity. Clinical Psychology: Science and Practice 1998;5:526–43.
64. Perri MG, McAdoo WG, McAllister DA, et al. Effects of peer support and therapist contact on long term weight loss. J Consult Clin Psychol 1987;55: 615–7.
65. Perri MG, McAdoo WG, McAllister DA, et al. Enhancing the efficacy of behavior therapy for obesity: effects of aerobic exercise and a multi-component maintenance program. J Consult Clin Psychol 1986;54:670–5.
66. Perri MG, McAdoo WG, Spevak PA, et al. Effect of a multi-component maintenance program on long-term weight loss. J Consult Clin Psychol 1984; 52:480–1.
67. Dunn AL, Anderson RE, Jakicic JM. Lifestyle physical activity interventions: history, short and long-term effects and recommendations. Am J Prev Med 1998;15:398–412.
68. Lindstrom LL, Balch P, Reese S. In person versus telephone treatment for obesity. J Behav Ther Exp Psychiatry 1976;7:367–9.
69. Tate DF, Jackvony EH, Wing RR. Effects of Internet behavioral counseling on weight loss in adults at risk for type 2 diabetes. JAMA 2003;289:1833–6.
70. Marcus GH, Lewis BA, Williams DM, et al. A comparison of Internet and print-based physical activity interventions. Arch Intern Med 2007;167:944–9.
71. Venditti EM. Efficacy of lifestyle behavior change programs in diabetes. Curr Diab Rep 2007;7:123–7.
72. Wing RR, Tate DF, Gorin AA. A self-regulation program for maintenance of weight loss. N Engl J Med 2006;355:1563–71.
73. Wing RR, Tate DF, Gorin AA, et al. STOP Regain: are there negative effects of daily weighing? J Consult Clin Psychol 2007;75:652–6.
74. Linde JA, Jeffery RW, French SA, et al. Self-weighing in weight gain prevention and weight loss trials. Ann Behav Med 2005;30:210–6.
75. Jeffrey RW, Bjornson-Benson WM, Rosenthal BS, et al. Effectiveness of monetary contracts with two repayment schedules on weight reduction in men and women from self-referred and population samples. Behav Ther 1984;15:273–9.
76. Jeffrey RW, Wing RR, Thorson C, et al. Use of personal trainers and financial incentives to increase exercise in a behavioral weight loss program. J Consult Clin Psychol 1998;66:777–83.

77. Brownell KD, Yopp-Cohen R, Stunkard AJ, et al. Weight loss competitions at the work site: impact on weight, morale, and cost-effectiveness. Am J Public Health 1984;74:1283–5.

78. Zandee GL, Oermann MH. Effectiveness of contingency contracting. AAOHN J 1996;44:183–8.

79. Beck AT. The current state of cognitive therapy: a 40-year perspective. Arch Gen Psychiatry 2005;62:953–9.

80. Beck AT, Weishar M, et al. Cognitive therapy. In: Freeman A, Simon KM, Beutler LE, et al, editors. Comprehensive handbook of cognitive therapy. New York: Plenum; 1989. p. 21–36.

81. Van Dorsten B. Amputation. In: Radnitz CL, editor. Cognitive-behavioral therapy for persons with disabilities. Northvale (NJ): Jason Aronson, Inc; 2000. p. 59–75.

82. Hollon SD. What is cognitive behavioural therapy and does it work? Curr Opin Neurobiol 1998;8:289–92.

83. Liao KL. Cognitive behavioral approaches and weight management: an overview. J R Soc Health 2000;120:27–30.

84. Stahre L, Tarnell B, Hakanson CE, et al. A randomized controlled trial of two weight-reducing short-term group treatment programs for obesity with an 18-month follow-up. Int J Behav Med 2007;14:48–55.

85. Cooper Z, Fairburn CG. A new cognitive behavioural approach to the treatment of obesity. Behav Res Ther 2001;30:499–511.

86. Cochrane G. Role for a sense of self-worth in weight-loss treatments. Can Fam Physician 2008;54:543–7.

87. Fabricatore AN. Behavior therapy and cognitive-behavioral therapy of obesity: is there a difference? J Am Diet Assoc 2007;107:92–9.

88. Miller WR, Rollnick S. Motivational interviewing: preparing people for change. New York: Guilford; 2002.

89. Prochaska JL, DiClemente CC, Norcross JC. In search of how people change: applications to addictive behaviors. Am Psychol 1992;47:1102–14.

90. Prochaska JL, Redding C, Evers K. The transtheoretical model of behavioral change. In: Glanz K, Lewis FM, Rimer BK, editors. Health behavior and health education: theory, research and practice. San Francisco: Jossey Bass; 1994. p. 60–84.

91. Van Dorsten B. The use of motivational interviewing in weight loss. Curr Diab Rep 2007;7:386–90.

92. Brodie DA, Inoue A. Motivational interviewing to promote physical activity for people with chronic heart failure. J Adv Nurs 2005;50:518–27.

93. DiLillo V, Siegfried NJ, Smith-West D. Incorporating motivational interviewing into behavioral obesity treatment. Cogn Behav Pract 2003;10:120–30.

94. Scales R, Miller JH. Motivational techniques for improving compliance with an exercise program: skills for primary care physicians. Curr Sports Med Rep 2003;2:166–72.

95. Hettema J, Steele J, Miller WR. Motivational interviewing. Annu Rev Clin Psychol 2005;1:91–111.

96. Smith D, Heckemeyer C, Kratt P, et al. Motivational interviewing to improve adherence to a behavioral weight-control program for older obese women with NIDDM. Diabetes Care 1997;20:52–8.

97. Foster GD, Wadden TA, Vogt RA, et al. What is reasonable weight loss? Patient's expectations and evaluations obesity treatment outcomes. J Consult Clin Psychol 1997;65:79–85.

98. Foster GD, Wadden TA, Phelan S, et al. Obese patient's perceptions of treatment outcomes and the factors that influence them. Arch Intern Med 2001; 161:2133–9.

99. Wadden TA, Berkowitz RI, Sarwer DB, et al. Benefits of lifestyle modification in the pharmacological treatment of obesity. Arch Intern Med 2001;161:218–27.

100. Wadden TA, Wombl L, Sarwer DB, et al. Great expectations: "I'm losing 25% of my weight no matter what you say". J Consult Clin Psychol 2003;71:1084–9.

101. Shaw K, O'Rourke P, Del Mar C, et al. Psychological interventions for overweight or obesity. Cochrane Database Syst Rev 2005;2:CD003818.

102. Norris SL, Zhang X, Avenell A, et al. Long-term non-pharmacological weight loss interventions for adults with type 2 diabetes mellitus. Cochrane Database Syst Rev 2005;2:CD004095.

103. Block J. Effects of rational emotive therapy on overweight adults. Psychology and Psychotherapy: Theory, Research, and Practice 1980;17:277–80.

104. Dennis K, Pane K, Adams B, et al. The impact of a shipboard weight control program. Obes Res 1999;7:60–7.

105. Painot D, Jotterand S, Kammer A, et al. Simultaneous nutritional cognitive-behavioural therapy in obese patients. Patient Educ Couns 2001;42:47–52.

106. Sbrocco T, Nedegaard R, Stone J, et al. Behavioral choice treatment promotes continued weight loss: preliminary results of a cognitive-behavioral decision-based treatment for obesity. J Consult Clin Psychol 1999;67:260–6.

107. Miller WC, Koceja DM, Hamilton EJ. A meta-analysis of the past 25 years of weight loss research using diet, exercise or diet plus exercise intervention. Int J Obes 1997;21:941–7.

108. Votruba SB, Horvitz MA, Schoeller DA. The role of exercise in the treatment of obesity. Nutrition 2000;16:179–88.

109. Diabetes Prevention Program Research Group. Reduction in the incidence of type 2 diabetes with lifestyle intervention and metformin. N Engl J Med 2002; 346:393–403.

110. Look AHEAD Research Group. Reduction in weight and cardiovascular disease risk factors in individuals with Type 2 diabetes: one year results of the Look-AHEAD trial. Diabetes Care 2007;30:1374–83.

111. Tuohimehto J, Lindstrom J, Eriksson JG, et al. Prevention of type 2 diabetes mellitus by changes in lifestyle among subjects with impaired glucose tolerance. N Engl J Med 2001;344:1343–9.

112. Stahre L, Hallstrom T. A short-term cognitive group treatment program gives substantial weight reduction up to 18 months from the end of treatment. A randomized controlled trial. Eat Weight Disord 2005;10:51–8.

113. Rapoport L, Clark M, Wardle J. Evaluation of a modified cognitive-behavioural programme for weight management. Int J Obes 2000;24:1726–37.

114. Kramer FM, Jeffery RW, Forster JL, et al. Long-term follow-up of behavioral treatment for obesity: patterns of weight regain among men and women. Int J Obes 1989;13:123–36.

115. Stunkard A, Mc Laren-Hume M. The results of treatment for obesity: a review of the literature and report of a series. AMA Arch Intern Med 1959;103:79–85.

116. Wing RR, Hill JO. Successful weight loss maintenance. Annu Rev Nutr 2001;21: 323–41.

117. Hill JO, Thompson H, Wyatt H. Weight maintenance: what's missing? J Am Diet Assoc 2005;105:S63–6.

118. Astrup A, Gotzsche PC, van de Werken K, et al. Meta-analysis of resting metabolic rate in formerly obese subjects. Am J Clin Nutr 1999;69:1117–22.

119. Doucet E, St-Pierre S, Almeras N, et al. Evidence for the existence of adaptive thermogenesis during weight loss. Br J Nutr 2001;85:715–23.

120. Franssila-Kallunki A, Rissanen A, Ekstrand A, et al. Effects of weight loss on substrate oxidation, energy expenditure, and insulin sensitivity in obese individuals. Am J Clin Nutr 1992;55:356–61.

121. Leibel RL, Rosenbaum M, Hirsch J. Changes in energy expenditure resulting from altered body weight. N Engl J Med 1995;332:621–8.

122. MacLean PS, Higgins JA, Jackman MR, et al. Peripheral metabolic responses to prolonged weight reduction that promote rapid, efficient regain in obesity-prone rats. Am J Physiol Regul Integr Comp Physiol 2006;290:R1577–88.

123. MacLean PS, Higgins JA, Johnson GC, et al. Enhanced metabolic efficiency contributes to weight regain after weight loss in obesity-prone rats. Am J Physiol Regul Integr Comp Physiol 2004;287:R1306–15.

124. MacLean PS, Higgins JA, Johnson GC, et al. Metabolic adjustments with the development, treatment, and recurrence of obesity in obesity-prone rats. Am J Physiol Regul Integr Comp Physiol 2004;287:R288–97.

125. Hill JO. Understanding and addressing the epidemic of obesity: an energy balance perspective. Endocr Rev 2006;27:750–61.

126. Catenacci VA, Ogden LG, Stuht J, et al. Physical activity patterns in the National Weight Control Registry. Obesity 2008;16:153–61.

127. Wyatt HR, Grunwald GK, Mosca CL, et al. Long-term weight loss and breakfast in subjects in the National Weight Control Registry. Obes Res 2002;10:78–82.

128. Rampersaud GC, Pereira MA, Girard BL, et al. Breakfast habits, nutritional status, body weight, and academic performance in children and adolescents. J Am Diet Assoc 2005;105:743–60.

129. Wing RR, Goldstein MG, Action KJ, et al. Behavioral science research in diabetes. Diabetes Care 2001;24:117–23.

130. Hill JO, Hauptman J, Anderson JW, et al. Orlistat, a lipase inhibitor, for weight maintenance after conventional dieting: A 1-year study. Am J Clin Nutr 1999; 69:1108–16.

131. Mauro M, Taylor V, Wharton S, et al. Barriers to obesity treatment. Eur J Intern Med 2008;19:173–80.

Medications for Weight Reduction

George A. Bray, MD

KEYWORDS

- Sympathomimetic drugs • Lipase inhibitor
- Cannabinoid receptor antagonists
- Glucagon-like peptide analogues

Obesity is often described as an epidemic.[1–3] In this context, it is essential to develop ways of preventing more people from becoming obese. When prevention fails, treatment may be necessary. Several different strategies have been used to treat obesity, including diet, exercise, behavior therapy, medications, and surgery. Criteria for selecting among these treatments involve evaluating the risks to the individual from obesity and balancing the risks against any possible problems with the treatment. Because all medications inherently have more risks than diet and exercise, the decision to use medications should only be made for people for whom the benefit justifies the risk.[4]

This process of evaluation is particularly important because drug treatment for obesity has been tarnished by several problems over the years. Since the introduction of thyroid hormone to treat obesity in 1893, almost every drug that has been tried in obese patients has caused undesirable outcomes necessitating its termination. Caution must be used in accepting any new drug for the treatment of obesity unless the safety profile makes it acceptable for almost everyone.[4]

Another issue surrounding drug treatment of obesity is the perception that, because patients regain weight when drugs are stopped, the drugs are ineffective; however, the contrary is true. Obesity is a chronic disease that has many causes. Because cure is rare, treatment is aimed at palliation, that is, producing and maintaining weight loss. Physicians do not expect to cure diseases such as hypertension or hypercholesterolemia with medications; rather, they expect to palliate them. When the medications for any of these chronic diseases are discontinued, the disease is expected to recur. This means that medications only work when they are used. The same argument applies for medications used to treat obesity.[4]

If an individual is to lose weight, he or she must go into "negative" energy balance in which the energy taken in as food is less, on average, than the energy needed for daily

A version of this article appeared in the 37:4 issue of the *Endocrinology and Metabolism Clinics of North America*.

The author has received research support from Merck and has served as a consultant to Sanofi-Aventis, Merck, Schering-Plough, Eli Lilly, Amgen, and Amylin.

Pennington Biomedical Research Center, 6400 Perkins Road, Baton Rouge, LA 70808, USA

E-mail address: brayga@pbrc.edu

Med Clin N Am 95 (2011) 989–1008

doi:10.1016/j.mcna.2011.06.009

medical.theclinics.com

activities. The current group of medications can be divided into two broad categories: (1) those that act primarily on the central nervous system to reduce food intake and (2) those that act primarily outside the brain. Regardless of the primary site of action, the net effect must be a reduction in food intake, an increase in energy expenditure, or both. Currently, several drugs are available in the United States to treat obesity.[5–10] **Table 1** summarizes these drugs.

APPROVED DRUGS THAT REDUCE FOOD INTAKE PRIMARILY BY ACTING IN THE CENTRAL NERVOUS SYSTEM

The drugs considered in this category are sibutramine, phentermine, and the other sympathomimetic drugs.

Sibutramine

Sibutramine is a serotonin-norepinephrine reuptake inhibitor that is approved by the US Food and Drug Administration (FDA) for long-term use. Sibutramine has been evaluated extensively in several placebo-controlled, double-blind multicenter clinical trials lasting 6 to 24 months and including men and women of all ethnic groups, with ages ranging from 18 to 65 years and body mass indices (BMI) between 27 and 40 kg/m^2.[5,7–9,11,12] In a clinical trial lasting 8 weeks, sibutramine produced a dose-dependent weight loss with doses of 5 and 20 mg per day.[9] In a 6-month dose-ranging study of 1047 patients, 67% of those treated with sibutramine achieved a 5% weight loss from baseline and 35% lost 10% or more.[9] There was a clear dose-response effect in this 24-week trial, and patients regained weight when the drug was stopped, indicating that the drug remained effective when used (**Fig. 1**).

In a 1-year trial of 456 patients who received sibutramine (10 or 15 mg/day) or placebo, 56% of those who stayed in the trial for 12 months lost at least 5% of their initial body weight, and 30% of the patients lost 10% of their initial body weight while taking the 10-mg dose.[13] In a third trial in patients who initially lost weight eating a very low-calorie diet before being randomized to sibutramine or placebo, sibutramine (10 mg/day) produced additional weight loss, whereas the placebo-treated patients regained weight.[14] The Sibutramine Trial of Obesity Reduction and Maintenance lasted 2 years and provided further evidence for weight maintenance.[15] Seven centers participated in this trial, in which patients were initially enrolled in a 6-month open-label phase and treated with 10 mg per day of sibutramine. Of the patients who lost more than 8 kg, two thirds were then randomized to sibutramine and one third to placebo. During the 18-month double-blind phase of this trial, the placebo-treated patients steadily regained weight, maintaining only 20% of their weight loss at the end of the trial. In contrast, the subjects treated with sibutramine maintained their weight for 12 months and then regained an average of only 2 kg, maintaining 80% of their initial weight loss after 2 years.[15] Despite the higher weight loss with sibutramine at the end of the 18 months of controlled observation, the blood pressure levels of the sibutramine-treated patients were still higher than in the patients treated with placebo.

The possibility of using sibutramine as intermittent therapy has been tested in a randomized, placebo-controlled trial lasting 52 weeks.[16] The patients randomized to sibutramine received one of two regimens. One group received continuous treatment with 15 mg per day for 1 year, whereas the other had two 6-week periods when sibutramine was withdrawn. During the periods when the drug was replaced by placebo, there was a small regain in weight that was lost when the drug was resumed. At the end of the trial, the continuous-therapy and intermittent-therapy groups had lost the same amount of weight.

Table 1
Drugs approved by the United States Food and Drug Administration for treatment of obesity

Generic Name	Trade Names	Status	Usual Dose	Comments
Drugs approved for long-term treatment of overweight patients				
Orlistat	Xenical	Not scheduled	120 mg three times a day	May have gastrointestinal side effects
Sibutramine	Meridia, Reductil	DEA-IV	5–15 mg/d	Raises blood pressure
Drugs approved for short-term treatment of overweight patients				
Benzphetamine	Didrex	DEA-III	25–50 mg one to three times/d	Short-term use only
Diethylpropion	Tenuate Tepanil Tenuate Dospan	DEA-IV	25 mg tid 25 mg tid 75 mg in AM	Short-term use only
Phendimetrazine	Standard release: Bontril PDM Plegine X-Trozine Slow release: Bontril Prelu-2 X-Trozine	DEA-III	35 mg tid before meals 105 mg/d in AM of slow-release	Short-term use only
Phentermine	Standard release: Adipex-P Fastin Obenix Oby-Cap Oby-Trim Zantryl Slow release: Ionamin	DEA-IV	18.75–37.5 mg tid 15–30 mg/d in AM of slow-release	Short-term use only

Some trials have reported the use of sibutramine to treat patients with hypertension. In a 52-week trial involving patients with hypertension whose blood pressure levels were controlled with calcium channel blockers with or without beta-blockers or thiazides,[17] sibutramine doses were increased from 5 to 20 mg per day during the first 6 weeks. Weight loss was significantly greater in the sibutramine-treated patients, averaging 4.4 kg (4.7%) as compared with 0.5 kg (0.7%) in the placebo-treated group. Diastolic blood pressure levels decreased 1.3 mm Hg in the placebo-treated group and increased 2 mm Hg in the sibutramine-treated group. The systolic blood pressure levels increased 1.5 mm Hg in the placebo-treated group and 2.7 mm Hg in the sibutramine-treated group. Heart rate was unchanged in the placebo-treated patients but increased by an average of 4.9 beats per minute in the sibutramine-treated patients.

In two studies, patients with diabetes were treated for 12 weeks or 24 weeks with sibutramine. In the 12-week trial, patients with diabetes treated with sibutramine at 15 mg per day lost 2.4 kg (2.8%) compared with 0.1 kg (0.12%) in the placebo group. Hemoglobin A_{1C} levels decreased 0.3% in the drug-treated group and remained stable in the placebo group. Fasting glucose values decreased 0.3 mg/dL in the

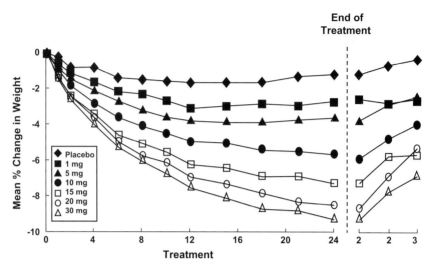

Fig. 1. Dose-dependent weight loss during 24-week trial of sibutramine. (*From* Bray GA, Blackburn GL, Ferguson JM, et al. Sibutramine: a dose-ranging and long-term efficacy study in the treatment of obesity. Obes Res 1999;7:193; with permission.)

drug-treated patients and increased 1.4 mg/dL in the placebo-treated group. In the 24-week trial, the dose of sibutramine was increased from 5 to 20 mg per day over 6 weeks.[18] Among those who completed the treatment, weight loss was 4.3 kg (4.3%) in the sibutramine-treated patients compared with 0.3 kg (0.3%) in placebo-treated patients. Hemoglobin A_{1C} levels decreased 1.67% in the drug-treated group compared with 0.53% in the placebo-treated group. These changes in glucose and hemoglobin A_{1C} levels were expected from the amount of weight loss associated with drug treatment.

Sibutramine has also been used in children.[19–22] In a large 12-month multicenter trial, 498 adolescents aged 12 to 16 years were randomized to treatment with placebo or sibutramine, 10 mg per day, which could be increased to 15 mg per day in those who had not lost greater than 10% of their body weight by 6 months.[21] After 12 months, the mean absolute change in BMI was -2.9 kg/m^2 (-8.2%) in the sibutramine group compared with -0.3 kg/m^2 (-0.8%) in the placebo group ($P<.001$). Triglycerides, high-density lipoprotein (HDL) cholesterol, and insulin sensitivity improved, and there was no significant difference in the changes in systolic or diastolic blood pressure.

Sibutramine has also been studied as part of a behavioral weight-loss program. With sibutramine alone and minimal behavioral intervention, the weight loss over 12 months was approximately -5.0 ± 7.4 kg. Behavior modification alone produced a weight loss of -6.7 ± 7.9 kg. Adding a brief behavioral therapy session to a group who also received sibutramine produced a slightly larger weight loss of -7.5 ± 8.0 kg. When the intensive lifestyle intervention was combined with sibutramine, the weight loss increased to -12.1 ± 9.8 kg.[23]

Sibutramine is available in 5, 10, and 15 mg doses. A single dose of 10 mg per day is the recommended starting level, with titration up or down depending on response. Doses higher than 15 mg per day are not recommended. Of the patients who lost 2 kg (4 lb) in the first 4 weeks of treatment, 60% achieved a weight loss of more than 5% compared with less than 10% of those who did not lose 2 kg (4 lb) in 4 weeks.

Combining data from the 11 studies on sibutramine showed a reduction in triglyceride, total cholesterol, and low-density lipoprotein (LDL) cholesterol levels and an increase in HDL cholesterol levels that were related to the magnitude of the weight loss.

Safety

Sibutramine increases blood pressure levels in normotensive patients or prevents the decrease that might have occurred with weight loss. Because the magnitude of the change may be dose related, lower doses are preferred. Systolic and diastolic blood pressure levels increase an average of +0.8 mm Hg and +0.6 mm Hg, respectively, and pulse increases approximately four to five beats per minute. Caution should be used when combining sibutramine with other drugs that may increase blood pressure levels. Sibutramine is contraindicated in patients with a history of coronary artery disease, congestive heart failure, cardiac arrhythmias, or stroke. Sibutramine should not be used with selective serotonin reuptake inhibitors or monoamine oxidase inhibitors, and there should be a 2-week interval between terminating monoamine oxidase inhibitors and beginning sibutramine. Because sibutramine is metabolized by the cytochrome P-450 enzyme system (isozyme CYP3A4), it may interfere with the metabolism of erythromycin and ketoconazole.

Sympathomimetic Drugs: Pharmacology and Efficacy

The sympathomimetic drugs benzphetamine, diethylpropion, phendimetrazine, and phentermine are grouped together because they act like norepinephrine. Drugs in this group work by a variety of mechanisms, including the blockade of norepinephrine reuptake from synaptic granules.[9]

All of these drugs are absorbed orally and reach peak blood concentrations within a short period. The half-life in blood also is short for all except the metabolites of sibutramine, which have a long half-life. The two metabolites of sibutramine are active, whereas this is not true for the metabolites of other drugs in this group. Liver metabolism inactivates a large fraction of these drugs before excretion. Side effects include dry mouth, constipation, and insomnia. Food intake is suppressed either by delaying the onset of a meal or by producing early satiety.

The efficacy of an appetite-suppressing drug can be established through randomized, double-blind clinical trials that show a significantly greater weight loss than in the placebo group and a weight loss that is more than 5% below that with placebo.[5,7,11] Clinical trials of sympathomimetic drugs conducted before 1975 were generally short because it was widely believed that short-term treatment would "cure" obesity. This belief was unfounded optimism, and because the trials had a short duration and often used a crossover design, they provided few long-term data. The focus herein is on longer-term trials lasting 24 weeks or more that included an adequate control group.

One of the longest of these clinical trials lasted 36 weeks and compared placebo treatment with continuous phentermine or intermittent phentermine.[9] Both continuous and intermittent phentermine therapy produced more weight loss than placebo. In the drug-free periods, the patients treated intermittently slowed their weight loss, only to lose weight more rapidly when the drug was reinstituted. Phentermine and diethylpropion are classified by the US Drug Enforcement Agency as schedule IV drugs; benzphetamine and phendimetrazine are schedule III drugs. This regulatory classification indicates the US government's belief that they have the potential for abuse, although this potential appears to be low. Phentermine and diethylpropion are approved for only a "few weeks," which is usually interpreted as up to 12 weeks. Weight loss with phentermine and diethylpropion persists for the duration of treatment, suggesting that tolerance does not develop to these drugs. If tolerance were to develop, the drugs would be expected to lose their effectiveness, and patients would require increased amounts of the drug to maintain weight loss, which does not occur.

Safety of sympathomimetic drugs

The side-effect profiles for sympathomimetic drugs are similar.[8,9] These agents produce insomnia, dry mouth, asthenia, and constipation. The safety of older sympathomimetic appetite suppressant drugs has been the subject of considerable controversy because dextroamphetamine is addictive. The sympathomimetic drugs phentermine, diethylpropion, benzphetamine, and phendimetrazine have little abuse potential, as assessed by the low rate of reinforcement when the drugs are self-injected intravenously by test animals.[9] Sympathomimetic drugs can also increase blood pressure levels.

APPROVED DRUGS THAT REDUCE FAT ABSORPTION
Orlistat: Pharmacology and Efficacy

Orlistat is a potent and selective inhibitor of pancreatic lipase that reduces the intestinal digestion of fat. The drug has a dose-dependent effect on fecal fat loss, increasing it to approximately 30% on a diet that has 30% of its energy as fat. Orlistat has little effect in subjects eating a low-fat diet, as might be anticipated from its mechanism of action.[9]

Several long-term clinical trials (1–4 years) of orlistat have been published.[5,7,11,12] The first published trial consisted of two parts. In the first year, patients received a hypocaloric diet calculated to be 500 kcal per day less than the patient's requirements.[24] During the second year, the diet was calculated to maintain weight. By the end of year 1, the placebo-treated patients lost 6.1% of their initial body weight and the drug-treated patients lost 10.2%. The patients were randomized at the end of year 1. Those switched from orlistat to placebo gained weight from −10% to −6% below baseline. Those switched from placebo to orlistat lost weight from −6% to −8.1% below baseline, which was essentially identical to the −7.9% loss in the patients treated with orlistat for the full 2 years (**Fig. 2**).

In a second 2-year study, 892 patients were randomized. One group remained on placebo throughout the 2 years (97 patients), and a second group remained on orlistat (120 mg three times per day) for 2 years (109 patients). At the end of 1 year, two thirds of the group treated with orlistat for 1 year were changed to orlistat (60 mg three times per day; 102 patients), and the others were switched to placebo (95 patients). After 1 year, the weight loss was −8.7 kg in the orlistat-treated group and −5.8 kg in the placebo group ($P<.001$). During the second year, those switched to placebo after 1 year reached the same weight as those treated with placebo for 2 years (−4.5% in those with placebo for 2 years and −4.2% in those switched to placebo during year 2).

In a third 2-year study, 783 patients remained in the placebo- or orlistat-treated groups at 60 mg or 120 mg three times per day for the entire 2 years. After 1 year with a weight-loss diet, the placebo group lost 7 kg, which was significantly less than the 9.6 kg lost by the group treated with orlistat 60 mg three times daily, or the 9.8 kg lost by the group treated with orlistat 120 mg three times daily. During the second year, when the diet was liberalized to a "weight maintenance" diet, all three groups regained some weight. At the end of 2 years, the patients in the placebo group were −4.3 kg below baseline, the patients treated with orlistat 60 mg three times per day were −6.8 kg below baseline, and the patients who took orlistat 120 mg three times per day were −7.6 kg below baseline.

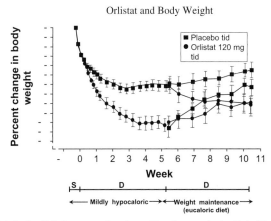

Orlistat and Body Weight

Legend:
■ Placebo tid
● Orlistat 120 mg tid

X-axis: Week (0 1 2 3 4 5 6 7 8 9 10 11)
Y-axis: Percent change in body weight

S — D ⟵ Mildly hypocaloric ⟶⟵ Weight maintenance ⟶ D
(eucaloric diet)

Fig. 2. Two-year trial of orlistat versus placebo with a hypocaloric diet. (*From* Sjostrom L, Rissanen A, Andersen T, et al. Randomized placebo-controlled trial of orlistat for weight loss and prevention of weight regain in obese patients: European Multicentre Orlistat Study Group. Lancet 1998;352(9123):169; with permission.)

The final 2-year trial evaluated 796 subjects in a general practice setting. After 1 year of treatment with orlistat 120 mg three times per day, the orlistat-treated patients (n = 117) had lost −8.8 kg compared with −4.3 kg in the placebo group (n = 91). During the second year, when the diet was liberalized to "maintain body weight," both groups regained some weight. At the end of 2 years, the orlistat group was −5.2 kg below their baseline weight compared with −1.5 kg below baseline for the group treated with placebo.

A 4-year double-blind, randomized, placebo-controlled trial with orlistat treated a total of 3304 overweight patients, 21% of whom had impaired glucose tolerance.[25] The lowest body weight was achieved during the first year and was more than −11% below baseline in the orlistat-treated group compared with −6% below baseline in the placebo-treated group. Over the remaining 3 years of the trial, there was a small regain in weight, such that by the end of 4 years, the orlistat-treated patients were −6.9% below baseline compared with −4.1% for those receiving placebo. The trial also showed a 37% reduction in the conversion of patients from impaired glucose tolerance to diabetes; essentially all of this benefit occurred in the patients with impaired glucose tolerance at enrollment into the trial.

Orlistat has also been used to treat obese children. A multicenter trial tested the effect of orlistat in 539 obese adolescents.[26] Subjects were randomized to placebo or orlistat 120 mg three times a day and a mildly hypocaloric diet containing 30% fat. By the end of the study, BMI had decreased −0.55 kg/m^2 in the drug-treated group but had increased +0.31 kg/m^2 in the placebo group. By the end of the study, weight had increased by only +0.51 kg in the orlistat-treated group compared with +3.14 kg in the placebo-treated group. This difference was due to differences in body fat. The side effects were gastrointestinal in origin as expected from the mode of action of orlistat.

Weight maintenance with orlistat was evaluated in a 1-year study. Patients were enrolled if they had lost more than 8% of their body weight over 6 months while eating a 1000 kcal per day (4180 kJ/d) diet. The 729 patients were randomized to receive placebo or orlistat at 30, 60, or 120 mg three times per day for 12 months. At the end of this time, the placebo-treated patients had regained 56% of their body weight compared with 32.4% regain in the group treated with orlistat 120 mg three times per day. The other two doses of orlistat were not different from placebo in preventing the regain of weight.

Patients with diabetes treated with orlistat 120 mg three times daily for 1 year lost −6.5% of their body weight compared with −4.2% in the placebo-treated group.[27–29] The subjects with diabetes also showed a significantly greater decrease in hemoglobin A_{1C} levels. In another study of orlistat and weight loss, investigators pooled data on 675 subjects from three of the 2-year studies described previously in which glucose tolerance tests were available.[30] During treatment, 6.6% of the patients taking orlistat converted from a normal to an impaired glucose tolerance test compared with 10.8% in the placebo-treated group. None of the orlistat-treated patients who originally had normal glucose tolerance developed diabetes compared with 1.2% in the placebo-treated group. Of those who initially had normal glucose tolerance, 7.6% in the placebo group but only 3% in the orlistat-treated group developed diabetes.

Safety of orlistat

Orlistat is not absorbed to any significant degree, and its side effects are related to the blockade of triglyceride digestion in the intestine.[31] Fecal fat loss and related gastrointestinal symptoms are common initially but subside as patients learn to use the drug. The quality of life in patients treated with orlistat may improve despite concerns about gastrointestinal symptoms. Orlistat can cause small but significant decreases in fat-soluble vitamins. Levels usually remain within the normal range, but a few patients may need vitamin supplementation. Because it is impossible to tell which patients need vitamins, it is wise to provide a multivitamin routinely with instructions to take it before bedtime. Orlistat does not seem to affect the absorption of other drugs, except acyclovir.

Combining orlistat and sibutramine

Because orlistat works peripherally to reduce triglyceride digestion in the gastrointestinal tract and sibutramine works on noradrenergic and serotonergic reuptake mechanisms in the brain, their mechanisms of action do not overlap, and combining them might provide additive weight loss. To test this possibility, researchers randomly assigned patients to orlistat or placebo after 1 year of treatment with sibutramine.[32] During the additional 4 months of treatment, there was no further weight loss; therefore, no data suggest that adding orlistat and sibutramine is beneficial.

DRUGS THAT HAVE BEEN USED TO TREAT OBESITY BUT ARE NOT APPROVED FOR THIS PURPOSE
Fluoxetine and Sertraline

Fluoxetine and sertraline are selective serotonin reuptake inhibitors that block serotonin transporters, prolonging the action of serotonin. These drugs reduce food intake. In a 2-week placebo-controlled trial, fluoxetine at a dose of 60 mg per day produced a 27% decrease in food intake.[33] Both fluoxetine and sertraline are approved by the FDA for treatment of depression. In clinical trials with depressed patients lasting 8 to 16 weeks, sertraline was associated with an average weight loss of −0.45 to −0.91 kg. Fluoxetine at a dose of 60 mg per day (three times the usual dose for treatment of depression) was effective in reducing body weight in overweight patients. A meta-analysis of six studies using fluoxetine showed a wide range of results, with a mean weight loss in one study of −14.5 kg and a weight gain of + 0.40 kg in another.[7] In the meta-analysis by Avenell and colleagues,[12] the weight loss at 12 months was −0.33 kg (95% CI, −1.49 to −0.82 kg). Goldstein and colleagues[34] reviewed the trials with fluoxetine, which included one 36-week trial in type 2 diabetic subjects, one 52-week trial in subjects with uncomplicated overweight, and two 60-week trials in subjects with dyslipidemia, diabetes, or both. A total of 719 subjects were randomized to fluoxetine and 722 to placebo. A total of 522 subjects on fluoxetine and 504 subjects on placebo completed 6 months of treatment. Weight losses in the placebo and fluoxetine groups at 6 months and 1 year were −2.2 and −4.8 and −1.8 and −2.4 kg, respectively. The regain of 50% of the lost weight during the second 6 months of treatment with fluoxetine makes this drug inappropriate for the long-term treatment of obesity. Fluoxetine and sertraline, although not good drugs for long-term treatment of obesity, may be preferred for the treatment of depressed obese patients over some of the tricyclic antidepressants that are associated with significant weight gain.

Bupropion

Bupropion is a norepinephrine and dopamine reuptake inhibitor that is approved for the treatment of depression and for help in smoking cessation. In one clinical trial, 50 overweight subjects were randomized to bupropion or placebo for 8 weeks with a blinded extension for responders to 24 weeks. The dose of bupropion was increased to a maximum of 200 mg twice daily in conjunction with a calorie-restricted diet. At 8 weeks, 18 subjects in the bupropion group lost −6.2 ± 3.1% of body weight compared with −1.6 ± 2.9% for the 13 subjects in the placebo group (P<.0001). After 24 weeks, the 14 responders to bupropion lost −12.9 ± 5.6% of initial body weight, of which 75% was fat as determined by dual x-ray absorptiometry (DXA).[35]

Two multicenter clinical trials, one in obese subjects with depressive symptoms and one in uncomplicated overweight patients, followed this study. In the study of overweight patients with depressive symptom ratings of 10 to 30 on a Beck Depression Inventory, 213 patients were randomized to 400 mg per day of bupropion and 209 subjects were assigned to placebo for 24 weeks. The 121 subjects in the bupropion group who completed the trial lost −6.0 ± 0.5% of initial body weight compared with −2.8 ± 0.5% in the 108 subjects in the placebo group (P<.0001).[36] The study in uncomplicated overweight subjects randomized 327 subjects to bupropion 300 mg per day, bupropion 400 mg per day, or placebo in equal proportions. At 24 weeks, 69% of those randomized remained in the study, and the percent losses of initial body weight were −5 ± 1%, −7.2 ± 1%, and −10.1 ± 1% for the placebo, bupropion 300 mg, and bupropion 400 mg groups, respectively (P<.0001). The placebo group was randomized to the 300- or 400-mg group at 24 weeks and the trial was extended to week 48. By the end of the trial, the dropout rate was 41%, and the weight losses in the bupropion 300 mg and bupropion 400 mg groups were −6.2 ± 1.25% and −7.2 ± 1.5% of initial body weight, respectively.[37] Nondepressed subjects may respond to bupropion with weight loss to a greater extent than those with depressive symptoms.

Topiramate

Topiramate is approved for the treatment of selected seizure disorders. It is a weak carbonic anhydrase inhibitor. Topiramate also modulates the effects at receptors for gamma-aminobutyric acid ($GABA_A$) and the AMPA (alpha-amino-3-hydroxy-5-methyl-4-isoxazolepropionic acid)/kainate subtype of the glutamate receptor. The drug also exhibits state-dependent blockade of voltage-dependent Na^+ or Ca^{2+} channels. These mechanisms are believed to contribute to its antiepileptic properties. The modulation of $GABA_A$ receptors may provide one potential mechanism to reduce food intake, although other mechanisms, yet to be described, may be more important in defining its effects on body weight.[38] Topiramate is an antiepileptic drug that was discovered to be associated with weight loss in the clinical trials for epilepsy. Weight losses of −3.9% of initial weight were seen at 3 months and losses of −7.3% of initial weight at 1 year.[39]

Bray and colleagues[40] reported the results of a 6-month, placebo-controlled, dose-ranging study of topiramate. A total of 385 obese subjects were randomized to placebo or topiramate at 64, 96, 192, or 384 mg per day. These doses were gradually reached by a tapering increase and were reduced in a similar manner at the end of the trial. Weight loss from baseline to 24 weeks was −2.6%, −5%, −4.8%, −6.3%, and −6.3% in the placebo, 64, 96, 192, and 384 mg groups, respectively. The most frequent adverse events were paresthesias, somnolence, and difficulty with concentration, memory, and attention. This trial was followed by two other multicenter trials. The first trial randomized 1289 obese subjects to placebo or topiramate 89, 192, or 256 mg per day. This trial was terminated early due to the sponsor's decision to pursue a time-release form of the drug. The 854 subjects who completed 1 year of the trial before it was terminated lost −1.7%, −7%, −9.1%, and −9.7% of their initial body weight in the placebo, 89, 192, and 256 mg groups, respectively. Subjects in the topiramate groups had significant improvement in blood pressure and glucose tolerance.[41] The second trial enrolled 701 subjects who were treated with a very-low-calorie diet to induce an 8% loss of initial body weight. The 560 subjects who achieved an 8% weight loss were randomized to topiramate 96 mg per day, 192 mg per day, or placebo. This study was also terminated early. At the time of termination, 293 subjects had completed 44 weeks. The topiramate groups lost 15.4% and 16.5% of their baseline weight while the placebo group lost 8.9%.[42] Although topiramate is still available as an antiepileptic drug, the development program to obtain an indication for overweight was terminated by the sponsor due to the associated adverse events.

Zonisamide

Zonisamide is an antiepileptic drug that has serotonergic and dopaminergic activity in addition to inhibiting sodium and calcium channels. Weight loss was noted in the clinical trials for the treatment of epilepsy, again suggesting a potential agent for weight loss. Gadde and colleagues[43] tested this possibility by performing a 16-week randomized controlled trial in 60 obese subjects. Subjects were placed on a calorie-restricted diet and randomized to zonisamide or placebo. The zonisamide was started at 100 mg per day and increased to 400 mg per day. At 12 weeks, the subjects who had not lost 5% of initial body weight were increased to 600 mg per day. The zonisamide group lost −6.6% of initial body weight at 16 weeks compared with −1% in the placebo group. Thirty-seven subjects completing the 16-week trial elected to continue for 32 weeks—20 in the zonisamide group and 17 in the placebo group. At the end of 32 weeks, the 19 subjects in the zonisamide group lost −9.6% of their initial body weight compared with −1.6% for the 17 subjects in the placebo group.

Lamotrigine

Lamotrigine is a third antiepileptic drug that has been evaluated for its effects on body weight.[44] In a double-blind randomized placebo-controlled trial, the dose of lamotrigine was escalated from 25 mg per day to 200 mg per day over 6 weeks. The effect on weight loss was compared with placebo treatment over 26 weeks in 40 healthy overweight (BMI, 30–40 kg/m^2) adults aged more that 18 years. At the end of the trial, body weight was marginally lower ($P = .062$) in the lamotrigine-treated group (−6.4 kg) when compared with the placebo-treated group (−1.2 kg).[45]

Metformin

Metformin is a biguanide that is approved for the treatment of diabetes mellitus. This drug reduces hepatic glucose production, decreases intestinal absorption from the gastrointestinal tract, and enhances insulin sensitivity. In clinical trials in which metformin was compared with sulfonylureas, it produced weight loss.[9] In one French trial, BIGPRO, metformin was compared with placebo in a 1-year multicenter study in 324 middle-aged subjects with upper body adiposity and the insulin resistance (metabolic) syndrome. The subjects on metformin lost significantly more weight (1–2 kg) than the placebo group, and the study concluded that metformin may have a role in the primary prevention of type 2 diabetes.[46] In a meta-analysis of three of these studies, Avenell and colleagues[12] reported a weighted mean weight loss at 12 months of −1.09 kg (95% CI, −2.29 to −0.11 kg).

The best trial of metformin for obesity is the Diabetes Prevention Program (DPP) study of individuals with impaired glucose tolerance. This study included a double-blind comparison of metformin 850 mg twice daily versus placebo. During the 2.8 years of this trial, the 1073 patients treated with metformin lost −2.5% of their body weight ($P<.001$) when compared with the 1082 patients treated with placebo, and the conversion from impaired glucose tolerance to diabetes was reduced by 31% in a comparison with the placebo group. In the DPP trial, metformin was more effective in reducing the development of diabetes in the subgroup who were most overweight and in the younger members of the cohort.[47] Although metformin does not produce enough weight loss (5%) to qualify as a "weight-loss drug" (FDA criteria require ≥5% weight loss), it would appear to be a useful choice for overweight individuals who have diabetes or are at high risk for diabetes. One area where metformin has found use is in treating overweight women with the polycystic ovary syndrome, in which the modest weight loss may contribute to increased fertility and reduced insulin resistance.[48]

Pramlintide

Amylin is a peptide found in the beta cells of the pancreas that is co-secreted along with insulin to circulate in the blood. Both amylin and insulin are deficient in type 1 diabetes where beta cells are immunologically destroyed. Pramlintide, a synthetic amylin analog, has a prolonged biologic half-life.[49] Pramlintide is approved by the FDA for the treatment of diabetes. Unlike insulin and many other diabetic medications, pramlintide is associated with weight loss. In a study in which 651 subjects with type 1 diabetes were randomized to placebo or subcutaneous pramlintide, 60 μg three or four times a day along with an insulin injection, the hemoglobin A_{1C} level decreased 0.29% to 0.34% and weight decreased −1.2 kg in comparison with the placebo group.[50] Maggs and colleagues[51] analyzed the data from two 1-year studies in insulin-treated type 2 diabetic subjects randomized to pramlintide, 120 μg twice a day or 150 μg three times a day. Weight decreased by −2.6 kg and hemoglobin A_{1C} decreased 0.5%. When weight loss was then analyzed by ethnic group, African Americans lost −4 kg, Caucasians lost −2.4 kg, and Hispanics lost −2.3 kg, and the improvement in diabetes correlated with the weight loss, suggesting that pramlintide is effective in ethnic groups with the greatest burden from overweight. The most common adverse event was nausea, which was usually mild and confined to the first 4 weeks of therapy.

Exenatide

Glucagon-like peptide-1 (GLP-1) is derived from processing of the proglucagon peptide which is secreted by L cells in the terminal ileum in response to a meal.

Increased GLP-1 inhibits glucagon secretion, stimulates insulin secretion, stimulates gluconeogenesis, and delays gastric emptying.[52] It has been postulated to be responsible for the superior weight loss and superior improvement in diabetes seen after gastric bypass surgery for overweight.[53,54] GLP-1 is rapidly degraded by dipeptidyl peptidase-4 (DPP-4), an enzyme that is elevated in the obese. Bypass operations for overweight increase GLP-1 but do not change the levels of DPP-4.[49,55]

Exenatide (exendin-4) is a 39–amino acid peptide that is produced in the salivary gland of the Gila monster lizard. It has 53% homology with GLP-1 but a much longer half-life. Exenatide decreases food intake and body weight gain in Zucker rats while lowering hemoglobin A_{1C}.[56] It also increases beta-cell mass to a greater extent than would be expected for the degree of insulin resistance.[57] Exendin-4 induces satiety and weight loss in Zucker rats with peripheral administration and crosses the blood-brain barrier to act in the central nervous system.[58,59] Exenatide is approved by the FDA for the treatment of type 2 diabetic patients who are inadequately controlled while being treated with either metformin or sulfonylureas.

In humans, exenatide reduces fasting and post-prandial glucose levels, slows gastric emptying, and decreases food intake by 19%.[60] The side effects of exenatide in humans are headache, nausea, and vomiting and are lessened by gradual dose escalation.[61] Several clinical trials of 30-week duration have been reported using exenatide at 10 μg subcutaneously per day or a placebo.[62–64] In one trial including 377 type 2 diabetic subjects who were failing maximal sulfonylurea therapy, exenatide produced a fall of 0.74% in hemoglobin A_{1C} when compared with placebo. Fasting glucose also decreased, and there was a progressive weight loss of 1.6 kg.[64] The interesting feature of this weight loss is that it occurred without lifestyle change, diet, or exercise. In a 26-week randomized control trial, exenatide produced a -2.3 kg weight loss compared with a gain of $+1.8$ kg in the group receiving insulin glargine.[65]

DRUGS WITH PHASE III CLINICAL TRIAL DATA
Rimonabant

Rimonabant is approved and marketed in Europe, but at an Advisory Committee meeting to the FDA in June 2007, the vote was not to approve rimonabant in the United States. The stimulation of food intake by tetrahydrocannabinol found in the marihuana plant occurs by stimulation of cannabinoid receptors. There are two cannabinoid receptors, CB-1 (470 amino acids in length) and CB-2 (360 amino acids in length), which respond to endogenous endocannabinoids, of which at least two have been found, anandamide and 2-arachidonoyl-glycerol. The CB-1 receptors are distributed throughout the brain in the areas related to feeding as well as on fat cells and in the gastrointestinal tract. Rimonabant is a specific antagonist of the CB-1 receptor and inhibits intake of sweet or palatable food in marmosets as well as high-fat food intake in rats but not in rats fed standard chow. In addition to inhibiting the intake of highly palatable food, rimonabant may increase energy expenditure in rodents. Genetically engineered mice that lack the CB-1 receptor are lean and resistant to diet-induced obesity.

The results of four phase III trials of rimonabant for the treatment of obesity have been published.[66–69] In a 1-year trial, 1507 patients with a BMI greater than 30 kg/m^2 (or >27 kg/m^2 with treated or untreated dyslipidemia, hypertension, or both) were randomly assigned to receive rimonabant (5 or 20 mg/day) or placebo in addition to a diet calculated to produce a 600 kcal per day deficit.[66] The mean weight loss ($\pm$ SD) at 1 year was -3.4 kg $\pm$ 5.7, -6.6 kg $\pm$ 7.2, and -1.8 kg $\pm$ 6.4 in the rimonabant 5 mg, 20 mg, and placebo groups, respectively. More patients in the group receiving 20 mg per day of rimonabant when compared with those receiving placebo achieved a weight loss of greater than 5% (51% vs 19%) or 10% (27% vs 7%). The 20 mg per day dose of rimonabant produced significantly greater improvements in waist circumference, HDL, triglycerides, insulin resistance, and prevalence of the metabolic syndrome than did placebo. Side effects, including mood changes, nausea and vomiting, diarrhea, headache, dizziness, and anxiety, were more frequent in the rimonabant 20-mg group than the 5-mg or placebo groups; however, dropout rates were similar in all three groups. Rimonabant 20 mg per day resulted in clinically meaningful weight loss, reduction in waist circumference, and improvements in several metabolic risk factors.

In a second 1-year study, 1018 obese subjects with dyslipidemia and a BMI between 27 and 40 kg/m^2 were randomized equally to placebo, rimonabant 5 mg per day, or rimonabant 20 mg per day.[67] Weight loss was 2% in the placebo group and 8.5% in the 20-mg rimonabant group. In the group receiving 20 mg per day of rimonabant, waist circumference was reduced 9 cm, triglycerides were reduced by 15%, and HDL cholesterol was increased by 23% compared with 3.5 cm, 3%, and 12%, respectively, in the placebo group. In the 20-mg per day group, the LDL particle size increased, adiponectin increased, glucose decreased, insulin decreased, C-reactive protein decreased, and the metabolic syndrome prevalence was cut in half. There was no increase in depression or anxiety, and neither pulse nor blood pressure increased.

The third study conducted in North America was a 2-year double-blind trial that randomized 3040 obese subjects without diabetes to placebo, 5 mg of rimonabant, or 20 mg of rimonabant.[68] At 1 year, half of the rimonabant groups were rerandomized to placebo. At 1 year, weight loss was 2.8 kg in the placebo group and 8.6 kg in the 20 mg per day rimonabant group (**Fig. 3**).

In the fourth study,[69] 1047 subjects with type 2 diabetes were randomized to 1 year of treatment. The weight losses were not as great as in the other three groups, but there was consistent improvement in the comorbid risk factors.

Safety

There were significantly more "psychiatric" side effects with the higher dose of rimonabant in the first year of treatment, and three suicides were reported to the FDA

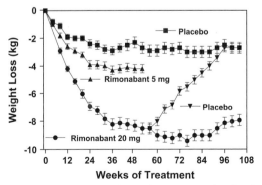

Fig. 3. Weight loss in obese subjects using rimonabant versus placebo. (*Data from* Pi-Sunyer FX, Aronne LJ, Heshmati HM, et al. Effect of rimonabant, a cannabinoid-1 receptor blocker, on weight and cardiometabolic risk factors in overweight or obese patients. RIO-North America: a randomized controlled trial. JAMA 2006;295(7):761–75.)

during clinical trials. Because patients with depression were excluded from the initial phase III studies, there is no information on how this drug works in depressed patients or those taking antidepressants.

Other cannabinoid receptor-1 modulators (antagonists or inverse agonists) are currently under trial. Taranabant is in a phase III trial. Abstract data on this drug show that it reduces food intake and increases energy expenditure in humans. A phase III trial for drug CP 945,598 is underway. Other cannabinoid receptor modulators are in phase II trials.

Neuropeptide Y Receptor Antagonists

Neuropeptide Y (NPY) is a widely distributed neuropeptide that has five receptors, Y-1, Y-2, Y-4, Y-5, and Y-6. NPY stimulates food intake, inhibits energy expenditure, and increases body weight by activating Y-1 and Y-5 receptors in the hypothalamus.[70] Levels of NPY in the hypothalamus are temporally related to food intake and are elevated with energy depletion. Surprisingly, NPY-knockout mice have no phenotype.

Several clinical trials with a selective Y-5 receptor antagonist have been completed. The first was a 2-year randomized, placebo-controlled trial that included two doses. The dose was selected based on displacement of brain receptor ligand in human positron emission tomography studies.[71] There was a significantly greater weight loss with the antagonist, indicating that NPY is involved in regulation of human body weight, but the magnitude of the effect was not deemed to be clinically significant. The second trial was designed to test the effect of the antagonist on the prevention of weight gain induced by providing patients with a very-low-calorie diet before randomization. Again, there was a significant effect, but it was not large enough to warrant continued pursuit of this drug.[71,72] Other drugs are under evaluation, but no data are available.

DRUGS WITH PHASE II CLINICAL DATA
Serotonin 2C Receptor Agonists

Mice lacking the 5HT-2C receptor have increased food intake because they take longer to be satiated. These mice also are resistant to fenfluramine, a serotonin agonist that causes weight loss. A human mutation of the 5HT-2C receptor is associated with early-onset increases in human body weight.[73,74] The precursor of serotonin, 5-hydroxytryptophan, reduces food intake and body weight in clinical studies.[75,76] Fenfluramine[77,78] and dexfenfluramine,[79] two drugs that act on the serotonin system but were withdrawn from the market in 1997 due to cardiovascular side effects, also reduce food intake in human studies. Meta-chlorophenylpiperazine, a direct serotonin agonist, reduces food intake by 28% in women and 20% in men.[80] Another serotoninergic drug, sumatriptan, which acts on the 5HT-1B/1D receptor, also reduces food intake in human subjects.[81]

The robust effects of agonists toward the HT-2C receptors in suppressing food intake have stimulated the development of several new compounds. Only one of these has advanced to formal clinical trials. The results of a phase II dose-ranging study for lorcaserin (APD356) have been presented. A total of 459 male and female subjects with a BMI between 29 and 46 kg/m^2 with an average weight of 100 kg were enrolled in a randomized, double-blind controlled trial comparing placebo against 10 and 15 mg given once daily and 10 mg given twice daily (20 mg/day). During the 12 weeks of the trial, the placebo group lost −0.32 kg (n = 88 completers) compared with −1.8 kg in the group given 10 mg once daily (n = 86), −2.6 kg in the group given 15 mg per day (n = 82 completers), and −3.6 kg in the group given 10 mg twice daily (20 mg total) (n = 77 completers). Side effects that were higher in the active treatment groups when compared with the placebo group were headache, nausea, dizziness, vomiting, and dry mouth. No cardiac valvular changes were noted.[82] Additional clinical trials are underway.

Cetilistat-A Pancreatic Lipase Inhibitor

Although orlistat, a lipase inhibitor, is already approved for the treatment of overweight, cetilistat (ATL-962), another gastrointestinal lipase inhibitor, is also in development. A 5-day trial of cetilistat in 90 normal volunteers was conducted on an inpatient unit. There was a three- to sevenfold increase in fecal fat that was dose dependent, but only 11% of subjects had more than one oily stool. It was suggested that this lipase inhibitor may have fewer gastrointestinal adverse events when compared with orlistat.[83,84] A 12-week randomized double-blind clinical trial of cetilistat showed a significantly greater decrease in body weight when compared with placebo (4.1 kg vs 2.4 kg, 120 mg three times per day). Weight loss with cetilistat was similar to that with orlistat, but there were fewer gastrointestinal side effects with cetilistat.

COMBINATIONS OF DRUGS THAT PRODUCE WEIGHT LOSS

The first important clinical trial combining drugs that act by separate mechanisms used phentermine and fenfluramine.[85] This trial showed a highly significant weight loss of nearly 15% below baseline with fewer side effects by using combination therapy. This combination became very popular,[86] but due to reports of aortic valvular regurgitation associated with its use, fenfluramine was withdrawn from the market worldwide on September 15, 1997.[87]

Several other combinations of existing drugs are under development. One of these is the combination of phentermine with topiramate (Qnexa) for which weight losses of over 10 kg have been reported. A second is the combination of phentermine with zonisamide. A third is the combination of naltrexone with bupropion for which additive weight loss has been noted. Initial data have been published on all of these combinations, but longer-term studies are needed to evaluate the potential drug-drug interactions and side effects produced.

DRUGS THAT INCREASE ENERGY EXPENDITURE

There are no effective drugs in this class, although several different molecules have been tested. Most of the early candidates were developed using receptors from experimental animals. When the human beta-3 receptor was cloned, it was sufficiently different that a new class of compounds was synthesized. The most recent of these molecules developed against the human beta-3 receptors is a Takeda compound (TAK-677, also AJ-9677 {[3-[(2R)-[[(2R)-(3-chlorophenyl)-2-hydroxyethyl]amino]propyl]-1H-indol-7-yloxy]-acetic acid}). Although developed against the human receptor, the drug was found to reduce body weight and glucose in experimental animals and to increase uncoupling protein-1.

A clinical trial with this compound enrolled 65 obese men and women (BMI 33.9 ± 2.1 kg/m^2) in a double-blind randomized placebo-controlled trial lasting 28 days, with subjects assigned to placebo, 0.1, or 0.5 mg twice daily.[88] There was a significant increase in heart rate with the 0.5-mg dose. The resting metabolic rate increased progressively in the treated group, rising by about 7% in the 0.5-mg twice daily dose and 3% in the 0.1-mg twice daily dose when compared with placebo. There was an acute rise in the resting metabolic rate and pulse rate that was related to plasma levels of TAK-677. Free fatty acids in the plasma also increased with the higher dose of TAK-677. There was no significant change in body weight or body fat during treatment.

SUMMARY

Comparatively few drugs are available for the treatment of overweight patients, and their effectiveness is limited to palliation of the chronic disease of obesity. Nevertheless, drug development that is now underway is more rapid than in the past, and we anticipate the discovery of safe and effective pharmacologic strategies for the management of obesity and its serious complications.

REFERENCES

1. World Health Organization. Obesity: preventing and managing the global epidemic. Geneva (Switzerland): World Health Organization; 1998.
2. NHLBI Obesity Education Initiative Expert Panel on the Identification, Evaluation, and Treatment of Overweight and Obesity in Adults. Clinical guidelines on the identification, evaluation, and treatment of overweight and obesity in adults—the evidence report. Obes Res 1998;6(Suppl 2):51S–209S.
3. Ogden CL, Yanovski SZ, Carroll MD, et al. The epidemiology of obesity. Gastroenterology 2007;132(6):2087–102.
4. Bray GA. The metabolic syndrome and obesity. Totowa (NJ): Humana Press; 2007.
5. Padwal R, Li SK, Lau DC. Long-term pharmacotherapy for overweight and obesity: a systematic review and meta-analysis of randomized controlled trials. Int J Obes Relat Metab Disord 2003;27(12):1437–46.
6. Shekelle PG, Hardy ML, Morton SC, et al. Efficacy and safety of ephedra and ephedrine for weight loss and athletic performance: a meta-analysis. JAMA 2003;289(12):1537–45.
7. Li Z, Maglione M, Tu W, et al. Meta-analysis: pharmacologic treatment of obesity. Ann Intern Med 2005;142(7):532–46.
8. Bray G, Greenway F. Pharmacological treatment of the overweight patient. Pharmacol Rev 2007;59(2):151–84.
9. Bray GA, Greenway FL. Current and potential drugs for treatment of obesity. Endocr Rev 1999;20(6):805–75.
10. Bray GA, Ryan DH. Drug treatment of the overweight patient. Gastroenterology 2007;132(6):2239–52.
11. Shekelle PG, Morton SC, Maglione M, et al. Pharmacological and surgical treatment of obesity. Evid Rep Technol Assess (Summ) 2004;(103):1–6.
12. Avenell A, Brown TJ, McGee MA, et al. What interventions should we add to weight reducing diets in adults with obesity? A systematic review of randomized controlled trials of adding drug therapy, exercise, behaviour therapy or combinations of these interventions. J Hum Nutr Diet 2004;7(4):293–316.
13. Smith IG, Goulder MA. Randomized placebo-controlled trial of long-term treatment with sibutramine in mild to moderate obesity. J Fam Pract 2001;50(6):505–12.
14. Apfelbaum M, Vague P, Ziegler O, et al. Long-term maintenance of weight loss after a very-low-calorie diet: a randomized blinded trial of the efficacy and tolerability of sibutramine. Am J Med 1999;106(2):179–84.
15. James WP, Astrup A, Finer N, et al. Effect of sibutramine on weight maintenance after weight loss: a randomised trial. STORM Study Group (Sibutramine Trial of Obesity Reduction and Maintenance). Lancet 2000;356(9248):2119–25.
16. Wirth A, Krause J. Long-term weight loss with sibutramine: a randomized controlled trial. JAMA 2001;286(11):1331–9.

17. McMahon FG, Fujioka K, Singh BN, et al. Efficacy and safety of sibutramine in obese white and African American patients with hypertension: a 1-year, double-blind, placebo-controlled, multicenter trial. Arch Intern Med 2000; 160(14):2185–91.
18. Fujioka K, Seaton TB, Rowe E, et al. Weight loss with sibutramine improves glycaemic control and other metabolic parameters in obese patients with type 2 diabetes mellitus. Diabetes Obes Metab 2000;2(3):175–87.
19. Berkowitz RI, Wadden TA, Tershakovec AM, et al. Behavior therapy and sibutramine for the treatment of adolescent obesity: a randomized controlled trial. JAMA 2003;289(14):1805–12.
20. Godoy-Matos A, Carraro L, Vieira A, et al. Treatment of obese adolescents with sibutramine: a randomized, double-blind, controlled study. J Clin Endocrinol Metab 2005;90(3):1460–5.
21. Berkowitz RI, Fujioka K, Daniels SR, et al. Effects of sibutramine treatment in obese adolescents: a randomized trial. Ann Intern Med 2006;145(2):81–90.
22. Daniels SR, Arnett DK, Eckel RH, et al. Overweight in children and adolescents: pathophysiology, consequences, prevention, and treatment. Circulation 2005; 111(15):1999–2012.
23. Wadden TA, Berkowitz RI, Womble LG, et al. Randomized trial of lifestyle modification and pharmacotherapy for obesity. N Engl J Med 2005;353(20):2111–20.
24. Sjostrom L, Rissanen A, Andersen T, et al. Randomised placebo-controlled trial of orlistat for weight loss and prevention of weight regain in obese patients: European Multicentre Orlistat Study Group. Lancet 1998;352(9123):167–72.
25. Torgerson JS, Hauptman J, Boldrin MN, et al. XENical in the prevention of diabetes in obese subjects (XENDOS) study: a randomized study of orlistat as an adjunct to lifestyle changes for the prevention of type 2 diabetes in obese patients. Diabetes Care 2004;27(1):155–61.
26. Chanoine JP, Hampl S, Jensen C, et al. Effect of orlistat on weight and body composition in obese adolescents: a randomized controlled trial. JAMA 2005; 293(23):2873–83.
27. Hollander PA, Elbein SC, Hirsch IB, et al. Role of orlistat in the treatment of obese patients with type 2 diabetes: a 1-year randomized double-blind study. Diabetes Care 1998;21(8):1288–94.
28. Kelley DE, Bray GA, Pi-Sunyer FX, et al. Clinical efficacy of orlistat therapy in overweight and obese patients with insulin-treated type 2 diabetes: a 1-year randomized controlled trial. Diabetes Care 2002;25(6):1033–41.
29. Miles JM, Leiter L, Hollander P, et al. Effect of orlistat in overweight and obese patients with type 2 diabetes treated with metformin. Diabetes Care 2002; 25(7):1123–8.
30. Heymsfield SB, Segal KR, Hauptman J, et al. Effects of weight loss with orlistat on glucose tolerance and progression to type 2 diabetes in obese adults. Arch Intern Med 2000;160(9):1321–6.
31. Zhi J, Mulligan TE, Hauptman JB. Long-term systemic exposure of orlistat, a lipase inhibitor, and its metabolites in obese patients. J Clin Pharmacol 1999; 39(1):41–6.
32. Wadden TA, Berkowitz RI, Womble LG, et al. Effects of sibutramine plus orlistat in obese women following 1 year of treatment by sibutramine alone: a placebo-controlled trial. Obes Res 2000;8(6):431–7.
33. Lawton CL, Wales JK, Hill AJ, et al. Serotoninergic manipulation, meal-induced satiety and eating pattern: effect of fluoxetine in obese female subjects. Obes Res 1995;3(4):345–56.

34. Goldstein DJ, Rampey AH Jr, Roback PJ, et al. Efficacy and safety of long-term fluoxetine treatment of obesity: maximizing success. Obes Res 1995;4(Suppl 3): 481S–90S.
35. Gadde KM, Parker CB, Maner LG, et al. Bupropion for weight loss: an investigation of efficacy and tolerability in overweight and obese women. Obes Res 2001; 9(9):544–51.
36. Jain AK, Kaplan RA, Gadde KM, et al. Bupropion SR vs placebo for weight loss in obese patients with depressive symptoms. Obes Res 2002;10(10):1049–56.
37. Anderson JW, Greenway FL, Fujioka K, et al. Bupropion SR enhances weight loss: a 48-week double-blind, placebo-controlled trial. Obes Res 2002;10(7):633–41.
38. Astrup A, Toubro S. Topiramate: a new potential pharmacological treatment for obesity. Obes Res 2004;12(Suppl):167S–73S.
39. Ben-Menachem E, Axelsen M, Johanson EH, et al. Predictors of weight loss in adults with topiramate-treated epilepsy. Obes Res 2003;11(4):556–62.
40. Bray GA, Hollander P, Klein S, et al. A 6-month randomized, placebo-controlled, dose-ranging trial of topiramate for weight loss in obesity. Obes Res 2003;11(6): 722–33.
41. Wilding J, Van Gaal L, Rissanen A, et al. A randomized double-blind placebo-controlled study of the long-term efficacy and safety of topiramate in the treatment of obese subjects. Int J Obes Relat Metab Disord 2004;28(11):1399–410.
42. Astrup A, Caterson I, Zelissen P, et al. Topiramate: long-term maintenance of weight loss induced by a low-calorie diet in obese subjects. Obes Res 2004; 12(10):1658–69.
43. Gadde KM, Franciscy DM, Wagner HR II, et al. Zonisamide for weight loss in obese adults: a randomized controlled trial. JAMA 2003;289(14):1820–5.
44. Devinsky O, Vuong A, Hammer A, et al. Stable weight during lamotrigine therapy: a review of 32 studies. Neurology 2000;54(4):973–5.
45. Merideth CH. A single-center, double-blind, placebo-controlled evaluation of lamotrigine in the treatment of obesity in adults. J Clin Psychiatry 2006;67(2):258–62.
46. Fontbonne A, Charles MA, Juhan-Vague I, et al. The effect of metformin on the metabolic abnormalities associated with upper-body fat distribution: BIGPRO study group. Diabetes Care 1996;19(9):920–6.
47. Knowler WC, Barrett-Connor E, Fowler SE, et al. Reduction in the incidence of type 2 diabetes with lifestyle intervention or metformin. N Engl J Med 2002; 346(6):393–403.
48. Ortega-Gonzalez C, Luna S, Hernandez L, et al. Responses of serum androgen and insulin resistance to metformin and pioglitazone in obese, insulin-resistant women with polycystic ovary syndrome. J Clin Endocrinol Metab 2005;90(3):1360–5.
49. Riddle MC, Drucker DJ. Emerging therapies mimicking the effects of amylin and glucagon-like peptide 1. Diabetes Care 2006;29(2):435–49.
50. Ratner RE, Dickey R, Fineman M, et al. Amylin replacement with pramlintide as an adjunct to insulin therapy improves long-term glycaemic and weight control in type 1 diabetes mellitus: a 1-year, randomized controlled trial. Diabet Med 2004;21(11):1204–12.
51. Maggs D, Shen L, Strobel S, et al. Effect of pramlintide on A1C and body weight in insulin-treated African Americans and Hispanics with type 2 diabetes: a pooled post hoc analysis. Metabolism 2003;52(12):1638–42.
52. Patriti A, Facchiano E, Sanna A, et al. The enteroinsular axis and the recovery from type 2 diabetes after bariatric surgery. Obes Surg 2004;14(6):840–8.
53. Small CJ, Bloom SR. Gut hormones as peripheral anti-obesity targets. Curr Drug Targets CNS Neurol Disord 2004;3(5):379–88.

54. Greenway SE, Greenway FL III, Klein S. Effects of obesity surgery on non–insulin-dependent diabetes mellitus. Arch Surg 2002;137(10):1109–17.
55. Lugari R, Dei Cas A, Ugolotti D, et al. Glucagon-like peptide 1 (GLP-1) secretion and plasma dipeptidyl peptidase IV (DPP-IV) activity in morbidly obese patients undergoing biliopancreatic diversion. Horm Metab Res 2004;36(2):111–5.
56. Szayna M, Doyle ME, Betkey JA, et al. Exendin-4 decelerates food intake, weight gain, and fat deposition in Zucker rats. Endocrinology 2000;141(6):1936–41.
57. Gedulin BR, Nikoulina SE, Smith PA, et al. Exenatide (exendin-4) improves insulin sensitivity and beta-cell mass in insulin-resistant obese fa/fa Zucker rats independent of glycemia and body weight. Endocrinology 2005;146(4): 2069–76.
58. Rodriquez de Fonseca F, Navarro M, Alvarez E, et al. Peripheral versus central effects of glucagon-like peptide-1 receptor agonists on satiety and body weight loss in Zucker obese rats. Metabolism 2000;49(6):709–17.
59. Kastin AJ, Akerstrom V. Entry of exendin-4 into brain is rapid but may be limited at high doses. Int J Obes Relat Metab Disord 2003;27(3):313–8.
60. Edwards CM, Stanley SA, Davis R, et al. Exendin-4 reduces fasting and post-prandial glucose and decreases energy intake in healthy volunteers. Am J Physiol Endocrinol Metab 2001;281(1):E155–61.
61. Fineman MS, Shen LZ, Taylor K, et al. Effectiveness of progressive dose-escalation of exenatide (exendin-4) in reducing dose-limiting side effects in subjects with type 2 diabetes. Diabetes Metab Res Rev 2004;20(5):411–7.
62. DeFronzo RA, Ratner RE, Han J, et al. Effects of exenatide (exendin-4) on glyce-mic control and weight over 30 weeks in metformin-treated patients with type 2 diabetes. Diabetes Care 2005;28(5):1092–100.
63. Kendall DM, Riddle MC, Rosenstock J, et al. Effects of exenatide (exendin-4) on glycemic control over 30 weeks in patients with type 2 diabetes treated with met-formin and a sulfonylurea. Diabetes Care 2005;28(5):1083–91.
64. Buse JB, Henry RR, Han J, et al. Effects of exenatide (exendin-4) on glycemic control over 30 weeks in sulfonylurea-treated patients with type 2 diabetes. Diabetes Care 2004;27(11):2628–35.
65. Heine RJ, Van Gaal LF, Johns D, et al. Exenatide versus insulin glargine in patients with suboptimally controlled type 2 diabetes: a randomized trial. Ann Intern Med 2005;143(8):559–69.
66. Van Gaal LF, Rissanen AM, Scheen AJ, et al. Effects of the cannabinoid-1 receptor blocker rimonabant on weight reduction and cardiovascular risk factors in overweight patients: 1-year experience from the RIO-Europe study. Lancet 2005;365(9468):1389–97.
67. Despres JP, Golay A, Sjostrom L. Effects of rimonabant on metabolic risk factors in overweight patients with dyslipidemia. N Engl J Med 2005;353(20): 2121–34.
68. Pi-Sunyer FX, Aronne LJ, Heshmati HM, et al. Effect of rimonabant, a cannabi-noid-1 receptor blocker, on weight and cardiometabolic risk factors in overweight or obese patients. RIO-North America: a randomized controlled trial. JAMA 2006; 295(7):761–75.
69. Scheen AJ, Finer N, Hollander P, et al. RIO-Diabetes Study Group. Efficacy and tolerability of rimonabant in overweight or obese patients with type 2 diabetes: a randomized controlled study. Lancet 2006;368:1660–72.
70. Parker E, Van Heek M, Stamford A. Neuropeptide Y receptors as targets for anti-obesity drug development: perspective and current status. Eur J Pharmacol 2002;440(2/3):173–87.

71. Erondu N, Gantz I, Musser B, et al. Neuropeptide Y5 receptor antagonism does not induce clinically meaningful weight loss in overweight and obese adults. Cell Metab 2006;4(4):275–82.

72. Erondu N, Wadden T, Gantz I, et al. Effect of NPY5R antagonist MK-0557 on weight regain after very-low-calorie diet-induced weight loss. Obesity (Silver Spring) 2007;15(4):895–905.

73. Gibson WT, Ebersole BJ, Bhattacharyya S, et al. Mutational analysis of the serotonin receptor 5-HT2C in severe early-onset human obesity. Can J Physiol Pharmacol 2004;82(6):426–9.

74. Nilsson BM. 5-Hydroxytryptamine 2C (5-HT2C) receptor agonists as potential antiobesity agents. J Med Chem 2006;49(14):4023–34.

75. Cangiano C, Ceci F, Cascino A, et al. Eating behavior and adherence to dietary prescriptions in obese adult subjects treated with 5-hydroxytryptophan. Am J Clin Nutr 1992;56(5):863–7.

76. Cangiano C, Laviano A, Del Ben M, et al. Effects of oral 5-hydroxy-tryptophan on energy intake and macronutrient selection in non–insulin-dependent diabetic patients. Int J Obes Relat Metab Disord 1998;22(7):648–54.

77. Rogers PJ, Blundell JE. Effect of anorexic drugs on food intake and the microstructure of eating in human subjects. Psychopharmacology (Berl) 1979;66(2):159–65.

78. Foltin RW, Haney M, Comer SD, et al. Effect of fenfluramine on food intake, mood, and performance of humans living in a residential laboratory. Physiol Behav 1996;59(2):295–305.

79. Drent ML, Zelissen PM, Koppeschaar HP, et al. The effect of dexfenfluramine on eating habits in a Dutch ambulatory android overweight population with an overconsumption of snacks. Int J Obes Relat Metab Disord 1995;19(5):299–304.

80. Walsh AE, Smith KA, Oldman AD, et al. m-Chlorophenylpiperazine decreases food intake in a test meal. Psychopharmacology (Berl) 1994;116:120–2.

81. Boeles S, Williams C, Campling GM, et al. Sumatriptan decreases food intake and increases plasma growth hormone in healthy women. Psychopharmacology (Berl) 1997;129(2):179–82.

82. Smith SR, Prosser W, Donahue D, et al. APD356, an orally-active selective 5-HT2C agonist reduces body weight in obese men and women. Diabetes Metab 2006;55(Suppl 1):A80.

83. Dunk C, Enunwa M, De La Monte S, et al. Increased fecal fat excretion in normal volunteers treated with lipase inhibitor ATL-962. Int J Obes Relat Metab Disord 2002;26(Suppl):S135.

84. Kopelman P, Bryson A, Hickling R, et al. Cetilistat (ATL-962), a novel lipase inhibitor: a 12-week randomized, placebo-controlled study of weight reduction in obese patients. Int J Obes (Lond) 2007;31(3):494–9.

85. Weintraub M. Long-term weight control: the National Heart, Lung, and Blood Institute funded multimodal intervention study. Clin Pharmacol Ther 1992;51(5):581–5.

86. Stafford RS, Radley DC. National trends in antiobesity medication use. Arch Intern Med 2003;163(9):1046–50.

87. Connolly HM, Crary JL, McGoon MD, et al. Valvular heart disease associated with fenfluramine-phentermine. N Engl J Med 1997;337(9):581–8.

88. Redman LM, de Jonge L, Fang X, et al. Lack of an effect of a novel beta-3-adrenoceptor agonist, TAK-677, on energy metabolism in obese individuals: a double-blind, placebo-controlled randomized study. J Clin Endocrinol Metab 2007;92(2):527–31.

Surgical Approaches to the Treatment of Obesity: Bariatric Surgery

Brian R. Smith, MD[a], Phil Schauer, MD[b], Ninh T. Nguyen, MD[c],*

KEYWORDS

- Bariatric surgery • Metabolic surgery • Obesity
- Metabolic syndrome • Diabetes resolution

As bariatric surgery for the treatment of morbid obesity enters its sixth decade, much has been and continues to be learned from the results of several key bariatric operations, particularly the Roux-en-Y gastric bypass. Because of the epidemic of obesity and development of the laparoscopic approach, bariatric procedures have increased exponentially in the past decade and are now among the more commonly performed gastrointestinal operations. In the United States, the laparoscopic adjustable gastric banding procedure was introduced in 2001 and has steadily gained popularity. With the introduction of the laparoscopic approach, the public now views bariatric surgery as a less-invasive procedure for treating a chronic disease that can threaten one's health and longevity. Along with the laparoscopic revolution, immense efforts were initiated to develop a new standard for safety, with a focus on improving outcomes. The concept of *centers of excellence* was developed, whereby centers performing bariatric surgery must adhere to a high standard with regard to the volume of surgery, the availability of a complete bariatric program, and maintenance of acceptable surgical outcomes. Emerging data support the role of bariatric surgery as an effective treatment for improvement or remission of type 2 diabetes, hypertension, dyslipidemia, and multiple other comorbid conditions that accompany obesity. The mechanisms involved in the remission of these conditions, however, remain poorly understood and constitute an exciting area of research. This article delineates the current types of bariatric surgery, their respective outcomes, and their impact on obesity-related medical comorbidities.

A version of this article appeared in the 37:4 issue of the *Endocrinology and Metabolism Clinics of North America*.

[a] University of California, Irvine Medical Center, Orange, CA, USA
[b] Cleveland Clinic Foundation, 9500 Euclid Avenue, M66-06, Cleveland, OH 44195, USA
[c] Division of Gastrointestinal Surgery, University of California, Irvine Medical Center, 333 City Boulevard West, Suite 850, Orange, CA 92868, USA
* Corresponding author.
E-mail address: ninhn@uci.edu

Med Clin N Am 95 (2011) 1009–1030
doi:10.1016/j.mcna.2011.06.010
0025-7125/11/$ – see front matter © 2011 Elsevier Inc. All rights reserved.

BARIATRIC SURGERY AS TREATMENT FOR SEVERE OBESITY

Obesity is a chronic disease that has become a major nutritional health problem in most industrialized countries, and its prevalence is increasing in the United States. A recent study involving data from the National Health and Nutrition Examination Survey (NHANES) from 2003 to 2004 indicates that obesity was present in 28.5% of adults aged 20 to 39 years, 36.8% aged 40 to 59 years, and 31.0% aged 60 years or older, with obesity defined as a body mass index (BMI) of 30.0 or higher.[1] The number of overweight children and adolescents in the United States is also increasing. According to the NHANES report, the prevalence of overweight individuals aged 12 to 19 years increased from 10.5% in 1988 to 1994 to 15.5% in 1999 to 2000.[2]

The health implications of obesity include increased risk for coronary artery disease, hypertension, hyperlipidemia, type 2 diabetes mellitus, sleep apnea, stroke, arthritis of the weight-bearing joints, and increased prevalence of selected types of cancer. Obesity contributes to approximately 300,000 premature deaths each year as a result of health-related complications.[3] The risk for developing these medical comorbidities is directly proportional to the degree of obesity.[4] Additionally, the relative risk for death increases substantially with increasing BMI, particularly for individuals who have BMI of 35 kg/m^2 or more.[5] Thus, severe obesity is somewhat arbitrarily defined as a BMI of 35 kg/m^2 or more, and morbid obesity is defined as a BMI of 40 kg/m^2 or more with coexistence of significant comorbidity.

The prevalence of severe obesity seems to be increasing at an even higher rate than moderate degrees of obesity.[1] Bariatric surgery, also known as *weight-loss surgery* or *obesity surgery*, is widely accepted as the only known effective treatment for severe obesity. This procedure was introduced in the 1950s and involves surgical manipulation of the gastrointestinal tract to induce long-term weight loss in severely obese individuals.

Bariatric surgery has been shown to substantially improve or resolve many common obesity-related comorbid conditions, including type II diabetes, hypertension, sleep apnea, and dyslipidemia. A recent report with 10-year outcome data from the observational Swedish Obese Subjects (SOS) study showed marked benefits in patients treated surgically compared with matched control subjects treated medically, including recovery from diabetes, lipid abnormalities, sleep apnea, and quality of life.[6] Several studies have also shown that bariatric surgery improves long-term survival.[7–13]

According to the 1991 National Institutes of Health (NIH) consensus conference,[14] bariatric surgery is an effective option for treating individuals categorized as having morbid obesity. Nonsurgical treatment options in the severely obese population include a combination of low-calorie diets, behavioral therapy, exercise programs, and pharmacotherapy. However, limited success has been reported. In long-term follow-up, most patients did not maintain their reduced body weight. Even with pharmacotherapy, patients who experienced response to therapy usually regained weight when treatment stopped. A randomized controlled trial comparing bariatric surgery with nonsurgical treatment showed that the mean difference in weight loss at 24 months of follow-up greatly favored surgical therapy.[15]

Surgery is currently the best-established and most successful method for sustained weight loss in the morbidly obese.[16,17] Several bariatric operations were introduced in the past 4 decades, encompassing a spectrum from primarily restrictive, to combined restrictive/malabsorptive, to purely malabsorptive operations. Roux-en-Y gastric bypass is currently the most commonly performed operation for treating morbid obesity, representing approximately 70% to 75% of all bariatric procedures. The past decade has seen a major growth in the number of bariatric operations performed in the United States. More patients are now seeking bariatric surgery, with the development of the laparoscopic approach an important factor in this growth. The public now views bariatric surgery as a less-invasive operation associated with less postoperative pain and a faster recovery. In addition, in June 2001 the U.S. Food and Drug Administration (FDA) approved laparoscopic adjustable gastric banding (LAGB; Lap-Band, Allergan, Irvine California) for clinical use. The LAGB represents approximately 20% to 25% of all bariatric operations in the United States and provides another minimally invasive surgical option that does not require gastric transection or gastrointestinal reconstruction. This article describes modern, commonly performed bariatric operations, outcomes of bariatric surgery regarding weight loss and morbidity and mortality, and the benefits of bariatric surgery for improvement or remission of obesity-related comorbidities.

PATIENT SELECTION AND WORKUP

Based on the 1991 NIH Consensus Development Conference Panel[14] for the treatment of severe obesity, individuals who have a BMI greater than 35 kg/m^2 with associated medical comorbidities or whose BMI is greater than 40 kg/m^2 qualify for bariatric surgery. Patients generally should have a chronic history of obesity with no underlying endocrine abnormality that can contribute to obesity. Nonsurgical means of weight loss should also have been attempted with failed results. These qualifications for bariatric surgery are endorsed by numerous professional societies and governmental agencies, including the Centers for Medicare and Medicaid Services.

Furthermore, numerous evidence-based reports support bariatric surgery as the preferred treatment for severe obesity.[18] However, most commercial insurance carriers currently do not cover or have very limited coverage of bariatric surgery. Thus, despite recent growth in bariatric surgery, patient access to the only known, broadly effective treatment for severe obesity is extremely limited.

Preoperative evaluation is considered critical to enhance outcomes. Most bariatric surgeons recommend psychological screening to ensure that patients have no severe, untreated psychological or psychosocial issues. In addition, most patients who have significant medical comorbidities often require preoperative cardiorespiratory clearance, because all medical conditions must be optimized before surgery. Other workup may include a sleep study to detect obstructive sleep apnea, arterial blood gas to detect obesity hypoventilation syndrome, and cardiac evaluation for patients suspected of having coronary heart disease.

Preoperative dietary education and the need for postoperative compliance with the comprehensive program are stressed in preoperative visits. Postoperative support group meetings are available and attendance is a common requirement among most bariatric practices, because patients who participate regularly in these meetings experience a significantly greater weight loss than those who do not.[19]

After appropriate patient selection, patients are counseled extensively on the various bariatric operations and the risks and benefits of each. The surgeon and patient select the appropriate bariatric procedure after extensive discussion of the pros and cons of each operation.

FACILITY REQUIREMENTS

For bariatric surgery to be safely performed, the health care facility must be able to accommodate morbidly obese patients in all aspects, starting with a system for evaluation through follow-up. The institution should have a bariatric surgical team, skilled staff, appropriate operating room equipment, and sufficient institutional resources. A bariatric surgical team consists of experienced surgeons and physicians, anesthesiologists, nurses, psychologists, and nutritionists. Specialists in the field of cardiology, pulmonology, rehabilitation, and endocrinology should be available. The operating room must have operating tables and ancillary equipment to accommodate morbidly obese patients, and the staff should be familiar with this equipment and how to care for these patients. The hospital facility should have beds, commodes, chairs, and wheelchairs to accommodate the morbidly obese. In addition, radiology facilities should be capable of handling the radiologic needs of morbidly obese patients.

SURGICAL OPERATIONS

Mason and Ito[20] conceived the original gastric bypass operation in the 1960s as a variation of gastric ulcer surgery. Weight loss was noted in a large percentage of patients who had undergone partial gastrectomy as primary treatment for peptic ulcer disease. The concept has since evolved through numerous modifications to achieve optimal weight loss while minimizing surgical morbidity and nutritional deficiency, with the emergence of a few safe operations. Although many surgical operations for weight loss currently exist, some have been relegated to historical perspective. Additionally, most modern bariatric surgery is performed laparoscopically unless it is revisional or cannot be performed for technical reasons.

Vertical Banded Gastroplasty

The vertical banded gastroplasty (VBG) consists of constructing a small gastric pouch based on the lesser curvature of the stomach, with the outlet restricted with a prosthetic band or mesh. The VBG is a purely restrictive bariatric procedure and the mechanism of weight loss is primarily related to caloric restriction. Although the NIH Consensus Panel proposed this operation as one of two acceptable bariatric procedures, it is not commonly performed because of its inferior weight loss compared with gastric bypass and its high incidence of late complications.

The VBG became popular because it is a simple operation and has a low perioperative risk profile. Although short-term results have been reported to be excellent, long-term results are less favorable.[21–25] The operative time for this procedure is generally short (1–2 hours), with an operative mortality of less than 1% in most series. Early complications included outlet stenosis and staple-line leak, whereas late complications included staple-line fistula, band erosion, stoma stenosis, food intolerance, and pouch dilation. Weight loss after VBG varies between reports. Morino and colleagues[24] reported a 61% excess weight loss at 4 years, whereas Kalfarentzos and colleagues[25] reported only a 37% excess weight loss at 5 years.

The advantages of VBG include its reversibility, preservation of the gastrointestinal tract, and maintained absorption of micronutrients. Disadvantages of VBG include lower weight loss compared with Roux-en-Y gastric bypass, long-term weight regain, high revisional rate, and development of maladaptive eating behavior.

Roux-en-Y Gastric Bypass

The modern Roux-en-Y gastric bypass operation is currently considered the safest and most efficacious operation combining a restrictive and malabsorptive component. It is the most widely performed bariatric operation today. The most common technique is the laparoscopic Roux-en-Y gastric bypass. Open surgery is reserved for difficult scenarios, such as patients who have high BMI, android body habitus, and a history of gastrointestinal surgery, and is also performed by surgeons who are not comfortable with the laparoscopic technique.

Laparoscopic gastric bypass is performed using five or six abdominal ports of variable sizes. A liver retractor is used to retract the left lobe of the liver to expose the entire stomach. One goal is to construct a small gastric pouch that can hold approximately 15 to 20 mL of solid or liquid. The gastric pouch is constructed immediately below the gastroesophageal junction by applying a linear stapler horizontally across the lesser curve, and then turning the staples in a cephalad direction to the angle of His (**Fig. 1**).

The proximal jejunum is then addressed, where the jejunum and its mesentery are divided at 30 to 40 cm distal to the ligament of Treitz. The distal jejunal limb is brought up toward the new gastric pouch as the Roux limb, and the omentum is divided to create a valley through which the Roux limb is brought antecolic into apposition with the new gastric pouch. The length of the Roux limb is carefully measured at 75 to 150 cm, at which point the biliopancreatic limb of the jejunum is anastomosed to the Roux limb, typically using a linear stapler. The mesenteric defects are closed to prevent internal herniation. Finally, an anastomosis is constructed between the gastric pouch and the Roux limb using a circular stapler, which is further reinforced with several interrupted sutures to relieve tension from the gastrojejunal staple-line. Intra-operative endoscopy is performed with air insufflation while the anastomosis is submerged under water to ensure the anastomosis is airtight. Operative time is generally 2 to 4 hours.

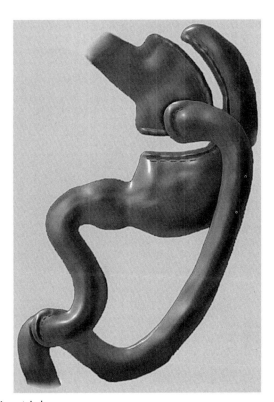

Fig. 1. Roux-en-Y gastric bypass.

Postoperatively, the authors' patients undergo an upper gastrointestinal contrast study with gastrograffin to check for leaks or obstructions before enteral feeds are initiated. Once the upper gastrointestinal study is negative, patients are started on a bariatric clear liquid diet consisting of no concentrated sweets and are instructed to ambulate extensively until discharge on postoperative day two or three. Follow-up is typically at 1 week postoperatively, at 1 month, and then at 3, 6, 9, and 12 months postoperatively.

Laparoscopic Adjustable Gastric Banding

The operation with the fastest rate of growth in recent years is LAGB. The two FDA-approved bands (Lap-Band, Allergan, Irvine, CA, USA, and Realize, Ethicon Endosurgery, Cincinnati, OH, USA) are made of silicone and have an inflatable ring on the inner surface that can be infused with saline (**Fig. 2**). Operative access is achieved with five abdominal ports. The band is placed around the proximal aspect of the stomach immediately below the gastroesophageal junction. Once in position, the band is tightened by closing the buckle and is secured through imbricating the band anteriorly with the gastric fundus to prevent band slippage or gastric herniation. The catheter attached to the band is then exteriorized through one of the port sites and connected to an infusion port, which is then secured to the rectus abdominus fascia. Operative time is usually approximately 1 to 2 hours.

Patients undergo a routine upper gastrointestinal study on the first postoperative day. After confirming easy passage of contrast through the band positioned at a 30° angle, patients are started on a bariatric clear liquid diet. They are typically discharged on postoperative day 1 when tolerating liquids and oral analgesics. Follow-up is similar to that for other bariatric operations; the first band adjustment occurs at 6 weeks postoperatively and then at 2- to 3-month intervals until the optimal level is achieved. Band

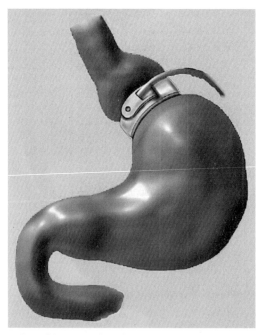

Fig. 2. Laparoscopic adjustable gastric banding.

adjustments are performed percutaneously in the office; however, some surgeons use fluoroscopy in the radiology suite.

Sleeve Gastrectomy

Sleeve gastrectomy has recently become an increasingly common and popular operation. The procedure originated as part of a duodenal switch operation and later evolved into a staging procedure for super-obese or high-risk patients. Patients in these categories would undergo an initial operation consisting entirely of a vertical resection of the lateral aspect of the gastric body and fundus (**Fig. 3**).

The operation begins with mobilization of the greater curvature of the stomach, with division of the short gastric vessels. Using the linear stapler, the greater curve of the stomach is transected approximately 6 cm proximal to the pylorus, and staples fired successively cephalad, parallel to the lesser curve and against a bougie, typically a 42-French. The resected stomach is removed through one of the large port sites. Operative time for this procedure is generally 1 to 2 hours. Postoperative course is similar to that of laparoscopic gastric bypass, with an upper gastrointestinal study on the first postoperative day and initiation of clear liquids when the study shows no leaks or obstruction. Patients typically are discharged on the first or second postoperative day after ambulating and tolerating oral analgesics.

Biliopancreatic Diversion and Duodenal Switch

The biliopancreatic diversion (BPD), developed by Scopinaro[26] in the late 1970s, is a malabsorptive operation whereby the small bowel is divided 250 cm proximal to the ileocecal valve and a subtotal gastrectomy performed, leaving a 400-mL gastric pouch. The distal (alimentary) limb is connected to the gastric pouch. The proximal (biliopancreatic) limb is connected end-to-side to the ileum 50 cm proximal to the ileocecal valve.

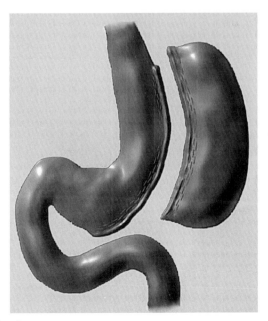

Fig. 3. Sleeve gastrectomy.

This operation is considerably more complex and technically more challenging than the previously described operations. The duodenal switch is a modification of the BPD, whereby a sleeve gastrectomy is performed rather than a subtotal gastrectomy. The duodenum is divided immediately beyond the pylorus. The alimentary limb is connected to the duodenum while the biliopancreatic limb is connected to the ileum 75 cm proximal to the ileocecal valve.

The role of malabsorptive procedures for treating morbid obesity is limited to selected centers. These procedures may have a role in treating patients who are extremely obese (BMI $\geq$60 kg/m^2) or for whom other bariatric operations have failed.

SURGICAL OUTCOMES

Bariatric surgical outcomes have become a significant area of scrutiny, predominately because of higher-than-expected morbidity and mortality rates that accompanied the introduction of laparoscopic gastric bypass at the turn of this century. It became evident that certain groups of patients, including men, elderly individuals, and the super-morbidly obese were at an increased risk for death from this operation, and a steep learning curve exists for laparoscopic gastric bypass.

Studies covering the early period of laparoscopic bariatric surgery tend to reflect higher morbidity and mortality rates, whereas more recent studies show improved perioperative outcomes. Recent national outcome data for bariatric surgery from the Agency for Health Research and Quality showed a 78% decrease in inpatient mortality from 1998 to 2004 (0.89%–0.19%).

For laparoscopic gastric bypass, most series report a mean BMI ranging between 44 and 51 kg/m^2.[27–35] The mean operative time ranges from 90 to 260 minutes, with a low conversion rate to open surgery in 0.5% to 2.0% of cases. The mortality rate after laparoscopic gastric bypass is between 0% and 1.1%.

Results of the recent national analysis of bariatric surgery performed by the University HealthSystem Consortium, a multi-institutional consecutive cohort study conducted among 29 academic institutions, are more reflective of current data for laparoscopic gastric bypass.[36] For gastric bypass procedures (n = 1049), the overall complication rate was 16%, with an anastomotic leak rate of 1.6% and a 30-day mortality rate of 0.4%. For restrictive procedures, the overall complication and 30-day mortality rates were 3.2% and 0%, respectively. Early perioperative complications included anastomotic leak, wound infection, early bowel obstruction, deep venous thrombosis, and gastrointestinal hemorrhage, whereas late complications included bowel obstruction from internal hernia, marginal ulcers, and anastomotic stricture.

Weight loss after laparoscopic gastric bypass is believed to be equivalent to that after open gastric bypass, because the only difference between the techniques is the method of access. Wittgrove and Clark[27] reported long-term weight loss after laparoscopic gastric bypass to be more than 80% of excess body weight loss at 5 years.

Data are emerging on the outcomes of laparoscopic gastric banding.[37–45] The operative time tends to be shorter than that of laparoscopic gastric bypass, ranging between 80 and 105 minutes. Conversion to open laparotomy is low (<1%), with a low mortality rate ranging from 0% to 0.5%. Perioperative complications included gastric or esophageal perforation and bleeding. Late complications included food intolerance, band slippage, pouch dilatation, and band erosion. Esophageal dilatation was also reported.[37] Weight loss after laparoscopic gastric banding was reported to be 56% to 59% at 5 years and 59% at 8 years.[37,39,40]

A recent study evaluated two multicenter, prospective trials that collectively evaluated 485 laparoscopic gastric banding procedures.[46] No perioperative mortalities were seen and complications averaged approximately 12% and consisted predominately of band slippage, stoma obstruction, port displacement, gastroesophageal reflux, esophageal dilation, and wound infections. Weight loss was excellent in both trials.[46]

For sleeve gastrectomy, the largest published study (n = 216) reported a 59% excess weight loss at 1 year,[47] with complications including leaks, nausea and vomiting, pulmonary embolism, and hemorrhage. No studies document long-term results for sleeve gastrectomy.

For malabsorptive operations, Rabkin and colleagues[26] reported the largest study of laparoscopic duodenal switch in 345 patients. The mean BMI in their study was 50 kg/m^2, with a mean operative time of 201 minutes. Conversion occurred in 2% of patients and no operative mortalities occurred. The mean percent of excess weight loss at 2 years was 91%.

COMPARISON OF GASTRIC BANDING, GASTRIC BYPASS, AND SLEEVE GASTRECTOMY

Three case-controlled studies have compared the outcomes of laparoscopic gastric banding with laparoscopic gastric bypass. Jan and colleagues[48] reported the outcomes of 219 patients who underwent laparoscopic gastric bypass compared with 154 patients who underwent Lap-Band. One death occurred in each group. The incidence of major and minor complications was similar, although the reoperation rate was higher in the Lap-Band group and weight loss was greater with gastric bypass.

In a matched control study of 103 patients undergoing Lap-Band and 103 undergoing laparoscopic gastric bypass, Weber and colleagues[49] reported that laparoscopic gastric bypass was superior to Lap-Band. BMI at 2 years decreased from 48.0 to 36.8 kg/m^2 in the Lap-Band group and from 47.7 to 31.9 kg/m^2 in the gastric bypass group. In addition, the gastric bypass procedure was associated with a significantly better reduction of medical comorbidities.

Lastly, in a comparative study of 1200 cases (456 gastric bypasses versus 805 Lap-Band procedures), Biertho and colleagues[32] reported that excess body weight loss at 18 months was superior in the gastric bypass group.

Only one prospective randomized trial has compared the outcomes of laparoscopic gastric banding to those of laparoscopic gastric bypass. Angrisani and colleagues[43] reported on 51 patients who were randomized to undergo laparoscopic gastric banding (n = 27) or laparoscopic gastric bypass (n = 24). At 5-year follow-up, patients who underwent laparoscopic gastric bypass had a higher percentage of excess body weight loss. Weight loss failure (BMI >35 kg/m^2) was observed in 35% of patients in the gastric banding group but only 4% of patients in the gastric bypass group.

In a randomized study comparing gastric banding with sleeve gastrectomy (n = 80), Himpens and colleagues[50] found that the median percentage of excess weight loss at 3 years was 48% for gastric banding and 66% for sleeve gastrectomy.

EFFECTS OF BARIATRIC SURGERY ON MORTALITY

Several studies have shown improved survival for patients who undergo bariatric surgery compared with a control cohort of severely obese patients who did not.[12,51,52] Christou and MacLean[51] compared a cohort of patients (n = 1035) who underwent bariatric surgery with a control cohort (n = 5746) of age- and gender-matched severely obese patients who did not undergo weight-reduction surgery. At a maximum of 5-year follow-up from inception, the mortality rate in the bariatric surgery cohort was 0.68% compared with 6.17% in controls, which translates to an 89% reduction in the relative risk for death.

In another study, Adams and colleagues[12] determined the long-term mortality of 7925 patients who underwent bariatric surgery and 7925 severely obese control subjects matched for age, sex, and BMI. During a mean follow-up of 7.1 years, adjusted long-term mortality from any cause decreased by 40% in the surgery group compared with the controls. Cause-specific mortality in the surgery group decreased by 56% for coronary artery disease, 92% for diabetes, and 60% for cancer.

Lastly, Sjostrom and colleagues[52] reported on the effects of bariatric surgery on mortality in 4047 obese subjects from the SOS study, of which 2010 underwent bariatric surgery and 2037 conventional treatment. During an average of 10.9 years of follow-up, 6.3% of subjects in the matched control group died, compared with 5% in the surgery group, representing a 29% adjusted (all-cause) mortality reduction associated with surgery.

EFFECTS OF BARIATRIC SURGERY ON OBESITY-RELATED COMORBIDITIES

In addition to the well-documented long-term efficacy of bariatric surgery in achieving sustainable weight loss, numerous studies have also evaluated the efficacy of bariatric surgery in ameliorating specific obesity-related comorbidities, particularly type 2 diabetes, hypertension, and dyslipidemia. However, because standards for evaluating the effect of surgery on metabolic diseases have not been established, results should be interpreted with the understanding that many studies lack important determinants, including designation of disease severity in the study population (eg, mild versus severe diabetes), uniform methods of measuring effect of surgery (eg, hemoglobin A1c [HbA1c] versus fasting plasma glucose versus medication withdrawal), and standard definitions of treatment end points (resolution versus remission versus improvement). Some studies, for example, define diabetes resolution as HbA1c of 7.0% or less, whereas others consider it as HbA1c of 6.0% or less. Because *resolution* implies cure, *remission* was chosen as a more accurate term in this article. *Remission* indicates absence of disease indicators, such as normal fasting plasma glucose and HbA1c, blood pressure recordings, and serum lipid levels, but does not imply that the normalization is necessarily permanent. Some of the more noteworthy and well-designed studies are reviewed briefly.

Few studies have examined outcomes of bariatric surgery for patients who have type 1 diabetics, presumably because of the relative infrequency of obesity in this population.[53] However, one small series examining obese patients who had type 1 diabetes showed significant reductions in insulin requirements and glycosylated Hb levels after surgical weight loss.[54]

Much more evidence exists to substantiate remission or improvement of type 2 diabetes after bariatric surgery. In the landmark prospective controlled SOS study involving obese subjects who underwent bariatric surgery and matched obese controls, the surgery group had lower 2- and 10-year incidence rates and remission rates of diabetes, hypertriglyceridemia, and hyperuricemia than the control group.[6] Multiple retrospective cohort studies have shown that all major bariatric procedures result in diabetes remission rates from 45% to nearly 100% (**Tables 1–3**)[55–65] with significant durability. These studies suggest that the bypass procedures (Roux-en-Y and BPD) yield greater weight loss and diabetes remission rates than the purely restrictive procedures.

Table 1
Laparoscopic adjustable gastric banding and type 2 diabetes mellitus

Author	N	Preoperative BMI	Type 2 Diabetes Mellitus Severity	Follow-up (y)	Weight Loss	Pre- versus Postoperative Fasting Plasma Glucose (mmol/L)	Pre- versus Postoperative Hemoglobin A1c	Response
Dixon et al,[55]	500	48	67 IGF 51 DC 4 IU	1	38% EWL	9.4 vs 6.2	7.8 vs 6.2	R = 64% I = 26% U = 10%
Pontiroli et al,[56]	143	45	47 IGF 19 T2DM	3	BMI (45–37)	6.2 vs 5.4	8.3 vs 5.3	R = 80%
Ponce et al,[57]	413	49	53 T2DM	3	52.6% EWL	N/A	7.2 vs 5.33	R = 80% I = 20%
Pontiroli et al,[58]	73	46	17 T2DM	4	BMI (46–38)	N/A	9.4 vs 8.0	R = 45%
LAGB	—	—	20 IGF	—	—	—	—	—
	49	45	20 T2DM	—	No change	—	8.6 vs 8.6	R = 4%
Controls	—	—	10 IGF	—	—	—	—	—

Abbreviations: BMI, body mass index; EWL, excess weight loss; I, improved; IGF, insulin-like growth factor; LAGB, laparoscopic adjustable gastric banding; N/A, not applicable; R, remission; T2DM, types 2 diabetes mellitus; U, unchanged.

Table 2
Roux-en-Y gastric bypass and type 2 diabetes mellitus

Author	N	Preoperative Weight	Type 2 Diabetes Mellitus Severity	Follow-up (y)	Weight Loss	Pre- versus Postoperative Fasting Plasma Glucose (mg/dL)	Pre- versus Postoperative Hemoglobin A1c	Response
Pories et al,[59]	608	134 kg	165 IGF 165 DC/OA	10	54% EWL	213 vs 117	12.3 vs 6.6	R = 89% I = 7% U = 4%
Schauer et al,[60]	1160	50.4 BMI	14 IGF 32 DC 93 OA 52 IU	4	60% EWL	180 vs 98	8.2 vs 5.6	R = 83% I = 17%
Torquati et al,[61]	117	49 BMI	117 T2DM	1	69% EWL	N/A	7.7 vs 6.0	R = 74% I = 26%
Morinigo et al,[62]	34	49 BMI	12 IGF 5 DC 4 OA 1 IU	1	32% IBW	155 vs 91	6.9 vs 4.6	R = 80% I = 20%

Abbreviations: BMI, body mass index; EWL, excess weight loss; I, improved; IBW, ideal body weight; IGF, insulin-like growth factor; N/A, not applicable; R, remission; T2DM, types 2 diabetes mellitus; U, unchanged.

Table 3
Biliopancreatic diversion and type 2 diabetes mellitus

Author	N	Weight (BMI)	Follow-up (y)	Weight Loss	Pre- versus Postoperative Fasting Plasma Glucose (mg/dL)	Pre- versus Postoperative Hemoglobin A1c	Response
Scopinaro et al,[63]	312	50.1	10	BMI (50–32)	178 vs 89	N/A	R = 98%
Marinari et al,[64]	268	49	5	BMI (49–31)	178 vs 86	N/A	R = 100% (71% follow-up)
Marceau et al,[65]	72	47	4	BPD = 61% EWL DS = 73% EWL	N/A	N/A	R = 96% I = 2.5% U = 1.5%

Abbreviations: BMI, body mass index; BPD, biliopancreatic diversion; EWL, excess weight loss; I, improved; IGF, insulin-like growth factor; N/A, not applicable; R, remission; U, unchanged.

The observation that the bypass procedures enable rapid remission before significant weight loss suggests the existence of an antidiabetic effect independent of weight loss. In one study by Schauer and colleagues,[60] 1160 patients underwent bypass, of which 240 (21%) had impaired fasting glucose or type 2 diabetes. Of the diabetic patients, fasting plasma glucose and glycosylated Hb concentrations returned to normal levels in 83% of patients or markedly improved in 17%. Factors found to be predictive of complete diabetes remission included duration of disease less than 5 years, mildest form of the disease (diet-controlled diabetes), and significant weight loss after surgery.[60]

MacDonald and colleagues[7] compared 154 patients who underwent gastric bypass with 78 control patients. With an average of 9 years of follow-up, the percentage of control subjects treated with oral hypoglycemics or insulin increased from 56% to 87%, whereas the percentage of surgical patients requiring medical management for diabetes decreased from 32% to 9%. In a systematic review of the literature involving 2738 citations and 22,094 patients between 1990 and 2002, Buchwald and colleagues[66] showed an overall diabetes remission rate of 48% for restrictive procedures, 84% for Roux-en-Y, and 98% for BPD.

In a recent randomized controlled trial, Dixon and colleagues[67] compared medical treatment of type 2 diabetes mellitus (eg, lifestyle modification and antidiabetic medications) with LAGB and equal medical treatment. All patients in the study had a BMI between 30 to 40 kg/m^2 and mild diabetes (<2-year history, no insulin requirement, and mean HbA1c of 7.7). After 2 years, the surgical group had a remission rate (normal fasting plasma glucose, HbA1c, and no medications) of 73% and weight loss of 20.7% of ideal body weight versus 13% and 1.7% of ideal body weight for the control group, respectively (P<.001). No serious side effects occurred in either group. This randomized controlled trial, along with the previous studies, provides strong evidence that bariatric surgery is an effective therapy for treating type 2 diabetes mellitus in patients who have mild to severe obesity.

Fewer data exist on amelioration of hypertension after bariatric surgery. A recent study from Michigan compared preoperative and postoperative diabetes, hypertension, lipids, and 10-year estimates of coronary heart disease based on Framingham risk scores.[68] Men and women were analyzed separately, and both groups and the collective group showed significant improvement in all categories. Another important study involving 1025 patients who underwent gastric bypass showed an average loss of 66% of excess body weight and hypertension remission in 69% of patients at 1-year follow-up. At 5-year follow-up, remission of hypertension was 66%.[69]

Data also support improvement and normalization of lipid profiles after bariatric surgery. In a group of 400 patients who underwent gastric bypass, hyperlipidemia either resolved or improved postoperatively in 80% to 100%,[70] whereas another group of 650 patients who underwent gastric banding showed a 72% rate of hypertriglyceridemia normalization within 18 months.[71] Across studies, however, the rates of normalization do not always reach statistical significance.[52]

Nevertheless, an important trend toward normalization is seen even in these data sets. When these data are considered collectively with the results of diabetes and hypertension remission rates, it becomes increasingly clear that bariatric surgery plays an important role in reversing the metabolic syndrome responsible for coronary heart disease. Many studies have documented the long-term efficacy of bariatric operations in treating the comorbidities of obesity, including sleep apnea, obesity hypoventilation, pseudotumor cerebri, nonalcoholic liver disease, polycystic ovary syndrome, gastroesophageal reflux, urinary incontinence, degenerative joint disease, and venous stasis disease.[72]

MECHANISMS FOR DIABETES REMISSION

Type 2 diabetes mellitus has long been and continues to be a significant source of morbidity and mortality and a substantial economic burden on worldwide health care.[73] Development of type 2 diabetes is rooted in two fundamental pathophysiologic processes: decreased production of endogenous insulin and cellular insulin resistance. Bariatric surgery has been shown to resolve or substantially improve glucose control.[60,74] Although no clear understanding exists of the mechanisms through which bariatric surgery facilitates remission of type 2 diabetes, numerous possible mechanisms for altering either insulin production or resistance have been proposed as potential explanations for improved or resolved diabetes after bariatric surgery. However, it is becoming increasingly clear that remission of diabetes is multifactorial.[60]

Caloric Restriction

Early improvement or remission of type 2 diabetes after bariatric surgery, before significant weight loss, support postoperative fasting and restriction of caloric intake as important mechanisms. Glucose and insulin requirements have been shown to significantly decline immediately after bariatric surgery.[75] Other small but similar studies showed comparable early changes in insulin resistance after gastric bypass, typically occurring within the first week postoperatively.[76] These results are consistent in most series, suggesting that weight loss alone is not the key factor in improving diabetes. Some authors have also noted a decline in glucose and insulin requirements that began 1 day before surgery,[76] providing the most compelling argument that caloric restriction that begins with the preoperative fast and continues with a bariatric clear liquid diet postoperatively results in significant normalization of these parameters. However, the lasting positive effects on the glucose profile at least partially suggest that the mechanism is far more complex than simply decreased caloric intake.

Weight Loss

The SOS study is one of the best-designed and most compelling studies supporting weight loss as the mechanism for improvement or remission of diabetes.[6] This study compared diabetes prevalence in patients who underwent bariatric surgery and controls, showing a steady prevalence in the former over 8 years, whereas controls had a significantly increased prevalence over the same period.

This finding suggests that in high-risk or early diabetic patients, weight loss from interventions such as bariatric surgery could potentially arrest progression of disease, and the type of bariatric operation is not critical. Compelling data also suggest a 58% reduction in new diabetes diagnoses in high-risk populations when modest weight loss is achieved.[77,78] Again, the data support the notion that weight loss ultimately halts progression of type 2 diabetes.

Conversely, a slightly more specific study evaluated improvement in glycemic control after laparoscopic gastric banding. This study showed a closer association with improved β cell function and duration of diabetes,[79] suggesting that a duration of the disease exists beyond which weight loss cannot overcome dysfunctional β-cell production of insulin. However, the same study also found weight loss to be more closely associated with improved insulin sensitivity,[79] suggesting that weight loss as a final end point can, when experienced sufficiently early in the disease process, reverse diabetes.

Several other studies have helped refute weight loss as the sole cause of diabetes remission. In a well-designed study with impressive long-term follow-up, Pories and colleagues[80] found significantly improved glycemic control within only 1 week of surgery, before any meaningful achievement in weight loss. These and other findings have prompted further research into hormonal and other factors as a mechanism for reversal of diabetes independent of any substantial weight loss.

Endocrine Changes

A substantial body of evidence shows improvement or remission of diabetes before significant weight loss after bariatric surgery.[6,75,81] These data support a mechanism of action mediated by hormonal changes that occur as a direct result of bypassing the fore- or midgut from feeding. Numerous studies have examined preoperative and postoperative gut hormone levels after bariatric surgery. The results have been somewhat mixed and resulted in even further speculation regarding interpretation of the results. A brief summary of hormonal changes after bariatric surgery is provided in the next sections.

Insulin

Good data show a significant decrease in postoperative circulating insulin levels after Roux-en-Y gastric bypass.[73,82] A corresponding decrease in insulin-like growth factor 1 (IGF-1) has also been shown. These hormone alterations occurred despite an expected incremental increase caused by surgical stress.[75] However, despite these changes, mean serum glucose levels decreased significantly to normal levels. These findings raise further questions regarding possible mechanisms and what role incretins play in these hormone alterations.

Incretins are gastrointestinal hormones that directly stimulate insulin release from β cells of the pancreas, and whose reduced secretion is theorized to significantly contribute to type 2 diabetes.[83] Two examples of incretins are gastric inhibitory peptide (GIP) and glucagon-like peptide-1 (GLP-1). Exenatide is the first drug in a new class of incretin-mimetics, and is administered as a twice-daily, long-acting subcutaneous injection.

Endogenous GLP-1 is made by L cells of the colon and ileum.[83] Mechanisms of action include direct stimulation of insulin secretion, inhibition of glucagon secretion, augmentation of the β cell mass, delayed gastric emptying and acid production, and increased satiety. Levels increase after carbohydrate intake and have been shown to increase in a nonstatistically significant way after gastric bypass.[75,83] This finding implies at least a partial role for GLP-1 in normalizing diabetes after surgery.

GIP is made by mucosal K cells of the duodenum and jejunum, and functions in a glucose-dependent manner to stimulate insulin release.[84,85] However, its stimulation of insulin secretion is blunted in patients who have diabetes, and serum levels after Roux-en-Y have been anything but consistent.[83,86,87] More recent data measuring levels of GLP-1 and GIP in response to both oral and intravenous glucose stimulation 1 month after gastric bypass showed significant increases in both hormone levels.[88] This finding corresponds to improved β cell function and resultant normalization of serum glucose, but fails to explain how bypassing the foregut, where GIP is synthesized, increases its secretion. Although much literature supports the notion that ablating the insulin-stimulating effects of GIP contributes to diabetes remission after gastric bypass, the mechanisms of incretin augmentation as a result of foregut bypass remain unclear.

Ghrelin

Ghrelin is produced by A cells in the gastric fundus and functions primarily to stimulate appetite. Other actions of ghrelin include stimulation of growth hormone and gastrointestinal motility. Levels of ghrelin decrease when insulin levels are elevated, and correspondingly increase with normalization of insulin. Receptors for ghrelin are predominately located in the brain, and a correlation seems to exist between serum levels and food intake.[89] However, obese patients have shown lower plasma levels, making the role of this hormone in weight management unclear. Reports have also conflicted on postbypass serum ghrelin levels,[90,91] further confusing its role in improving diabetes after surgery. Despite these findings, ongoing interest and research continues to attempt to clarify the role of this apparent key hormone in both pre- and post–bariatric surgery weight management.

Peptide YY

Peptide YY (PYY) is a peptide derived from intestinal endocrine L cells, which predominately line the distal small intestine and colon.[92] Most studies in animals and humans have shown reduced food intake through PYY stimulation of hypothalamic neuropeptide Y receptors.[93] The anorexic properties of this hormone are currently theorized to play a role in the termination of feeding. Recent work by le Roux and colleagues[94] showed attenuated levels of fasting and postprandial PYY in obese humans and rodents, who also had diminished plasma levels of PYY in response to graded oral challenges. The authors concluded that obese individuals have a PYY deficiency that effectively reduces postprandial satiety, and that this deficiency may be a consequence of obesity rather than a cause.

Leptin

Leptin is an adipose-derived hormone that functions to decrease appetite and inhibits glucose-stimulated insulin secretion.[93] Receptors for leptin reside in the hypothalamus, and levels have been shown to significantly and consistently decrease after gastric bypass.[76,82,88] Neuropeptide Y is believed to be the effector of leptin stimulation of the hypothalamus, and its levels markedly decrease and result in appetite reduction with elevated leptin levels.[94] Increased serum leptin also significantly inhibits glucose-induced insulin secretion and promotes insulin resistance, providing an important potential explanation for the diabetogenic nature of obesity.[83] Therefore, relative decreases in leptin levels from moderate weight loss would rapidly improve diabetes and promote sustained remission. However, definitive data sustaining this theory remain to be seen.

On a collective and larger scale, it is entirely conceivable that hormonal changes are what permit long-term maintenance of weight loss after surgery. Given the relatively poor longevity of diet-induced weight loss, it is certainly intuitive that these hormonal changes, which result from alterations in native intestinal anatomy, result in lasting endocrine changes that promote normalization of the enteroendocrine axis and sustained weight loss.

SUMMARY

As the obesity epidemic continues to grow in the Unites States, so does the search for the ideal nonsurgical or surgical solution. Bariatric surgery continues to be the most sustainable form of weight loss available to morbidly obese patients. In addition, bariatric surgery has established an acceptable safety profile with respect to morbidity and mortality. With the number of elective bariatric cases growing in recent years, it is unsurprising that results have improved and better data are emerging regarding improvement of obesity-related comorbid conditions. Additionally, ample evidence suggests that bariatric surgery may increase longevity, particularly through reducing cardiovascular deaths.

Although the specific mechanisms involved in the remission of these medical conditions remain to be fully elucidated, it has become clear that bariatric surgery has established a significant and firm role in the treatment of medical comorbidities that result directly from obesity. However, until commercial insurance carriers provide improved coverage for bariatric surgery, patient access to these treatments will remain limited.

REFERENCES

1. Ogden CL, Carroll MD, Curtin LR, et al. Prevalence of overweight and obesity in the United States, 1999–2004. JAMA 2006;295:1549–55.
2. Ogden CL, Flegal KM, Carroll MD, et al. Prevalence and trends in overweight among US children and adolescents, 1999–2000. JAMA 2002;288:1728–32.
3. Wolf AM. What is economic case for treating obesity? Obes Res 1998;6:2S–7S.
4. Must A, Spadano J, Coakley EH, et al. The disease burden associated with overweight and obesity. JAMA 1999;282:1523–9.
5. Allison DB, Fontaine KR, Manson JE, et al. Annual deaths attributable to obesity in the United States. JAMA 1999;282:1530–8.
6. Sjostrom CD, Lissner L, Wedel H, et al. Reduction in incidence of diabetes, hypertension and lipid disturbances after intentional weight loss induced by bariatric surgery: the SOS intervention study. Obes Res 1999;7:477–85.
7. MacDonald K, Long S, Swanson M, et al. The gastric bypass operation reduces the progression and mortality of non-insulin-dependent diabetes mellitus. J Gastrointest Surg 1997;1:30–7.
8. Flum DR, Dellinger EP. Impact of gastric bypass operation on survival: a population-based analysis. J Am Coll Surg 2004;199(4):543–51.
9. Christou NV, Sampalis JS, Liberman M, et al. Surgery decreases long-term mortality, morbidity, and health care use in morbidly obese patients. Ann Surg 2004;240(3):416–23 [discussion: 423–4].
10. Sowemimo OA, Yood SM, Courtney J, et al. Natural history of morbid obesity without surgical intervention. Surg Obes Relat Dis 2007;3(1):73–7.
11. O'Brien PE, Dixon JB, Laurie C, et al. Treatment of mild to moderate obesity with laparoscopic adjustable gastric banding or an intensive medical program: a randomized trial. Ann Intern Med 2006;144(9):625–33.
12. Adams TD, Gress RE, Smith SC, et al. Long-term mortality after gastric bypass surgery. N Engl J Med 2007;357(8):753–61.
13. Sjöström L, Narbro K, Sjöström CD, et al. Effects of bariatric surgery on mortality in Swedish obese subjects. N Engl J Med 2007;357(8):741–52.
14. NIH Conference: gastrointestinal surgery for severe obesity: consensus development conference panel. Ann Intern Med 1991;115:956–61.
15. Andersen T, Stokholm KH, Backer OG, et al. Long-term (5-year) results after either horizontal gastroplasty or very-low-calorie diet for morbid obesity. Int J Obes 1988;12:277–84.
16. Brolin RE. Update: NIH consensus conference. Gastrointestinal surgery for severe obesity. Nutrition 1996;12:403–4.
17. Buchwald H. Overview of bariatric surgery. J Am Coll Surg 2005;194:367–75.
18. Shekelle PG, Morton SC, Maglione M, et al. Pharmacological and surgical treatment of obesity [review]. Evid Rep Technol Assess (Summ) 2004;(103):1–6.
19. Elakkary E, Elhorr A, Aziz F, et al. Do support groups play a role in weight loss after laparoscopic adjustable gastric banding? Obes Surg 2006;16:331–4.
20. Mason EE, Ito C. Gastric bypass in obesity. Surg Clin North Am 1967;47:1345–51.

21. Azagra JS, Goergen M, Ansay J, et al. Laparoscopic gastric reduction surgery: preliminary results of a randomized, prospective trial of laparoscopic vs open vertical banded gastroplasty. Surg Endosc 1999;13:555–8.
22. Suter M, Giusti V, Heraief E, et al. Early results of laparoscopic gastric banding compared with open vertical banded gastroplasty. Obes Surg 1999;9:374–80.
23. Gerhart CD. Hand-assisted laparoscopic vertical banded gastroplasty: report of a series. Arch Surg 2000;135:795–8.
24. Morino M, Toppino M, Bonnet G, et al. Laparoscopic vertical banded gastroplasty for morbid obesity: assessment of efficacy. Surg Endosc 2002;16:1566–72.
25. Kalfarentzos F, Kechagias L, Soulikia K, et al. Weight loss following vertical banded gastroplasty: intermediate results of a prospective study. Obes Surg 2001;11:265–70.
26. Rabkin RA, Rabkin JM, Metcalf B, et al. Laparoscopic technique for performing duodenal switch with gastric reduction. Obes Surg 2003;13:263–8.
27. Wittgrove AC, Clark GW. Laparoscopic gastric bypass, Roux-en-Y 500 patients: technique and results, with 3–60 month follow-up. Obes Surg 2000;10:233–9.
28. Marema RT, Perez M, Buffington CK. Comparison of the benefits and complications between laparoscopic and open Roux-en-Y gastric bypass surgeries. Surg Endosc 2005;19:525–30.
29. Oliak D, Ballantyne GH, Davies RJ, et al. Short-term results of laparoscopic gastric bypass in patients with BMI > 60. Obes Surg 2002;12:643–7.
30. Higa KD, Ho T, Boone KB. Laparoscopic Roux-en-Y gastric bypass: technique and 3-year follow-up. J Laparoendosc Adv Surg Tech 2001;11:377–82.
31. Ballesta-Lopez C, Poves I, Cabrera M, et al. Learning curve for laparoscopic Roux-en-Y gastric bypass with totally hand-sewn anastomosis: analysis of first 600 consecutive patients. Surg Endosc 2005;19:519–24.
32. Biertho L, Steffen R, Ricklin T, et al. Laparoscopic gastric bypass versus laparoscopic adjustable gastric banding: a comparative study of 1,200 cases. J Am Coll Surg 2003;197:536–47.
33. Westling A, Gustavsson S. Laparoscopic vs open Roux-en-Y gastric bypass: a prospective, randomized trial. Obes Surg 2001;11:284–92.
34. Lugan JA, Frutos D, Hernandez Q, et al. Laparoscopic versus open gastric bypass in the treatment of morbid obesity: a randomized prospective study. Ann Surg 2004;239:433–7.
35. Sundbom M, Gustavsson S. Randomized clinical trial of hand-assisted laparoscopic versus open Roux-en-Y gastric bypass for the treatment of morbid obesity. Br J Surg 2004;91:418–23.
36. Nguyen NT, Silver M, Robinson M, et al. Result of a national audit of bariatric surgery performed at academic centers. Arch Surg 2006;141:445–50.
37. Dargent J. Laparoscopic adjustable gastric banding: lessons from the first 500 patients in a single institution. Obes Surg 1999;9(5):446–52.
38. O'Brien PE, Dixon JB. Lap-Band®: outcomes and results. J Laparoendosc Adv Surg Tech 2003;13:265–70.
39. Weiner R, Blanco-Engert R, Weiner S, et al. Outcome after laparoscopic adjustable gastric banding—8 years experience. Obes Surg 2003;13:427–34.
40. Ceelen W, Walder J, Cardon A, et al. Surgical treatment of severe obesity with a low-pressure adjustable gastric band: experimental data and clinical results in 625 patients. Ann Surg 2003;237:10–6.
41. Zinzindohoue F, Chevallier JM, Douard R, et al. Laparoscopic gastric banding: a minimally invasive surgical treatment for morbid obesity: prospective study of 500 consecutive patients. Ann Surg 2003;237:1–9.

42. Cadiere GB, Himpens J, Vertruyen M, et al. Laparoscopic gastroplasty (adjustable silicone gastric banding). Semin Laparosc Surg 2000;7:55–65.
43. Angrisani L, Furbetta F, Doldi SB, et al. Lap Band® adjustable gastric banding system: the Italian experience with 1863 patients operated on 6 years. Surg Endosc 2003;17:409–12.
44. Favretti F, Cardiere GB, Segato G, et al. Laparoscopic banding: selection and technique in 830 patients. Obes Surg 2002;12:385–90.
45. Szold A, Abu-Abeid S. Laparoscopic adjustable silicone gastric banding for morbid obesity: results and complications in 715 patients. Surg Endosc 2002; 16:230–3.
46. Martin LF, Smits GJ, Greenstein RJ. Treating morbid obesity with laparoscopic adjustable gastric banding. Am J Surg 2007;194:333–43.
47. Lee CM, Cirangle PT, Jossart GH. Vertical gastrectomy for morbid obesity in 216 patients: report of 2-year results. Surg Endosc 2007;21:1810–6.
48. Jan JC, Hong D, Pereira N, et al. Laparoscopic adjustable gastric banding versus laparoscopic gastric bypass for morbid obesity: a single-institution comparison study of early results. J Gastrointest Surg 2005;9:30–41.
49. Weber M, Muller MK, Bucher T, et al. Laparoscopic gastric bypass is superior to laparoscopic gastric banding for treatment of morbid obesity. Ann Surg 2004; 240:975–83.
50. Himpens J, Dapri G, Cadiere GB. A prospective randomized study between laparoscopic gastric banding and laparoscopic isolated sleeve gastrectomy: results after 1 and 3 years. Obes Surg 2006;16:1450–6.
51. Christou NV, MacLean LD. Effect of bariatric surgery on long-term mortality. Adv Surg 2005;39:165–79.
52. Sjostrom L, Lindroos AK, Peltonen M, et al. Lifestyle, diabetes, and cardiovascular risk factors 10 years after bariatric surgery. N Engl J Med 2004;351: 2683–93.
53. Greenfield JR, Samaras K, Campbell LV, et al. Type 1 diabetes is not associated with increased central abdominal obesity [letter]. Diabetes Care 2003;26:2703.
54. Czupryniak L, Strzelczyk J, Cypryk K, et al. Gastric bypass surgery in severely obese type 1 diabetic patients [letter]. Diabetes Care 2004;27:2561–2.
55. Dixon JB, O'Brien PE. Health outcomes of severely obese type 2 diabetic subjects 1 year after laparoscopic adjustable gastric banding. Diabetes Care 2002;25:358–63.
56. Pontiroli AE, Pizzocri P, Librenti MC, et al. Laparoscopic adjustable gastric banding for the treatment of morbid (grade 3) obesity and its metabolic complications: a three-year study. J Clin Endocrinol Metab 2002;87(8):3555–61.
57. Ponce J, Haynes B, Paynter S, et al. Effect of Lap-Band-induced weight loss on type 2 diabetes mellitus and hypertension. Obes Surg 2004;14(10):1335–42.
58. Pontiroli AE, Folli F, Paganelli M, et al. Laparoscopic gastric banding prevents type 2 diabetes and arterial hypretension and induces their remission in morbid obesity: a 4-year case-controlled study. Diabetes Care 2005;28(11):2703–9.
59. Pories WJ, Swanson M, MacDonald KG, et al. Who would have though it? An operation proves to be the most effective therapy for adult onset diabetes mellitus. Ann Surg 1995;222:339–52.
60. Schauer PR, Burguera B, Ikramuddin S, et al. Effect of laparoscopic Roux-en Y gastric bypass on type 2 diabetes mellitus. Ann Surg 2003;238:467–85.
61. Torquati A, Lutfi R, Abumrad N, et al. Is Rouz-en-Y gastric bypass surgery the most effective treatment for type 2 diabetes mellitus in morbidly obese patients? J Gastrointest Surg 2005;9(8):1112–8 [discussion: 1117–8].

62. Moringo R, Lacy AM, Casamitjana R, et al. GLP-1 and changes in glucose tolerance following gastric bypass surgery in morbidly obese subjects. Obes Surg 2006;16(12):1594–601.
63. Scopinaro N, Marinari GM, Camerini GB, et al. Specific effects of biliopancreatic diversion on the major components of metabolic syndrome: a long-term follow-up study. Diabetes Care 2005;28(10):2406–11.
64. Marinari GM, Papadia FS, Briatore L, et al. Type 2 diabetes and weight loss following biliopancreatic diversion for obesity. Obes Surg 2006;16(11):1440–4.
65. Marceau P, Hould FS, Simard S, et al. Biliopancreatic diversion and duodenal switch. World J Surg 1998;22(9):947–54.
66. Buchwald H, Avidor Y, Braunwald E, et al. Bariatric surgery: a systematic review and meta-analysis. JAMA 2004;292:1724–34.
67. Dixon JB, O'Brien PE, Playfair J, et al. Adjustable gastric banding and conventional therapy for type 2 diabetes: a randomized controlled trial. JAMA 2008; 299:316–23.
68. Vogel JA, Franklin BA, Zalesin KC, et al. Reduction in predicted coronary heart disease risk after substantial weight reduction after bariatric surgery. Am J Cardiol 2007;99:222–6.
69. Sugerman HJ, Wolfe LG, Sica DA, et al. Diabetes and hypertension in severe obesity and effects of gastric bypass-induced weight loss. Ann Surg 2003;237: 751–8.
70. Peluso L, Vanek VW. Efficacy of gastric bypass in the treatment of obesity-related comorbidities. Nutr Clin Pract 2007;22:22–8.
71. Busetto L, Sergi G, Enzi G, et al. Short-term effects of weight loss on the cardiovascular risk factors in morbidly obese patients. Obes Res 2004;121:1256–63.
72. Sugerman HJ. The pathophysiology of severe obesity and the effects of surgically induced weight loss. Surg Obes Relat Dis 2005;1:109–19.
73. Rubin R, Altman W, Mendelson D. Health care expenditures for people with diabetes mellitus. J Clin Endocrinol Metab 1994;78. 809A–F.
74. Pinkney J, Kerrigan D. Current status of bariatric surgery in the treatment of type 2 diabetes. Obes Rev 2004;5:69–78.
75. Hickey MS, Pories WJ, MacDonald KG, et al. A new paradigm for type 2 diabetes mellitus. Ann Surg 1998;227:637–44.
76. Wickremesekera K, Miller G, Naotunne T, et al. Loss of insulin resistance after Roux-en-Y gastric bypass surgery: a time course study. Obes Surg 2005;15:474–81.
77. Knowler WC, Barret-Connor E, Fowler SE, et al. Reduction in the incidence of type 2 diabetes with lifestyle intervention or metformin. N Engl J Med 2002;346: 393–403.
78. Tuomilehto J, Lindstrom J, Eriksson JG, et al. Finnish Diabetes Prevention Study Group. Prevention of type 2 diabetes mellitus by changes in lifestyle among subjects with impaired glucose tolerance. N Engl J Med 2001;344:1390–2.
79. Rubino F, Gagner M, Gentileschi P, et al. The early effect of the Roux-en-Y gastric bypass on hormones involved in body weight regulation and glucose metabolism. Ann Surg 2004;240:236–42.
80. Clements RH, Gonzalez QH, Long CI, et al. Hormonal changes after Roux-en Y gastric bypass for morbid obesity and the control of type-II diabetes mellitus. Am Surg 2004;70:1–4.
81. Kreymann B, Williams G, Ghatei MA, et al. Glucagon-like peptide-1 7-36: a physiological incretin in man. Lancet 1987;2:1300–4.
82. Flatt PR. Effective surgical treatment of obesity may be mediated by ablation of the lipogenic gut hormone gastric inhibitory peptide (GIP): evidence and clinical

opportunity for development of new obesity-related drugs? Diab Vasc Dis Res 2007;4:150–2.

83. Bloom SR, Polak JM. Gut hormones. Adv Clin Chem 1980;21:177–244.

84. Rubino F, Marescaux J. Effect of duodenal–jejunal exclusion in a non-obese animal model of type 2 diabetes: a new perspective for an old disease. Ann Surg 2004;239:1–11.

85. Naslund E, Backman L, Holst JJ, et al. Importance of small bowel peptides for the improved glucose metabolism 20 years after jejuno–ileal bypass for obesity. Obes Surg 1998;8:253–60.

86. Laferrere B, Heshka S, Wang K, et al. Incretin levels and effect are markedly enhanced 1 month after Roux-en-Y gastric bypass surgery in obese patients with type 2 diabetes. Diabetes Care 2007;30:1709–16.

87. Korner J, Inabnet W, Conwell IM, et al. Differential effects of gastric bypass and banding on circulating gut hormone and leptin levels. Obesity 2006;14:1553–61.

88. Cummings DE, Shannon MH. Ghrelin and gastric bypass: is there a hormonal contribution to surgical weight loss? J Clin Endocrinol Metab 2003;88:2999–3002.

89. Korner J, Bessler M, Cirilo LJ, et al. Effects of laparoscopic Roux-en-Y gastric bypass surgery on fasting and postprandial concentrations of plasma ghrelin, PYY and insulin. J Clin Endocrinol Metab 2005;90:359–65.

90. Pfluger PT, Kampe J, Cassaneda TR, et al. Effect of human body weight changes on circulating levels of Peptide YY and Peptide YY_{3-36}. J Clin Endocrinol Metab 2006;92:583–8.

91. Chan JL, Mun ED, Stoyneva V, et al. Peptide YY levels are elevated after gastric bypass surgery. Obesity 2006;14:194–8.

92. Le Roux CW, Batterham RL, Aylwin SJ, et al. Attenuated Peptide YY release in obese subjects is associated with reduced satiety. Endocrinology 2006;147:3–8.

93. Abbas SM. Reviewer summary of plasma ghrelin levels after diet-induced weight loss or gastric bypass surgery. Curr Surg 2006;63:94–5.

94. Cases JA, Gabrietly I, Ma XH, et al. Physiological increase in plasma leptin markedly inhibits insulin secretion in vivo. Diabetes 2001;50:348–52.

Index

Note: Page numbers of article titles are in **boldface** type.

A

Abdominal obesity
    definition of, 921
    insulin resistance relationship with, 878–884
Adipocytes
    dysfunction of, in obesity, 897–898
    in hypertension, 908
Adiponectin
    in dyslipidemia, 897–898
    in hypertension, 910–911
    in metabolic syndrome, 863–864
Agouti-related peptide, in lipid metabolism, 898
Akt protein, in metabolic syndrome, 861
Albuminemia, cardiovascular disease in, 929–930
Aldosterone, in hypertension, 905–906, 912
American Association of Clinical Endocrinologists, metabolic syndrome
    definition of, 856–857
American Heart Association, metabolic syndrome criteria of, 857–858
AMPK-sensitive protein kinase, in exercise, 955, 958
Angiotensin, in hypertension, 905–906, 912
Angiotensinogen, in hypertension, 908
Arcuate nucleus, lipid metabolism regulation in, 898
Atkins diet, 941–943
Atrial fibrillation, 923–924

B

Banting diet, 941–943
Bariatric surgery, **1009–1030**
    diabetes remission after, 1023–1025
    effect on obesity-related comorbidities, 1018–1022
    facility requirements for, 1011–1012
    impact on mortality, 1017–1018
    outcomes of, 1016–1022
    patient selection for, 1011
    procedures for, 1012–1016
    results of, 1010–1011
Baroreflex dysfunction, in hypertension, 906
Behavioral modification. *See* Cognitive-behavioral therapy.
Behavioral Risk Factor Surveillance System data, on weight loss, 972
Benzphetamine, 991, 993–994

Med Clin N Am 95 (2011) 1031–1040
doi:10.1016/S0025-7125(11)00078-2
0025-7125/11/$ – see front matter © 2011 Elsevier Inc. All rights reserved.

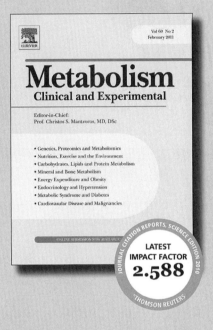
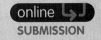

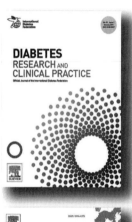
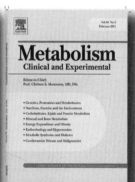
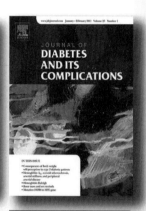
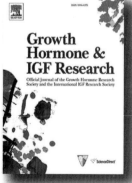
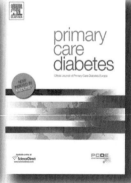
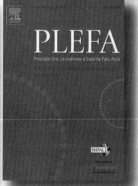

Moving?

Make sure your subscription moves with you!

To notify us of your new address, find your **Clinics Account Number** (located on your mailing label above your name), and contact customer service at:

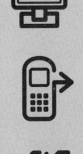

Email: journalscustomerservice-usa@elsevier.com

800-654-2452 (subscribers in the U.S. & Canada)
314-447-8871 (subscribers outside of the U.S. & Canada)

Fax number: 314-447-8029

Elsevier Health Sciences Division
Subscription Customer Service
3251 Riverport Lane
Maryland Heights, MO 63043

*To ensure uninterrupted delivery of your subscription, please notify us at least 4 weeks in advance of move.